ESSENTIAL JUICES AND SMOOTHIES

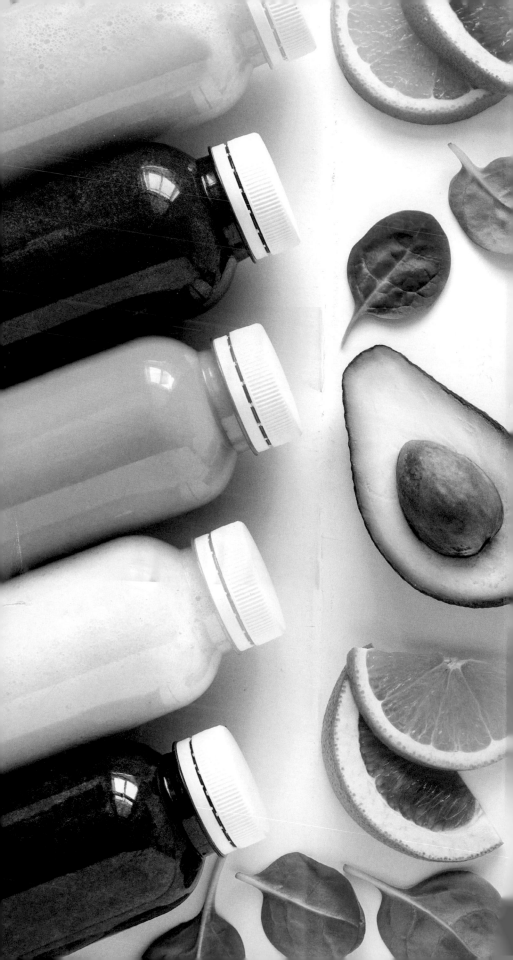

ESSENTIAL JUICES AND SMOOTHIES

The ultimate recipe guide to natural health drinks and bowls

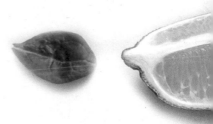

Charlotte van Aussel

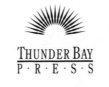

THUNDER BAY
P·R·E·S·S

San Diego, California

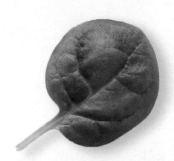

Thunder Bay Press
An imprint of Printers Row Publishing Group
10350 Barnes Canyon Road, Suite 100, San Diego, CA 92121
www.thunderbaybooks.com

Thunder Bay Press
Publisher: Peter Norton
Associate Publisher: Ana Parker
Publishing/Editorial Team: April Farr, Vicki Jaeger, Kelly Larsen, Stephanie Romero,
Kathryn C. Dalby, Carrie Davis
Editorial Team: JoAnn Padgett, Melinda Allman
Production Team: Jonathan Lopes, Rusty von Dyl

Produced by Moseley Road Inc., www.moseleyroad.com
President: Sean Moore
Art and Editorial Director: Lisa Purcell
Cover Designer: Lisa Purcell
Supplemental Writers: Jill Hamilton, Lisa Purcell, Karen Inge, Luisa Adam

Library of Congress Cataloging-in-Publication Data

Names: Van Aussel, Charlotte, author.
Title: Essential juices and smoothies / Charlotte van Aussel.
Description: San Diego, CA : Printers Row Publishing Group, 2019. | Includes index.
Identifiers: LCCN 2018031601 | ISBN 9781684126361
Subjects: LCSH: Detoxification (Health)--Recipes. | Self-care, Health--Popular works. | Fruit juices. |
        Vegetable juices. | Smoothies (Beverages)
Classification: LCC RA784.5 .V36 2019 | DDC 641.3/4--dc23
LC record available at https://lccn.loc.gov/2018031601

Printed in China

23 22 21 20 19   1 2 3 4 5

CONTENTS

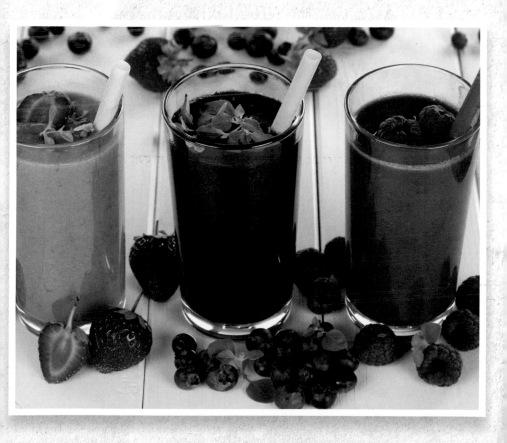

DRINK FOR HEALTH

In recent decades, researchers have developed a solid base of science to back up the mantra that generations of parents have preached to their recalcitrant kids: "Eat your greens, they're good for you!" According to the World Health Organization (WHO), "unhealthy diets and physical inactivity are key risk factors for the major noncommunicable diseases such as cardiovascular diseases, cancer, and diabetes." Like the overwhelming majority of reputable nutrition experts around the world, the WHO comes to the same conclusion as our mothers and grandmothers: the best way to ward off the twin evils of fast food and sluggish feet is to eat your fruits and veggies.

5-A-DAY

The now ubiquitous 5-a-day campaign seen on food packaging, along produce aisles in supermarkets, and in schools everywhere is based on the WHO's recommendation that we should all consume a minimum of 14 ounces of fruit and vegetables each day as part of an average, healthy, balanced diet. By improving our diet, we increase our energy levels and are more likely to perform and enjoy physical activity—kicking off a virtuous cycle of ever-improving health and fitness. It's that simple! And that's where juices and smoothies come into the picture. They are healthy, quick to make, and delicious—a great way to get those nutritious greens (and reds, yellows, purples, and pinks!).

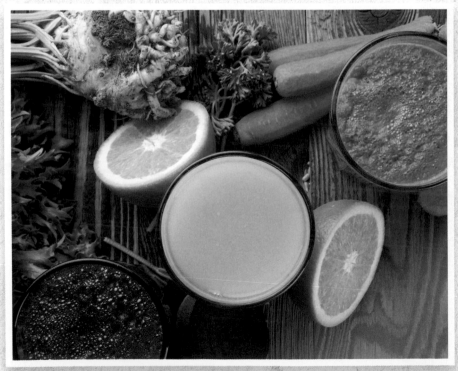

There is a vast selection of fruits and vegetable to choose from when juicing or making smoothies, from root veggies like carrots and beets to citrus fruits and healthy greens.

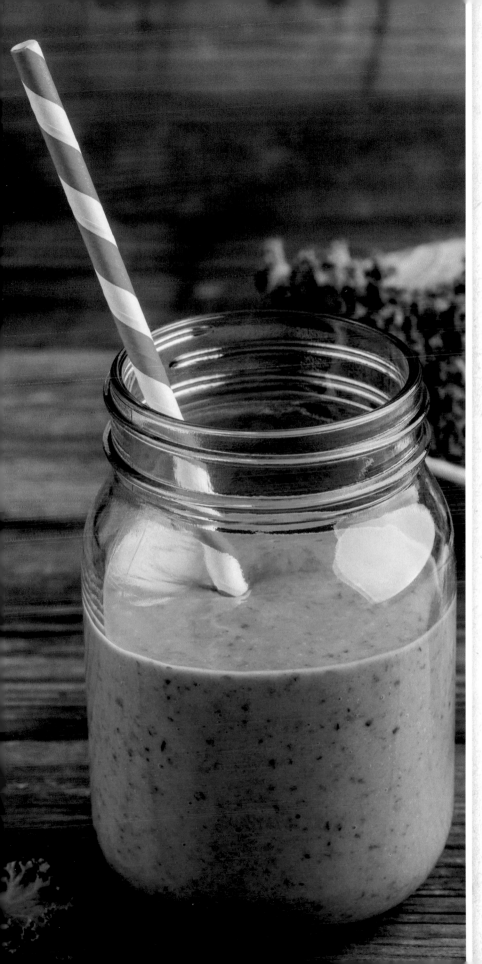

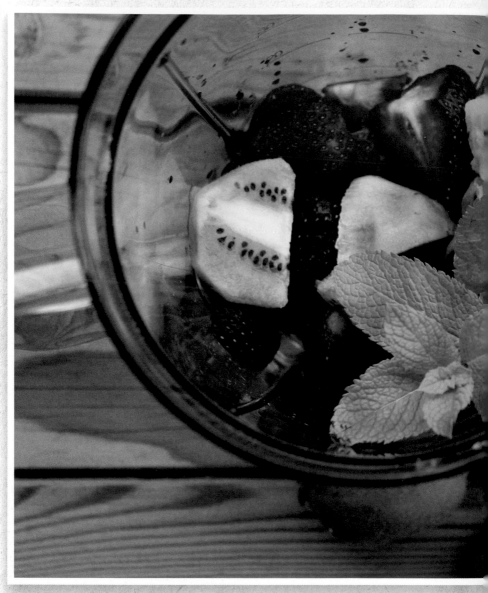

For a fast, nutritious meal, just drop your favorite fruits and milk in the blender.

DRINK YOUR GREENS, THEY'RE GOOD FOR YOU

We all know that food is our body's fuel, but many of us don't realize that certain foods—such as acid-promoting refined carbs, some grains, and refined sugars—are actually energy draining. Fatty foods have similar energy-sapping effects because the digestive system must work overtime to process fats. Foods that energize are the high-alkaline foods, such as fruits and vegetables, that are packed with nutrients—especially antioxidants. Start off each day with a high-power fruit juice and you will feel instantly energized.

It is worth noting that overindulging in any food will make you feel lethargic, and more and more experts are recommending that we take our fuel on board in smaller quantities at more regular intervals. A green smoothie, perhaps made with an energy-packed green-leaf vegetable such as spinach or kale, will provide a perfect energy boost at any time of day, so that we need never . . . well . . . run out of "juice"!

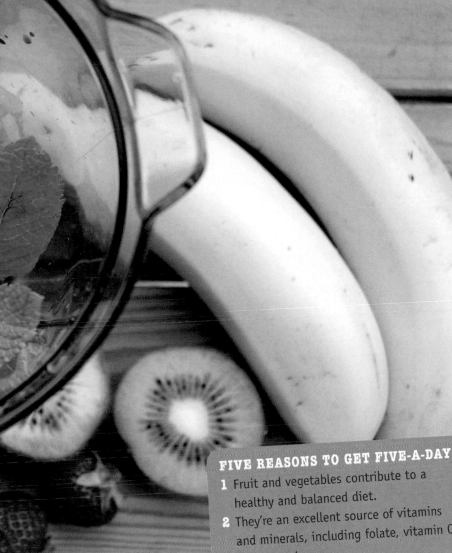

FIVE REASONS TO GET FIVE-A-DAY

1 Fruit and vegetables contribute to a healthy and balanced diet.
2 They're an excellent source of vitamins and minerals, including folate, vitamin C, and potassium.
3 Fruit and vegetables are low in fat and an excellent source of dietary fiber, which helps maintain a healthy gut and prevent digestive problems.
4 They can help reduce the risk of heart disease, stroke, and some cancers.
5 They taste delicious and there's a vast variety to choose from.

FAST FOOD

Juices and smoothies are incredibly easy to make (no recipe should take longer than ten minutes to prepare). The ever-rising tide of health consciousness has led to a raft of super-efficient food processors, blenders, and juicers that make the production of deliciously tempting health drinks easier than ever. Energy-boosting berries—and other fruits and vegetables suitable for juices and smoothies—can be bought frozen from the supermarket, so they can be conveniently stored in the freezer with no need to dilute your ingredients with ice to enjoy a refreshingly chilled health drink every morning.

TASTY TREATS

Juices and smoothies are genuinely delicious as well as nutritious. Fruit juices are naturally sweet, so few children need coaxing to enjoy a fruit juice—especially if strawberries or raspberries are in the mix. Even the dreaded green vegetables can be made more appetizing when combined with naturally sweet carrot juice. Presented in a sparkling glass with a suitable garnish, juices and smoothies can be quite beautiful to look at, too—a far cry from the sorrowful side portion of spinach that kids of previous generations poked around their plates with expressions of loathing. They are fun creations to be positively relished!

FINISHING TOUCHES

Just like alcoholic cocktails, fruit and vegetable juices and smoothies can be decorated with subtle or not-so-subtle embellishments that add to the sense of occasion when presented to your dinner guests (or even just to brighten your family breakfast). You can wedge slices of citrus fruit such as lemon or lime onto the edge of the glass (or use cucumber on a veggie juice); impale olives, grapes, or cherry tomatoes on cocktail sticks; drop whole berries or fruit segments into a transparent juice or float them on top of a creamy smoothie; sprinkle chopped nuts (like almonds or walnuts) and seeds (such as flaxseeds or chia) over a smoothie bowl, and add sprigs of mint, parsley, or other herbs to add texture and color. And why stop there? Straws, umbrellas, and even sparklers can all add to the fun.

Flip through the pages of this book and select a recipe that appeals to you, whether to quench your thirst, boost your energy, improve your health, or indulge your taste buds. And don't feel the need to stick rigidly to a recipe—improvisation and experimentation are a major part of the fun of juicing and making smoothies. Good health!

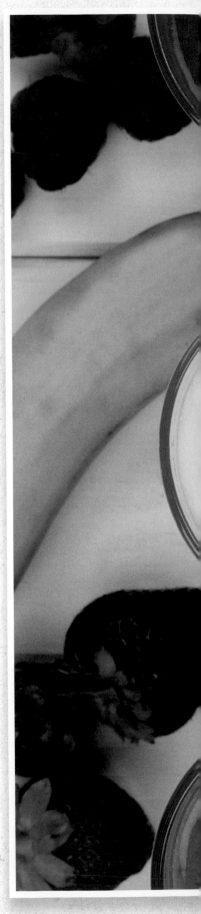

Raspberry, banana, and strawberry smoothies

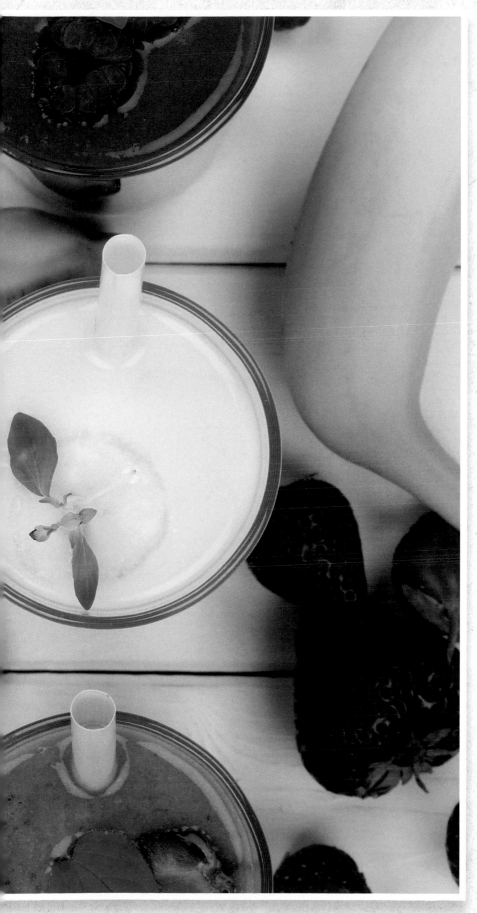

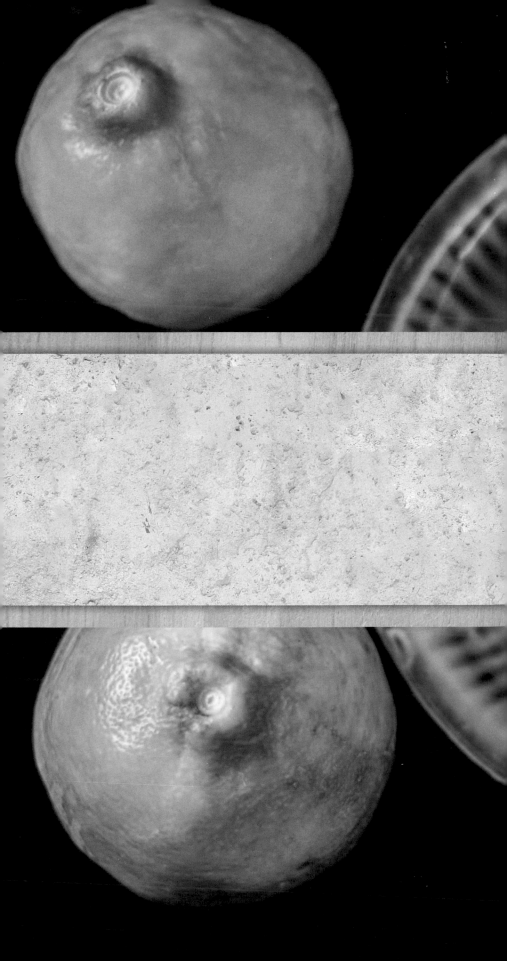

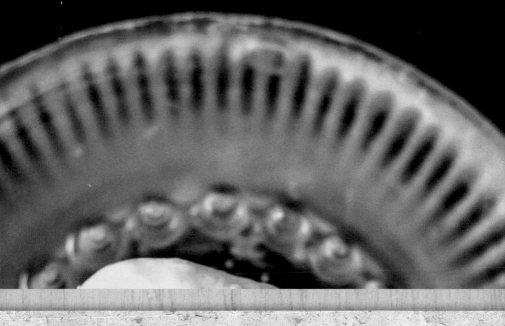

CHAPTER 1

JUICE AND SMOOTHIE BASICS

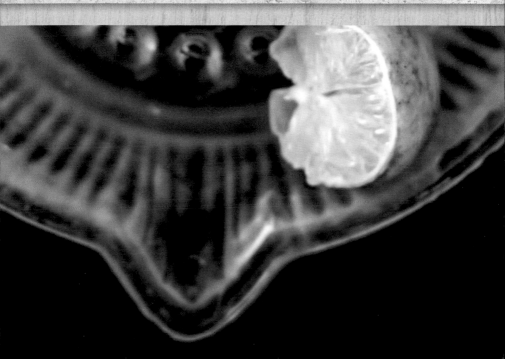

JUICE AND SMOOTHIE BASICS

Your first step to taking advantage of the many benefits of juices and smoothies is learning the essential information about nutrition. From there, you can decide how to stock up your kitchen with all the equipment you'll need to make these healthy beverages.

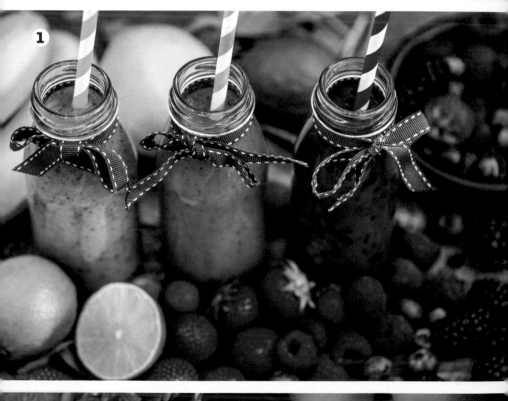

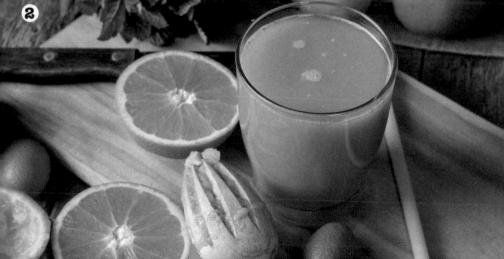

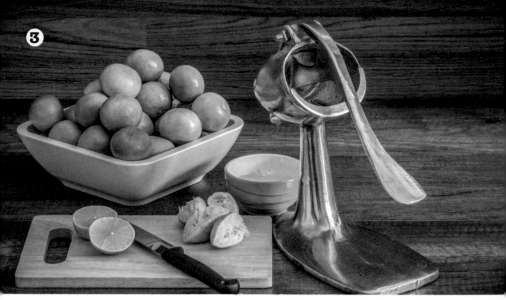

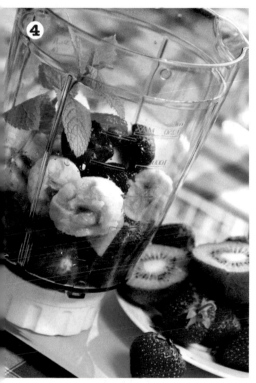

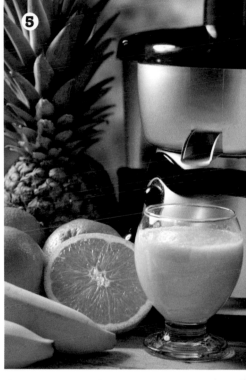

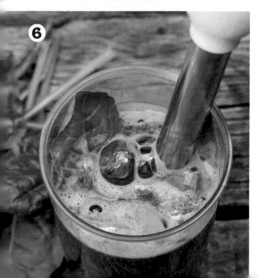

1 A rainbow of fresh-fruit smoothies
2 Fresh orange and kumquat juice extracted with a citrus reamer
3 Lime juice extracted with a tabletop lemon squeezer
4 Kiwi-strawberry-banana smoothie prepared in a blender
5 A blend of pineapple, orange, and banana juice extracted from a centrifugal juicer
6 Spinach smoothie prepared with a handheld blender

WHY JUICES AND SMOOTHIES?

Why? Because these are the easiest ways to ensure that you and your entire family consume the recommended daily allowance of vegetables and fruits—a whopping five servings a day, which can be difficult if you can't talk your child into a single carrot. And, for adults, juices and smoothies are the best and most nutritious way to cleanse and detoxify the body or to go on a diet. So, set up your equipment and get a selection of fruits and vegetables.

Fresh mango juice

JUICES

Munching on an apple or a carrot to extract a host of vital nutrients direct from the raw material is all well and good, but for those of us who can't get excited about fruits and veggies, juices are a lifesaver. Much of the goodness of the fruit is converted into an appetizing and easily digestible drink that can be enjoyed at breakfast or as an energy-boosting treat at any time of day.

HOMEMADE HEALTH
Provide your family with homemade juice from locally grown, organic produce rather than offering them many of the off-the-shelf juices that usually contain added sugar and are relatively low in nutrient value. This is especially true in the case of some popular carbonated drinks and "juices," which may actually contain very little fruit juice at all. With homemade juices, you know that the fruit is fresh and nutritious, and by selecting organic fruit, you can avoid residue from the pesticides that are used in many intensive farming methods.

FREEZING FRUIT

When you do buy (or pick) a fine crop of fresh fruits, conserve surplus fruit by peeling and chopping as you would in preparation for the juicer (or leave them whole in the case of many berries) and immediately store the fruit in plastic bags in your freezer for use at a later date. Fruit added to the juicer straight from the freezer is far preferable to fruit that has been left lying around for a few days, losing its goodness. Frozen fruit retains most of its nutrients and there's no need to dilute and chill the drink with additional ice. It emerges deliciously chilled straight from the juicer.

FUN FOR KIDS

For kids especially, the process of creating a juice from scratch is fascinating in itself. They love to watch as the often-uninspiring raw material is transformed in a matter of seconds into a sparkling, silky-smooth, or crystal-clear drink that tastes every bit as good as it looks.

Juices are often so delicious because the super-efficient modern juicer lives up to its name and removes all the bitter pith and pips, leaving only the sweet, sugar-rich juice. Juices are a great way to get a healthy dose of vitamin C and other vital vitamins and minerals into your kids, but they should be enjoyed in moderation. The dietary fiber and other goodness that is lost in the juicing process will have to be replaced elsewhere in your child's diet.

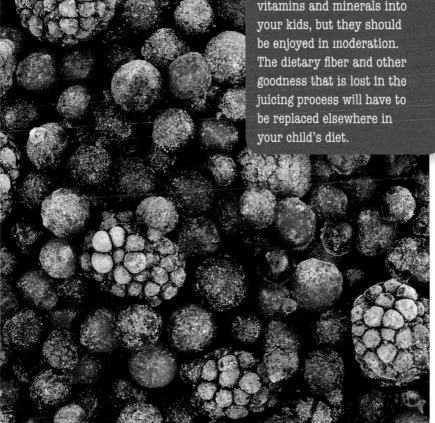

Frozen black and red currants, cranberries, raspberries, blackberries, bilberries, and blueberries. You can freeze berries whole to later drop into the blender to make smoothies and smoothie bowls that retain the berries' nutritional benefits.

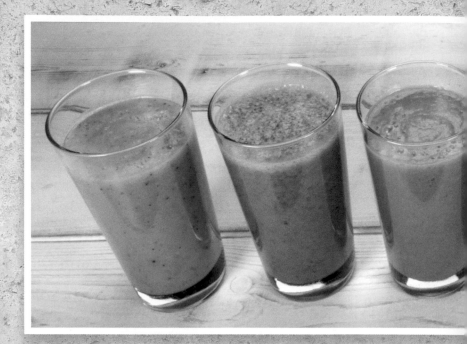

SMOOTHIES

Smoothies are made in a simple blender rather than with a specialist juicer—in many cases, the fruit or veggies can simply be washed, chopped up, and dropped into the blender, retaining all the goodness of the raw material. Sometimes, however, a little more preparation is required because peels, stones, and cores have to be removed before blending begins.

PACKED WITH GOODNESS

The health benefits of smoothies are substantial. Certain fruits and vegetables contain vital nutrients that are particularly recommended for preventing common illnesses and maintaining the health of the cardiovascular system, cleansing the digestive system, or promoting the growth of healthy bones. Their vitamins help enzymes in your body process food into energy, maintain your body's hormonal balance, and protect the immune system. Meanwhile, the many vital minerals found in fruit and vegetables—such as calcium, iron, and magnesium—help protect the nervous system and build strong muscles, bones, teeth, and hair. Fruits also contain powerful antioxidants that combat the effects of aging and protect the body against chronic illnesses. This book contains a whole host of recipes designed for their targeted health benefits.

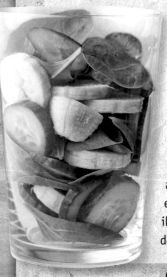

Banana in a green smoothie adds a soft sweetness to the bite of many green veggies.

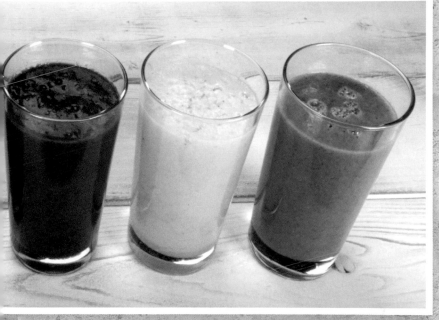

From left to right: apple, strawberry, carrot, blueberry, banana, and kale smoothies

SMOOTHIE BOWLS

Smoothie bowls offer all the benefits of smoothies served in a glass, but their slightly thicker texture makes them perfect spoonable meals or high-energy snacks. Blend up your choice of fruits and veggies, and add further texture, color, flavor, and nutrients with a wide range of toppings, such as sliced fruit, whole berries, seeds, chopped nuts, coconut shavings, and raw or toasted granola.

INDULGENT DELIGHTS

Pure-fruit smoothies and pure-vegetable, or "green," smoothies are usually high in dietary fiber and are more wholesome than juices from which the "pulp" is extracted. Generally speaking, smoothies can be enjoyed more frequently than juices; however, as well as being a nutrient-packed health drink, smoothies can be a sumptuous, creamy indulgence. By blending with milk, cream, or ice cream, you can create deliciously tempting (and high-calorie) desserts. Such concoctions should be saved as special treats rather than being served up every day. For those who enjoy more savory foods, herbs and spices such as ginger or cinnamon can liven up a smoothie. You can add alcohol to inject a bit of sparkle to a dinner-party dessert smoothie. There is a smoothie out there for everyone.

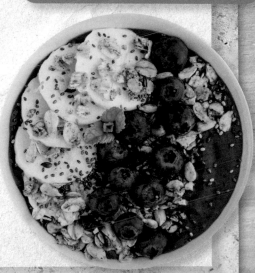

Blueberry smoothie bowl topped with fresh fruit, granola, and chia seeds

NUTRITION, CLEANSING, AND DETOXING

The terms *cleansing* and *detoxing* mean different things to different people. It may refer to your body's own ability, when it is properly nourished, to efficiently rid itself of the substances it does not need and utilize the substances it does need.

Raw celery provides a wide range of detox benefits.

CLEAN NUTRITION

Juices are key components of most cleansing and detoxing programs. Smoothies are also beneficial. When made from fresh fruit and veggies, perhaps with some grains and milk or yogurt added, smoothies are an extremely effective and simple way of increasing your intake of nutrients.

Nutrients found in food enable the systems and organs of the body to function in their intended ways. These include the digestive tract, kidneys, lungs, skin, liver, lymphatic system, and respiratory system, which are each directly involved in the body's own detoxification processes. They cleanse the body by breaking down compounds into other forms that are then excreted through waste, sweat, and breathing. Certain nutrients also promote the health of the cardiovascular system in various ways. For example, some help to keep arteries clean and flexible by preventing plaque from building up in them.

Vitamins, minerals, and phytonutrients are vitally important to the body's own cleansing processes. These are the minute substances found in food that enable chemical processes to occur within the body's systems and organs.

> **THINK ABOUT IT!**
> There is no one diet or food that can promise a body that functions at its optimum, and the issue is further complicated by the fact that what may be "toxic" to one person may be highly beneficial to another. Furthermore, some essential nutrients are paradoxically toxic if consumed in high quantities. It might also be true that such programs may be less likely to introduce so-called "toxins" into the body in the first place.

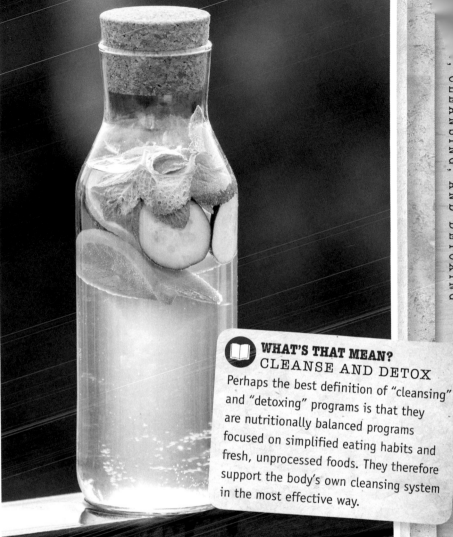

Detox drink of water infused with lemon and cucumber with mint

- Many of these substances support the immune system, protect cells, reduce or prevent inflammation, and help fight infection. Some are even thought to help ward off certain cancers.
- Others facilitate the release of energy, which is one of many reasons why eating fresh, unprocessed, natural foods helps boost energy levels.
- Some are needed for the effective metabolism of fats and carbohydrates, and for the building of healthy cells.
- Others facilitate production of hormones and enable their functioning, including some directly related to detoxification.

The list is seemingly endless, the processes complex, and yet the easiest and most effective way to support the body's own cleansing system is through good nutrition.

ESSENTIAL NUTRITION

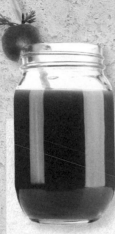

Carrot juice

To understand why juices and smoothies are so healthy for you, it helps to have a basic understanding of nutrition.

WHAT ARE NUTRIENTS?

Nutrients are the substances found in food that support and enable life. They enter the body through food and are not made by the body itself. Once absorbed into the body, they work alone or in combination with other substances to facilitate all the chemical interactions and bodily functions that occur within. Without nutrients, we could not grow, think, or otherwise exist. They are essential for the functioning of the human body and for its maintenance and repair.

There seems to be an infinite number of nutrients in food, including the fat-soluble vitamins A, D, E, and K as well as the water-soluble vitamins B complex and C; minerals such as calcium, magnesium, iron, and zinc; fats such as omega-3; proteins such as the amino acids found in legumes, meat, and dairy products; and carbohydrates, including the sugars found in fruit. Fiber and water are also considered nutrients.

Nutrients are found in all foods, including meat, grains, fats, and produce. Of course, overconsumption of certain nutrients such as saturated fats, sugars, and sodium is not beneficial for our health. Some foods, like sugary drinks and chips, have a low nutrient density,

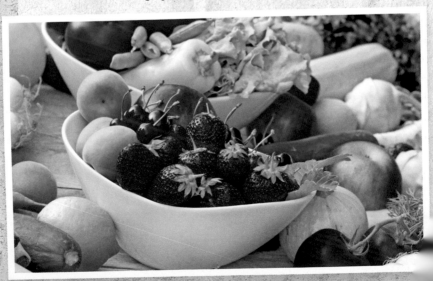

Fresh fruits and vegetables—the ingredients in juices and smoothies—are nutrient (

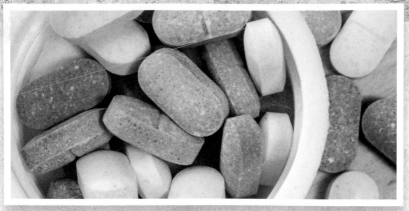

Ideally, vitamin supplements are just that—supplements to a healthy diet.

which means that even though they supply calories (energy), they provide little or no nutritional value. If you want to have a healthy diet then it is important to eat foods that have a high nutrient density— lots of nutrients for the calories. Fresh fruits and vegetables are good examples of foods that have a high nutrient density.

ESSENTIAL NUTRIENTS

There are seven categories of nutrients that are known as "essential" because they are necessary for health, growth, and life itself. Without them, we would not exist. They are:

- Vitamins
- Minerals
- Carbohydrates
- Proteins
- Fats (including oils)
- Fiber
- Water

Vitamins and minerals are known as micronutrients because only minute quantities are needed to enable the proper functioning of the body. Carbohydrates, proteins, and fats are known as macronutrients and are needed in larger quantities. Individual foods contain both macronutrients and micronutrients. For example, carrots are a good source of the macronutrient carbohydrate and also of vitamin A, a micronutrient. Fiber may also be classified as a macronutrient; it is needed in large amounts for the body to function properly. Water is in a class of its own because it is found in every cell in the body, is essential for the transportation of fluids within the body, and enables chemical reactions to occur, among a whole range of other functions.

VITAMINS AND MINERALS

Vitamins and minerals are chemical substances found in food. They support and maintain health and enable chemical processes to occur, including the conversion of carbohydrates into energy and the production of hormones by the body's glands. In some cases, they have preventative role, helping to protect the body from disease.

A varied and nutritious diet should, for the most part, provide all the vitamins and minerals that our bodies need. In certain situations, manufactured vitamin and mineral supplements are useful—for example, in cases of severe deficiency, when higher doses are required for the treatment of certain conditions, if people are following very restricted diets, or if locally available foods are deficient in specific nutrients. As the name itself implies, however, supplements should be used only to supplement rather than replace the vitamins and minerals sourced through fresh food.

The range of nutrients available through manufactured supplements is also limited by the extent of our knowledge. There is a wealth of both scientifically proven and folk knowledge about specific vitamins and minerals, but it is nonetheless still evolving—with no signs of an ending in sight. Continuing research is constantly revealing the myriad of ways that vitamins and minerals interact with our bodies, both on their own and in combination with other nutrients and substances in the body.

Vitamins and minerals are, of course, also found in other foods, but fresh produce offers a great variety, together with other valuable components such as phytonutrients, fatty acids, and all-important fiber. Fruit and vegetables are also relatively cheap, readily available, delicious, and easy to prepare.

Vitamins are needed in minute quantities in the body to ensure its proper functioning. They are classified into two groups: water soluble and fat soluble.

Fat-soluble vitamins: These vitamins—A, D, E, and K—are stored in the body. This means they are less susceptible to deficiencies than water-soluble vitamins, but at the same time, excesses building up in the body over time can result in unpleasant side effects.

Water-soluble vitamins: These vitamins—B-group and C—dissolve in the body's fluids, and excesses are excreted in urine. Because water-soluble vitamins are not stored in the body, they must be replenished frequently. The following tables outline some important vitamins.

CARBOHYDRATES

The main role of carbohydrates is to provide energy to the body. They come mainly from plants, including fruits, starchy vegetables, grains, and legumes. Although fats and proteins can also be used for energy, carbohydrates are the primary source.

Carbohydrates are broken down to glucose before being absorbed into the bloodstream. Glucose then circulates in the blood, providing fuel to the brain, and energy to the body and muscles, among other things. Importantly, not all carbohydrates are broken down by the body at the

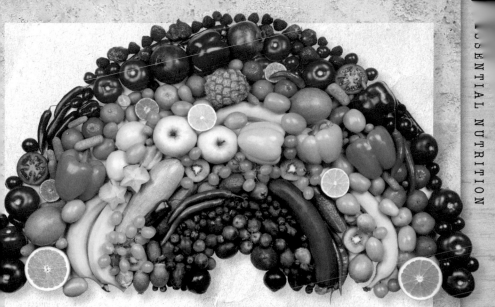

Think "food rainbow" when choosing fruits and vegetables. A wide range of colors ensures that you get a variety of important phytonutrients.

WHAT ABOUT PHYTOCHEMICALS?

There is an emergent group of micronutrients that is referred to as "phytonutrients," "phytochemicals," and "phytofoods." This book calls them phytonutrients or phytochemicals.

Phytochemicals are naturally occurring substances found in plants. They appear to be extremely beneficial to health but are in the early stages of scientific validation and have not, as yet, been classified as essential nutrients. Nonetheless, indications are that this is a promising area of research that is likely to have huge implications in preventative health practices (as people make lifestyle and dietary changes), as well as in treatments and remedies, and may eventually revolutionize our understanding of the health benefits of fresh fruit and vegetables.

Many phytonutrients have antioxidant properties, meaning they minimize damage caused to the body by harmful molecules called free radicals. Phytonutrients include beta-carotene (one of many carotenoids, which are the plant pigments that give carrots and other red-orange-yellow produce their color), anthocyanins (the blue pigment that colors berries and beets), chlorophyll (the green pigment in green fruits and vegetables), and the catechins found in black and green tea. Other phytonutrients are phytates (found in beans, brans, and whole grains), curcumins (found in turmeric and mustard), lignans (found in plant seeds such as flaxseed and certain produce), allicin (found in garlic and onion), and ellagic acid (found in grapes, strawberries, apples, and other fruit). A good rule of thumb is to eat a wide range of colored fruits and vegetables— sometimes described as a "food rainbow"—because the yellows, purples, and greens are indicative of the phytochemicals within.

GI INDEX LEVEL

The GI level in foods is classified into three groups. Low-GI foods have a GI of 55 or less, intermediate-GI foods have a GI between 55 and 70, and high-GI foods have a GI of 70 or above.

same rate. Those that break down more slowly are said to have a low glycemic index, or low GI.

Low GI foods are healthier for a number of reasons. In particular, they provide a steady but slow release of glucose into the bloodstream that results in smaller fluctuations in blood glucose and insulin levels. This in turn helps sustain energy over longer periods and also helps control appetite while promoting feelings of satiety and fullness for longer. These have obvious implications for weight management, but also in a wide range of other areas, such as helping to alleviate mood swings and to treat conditions such as diabetes and hyperglycemia.

Many fruits and some starchy vegetables are marvelous sources of low-GI carbs, providing high-quality, slow-release energy. Their fiber content also helps to make you feel full and staves off hunger longer.

PROTEIN

The main role of protein is to build, maintain, and repair our bodies. The amino acids found in proteins are called the "building blocks" of our bodies. When protein is digested, it is broken down into amino acids that are then reassembled in different configurations and used to rebuild the physical components of the body. Amino acids make up a large portion of our muscles and body tissues, and give structure to cells. Enzymes and other blood compounds are also built from amino acids, and they are essential for the building of bone and cartilage.

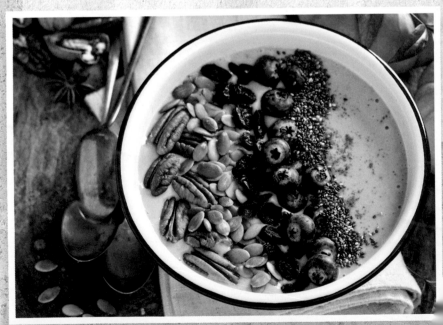

A pumpkin-based smoothie bowl gets a protein boost from a topping of berries, pecans, and pumpkin and chia seeds, making it a nutritious autumn lunch or dinner

There are at least 20 known amino acids, some of which we are able to source from food or produce ourselves, and others that must be sourced through food. Good sources of plant protein, and hence amino acids, include grains, legumes, and nuts. As some are lacking in certain amino acids but not in others, it is worth mixing the different sources of plant proteins so shortfalls in one food are corrected by the amino acids in another. Smoothies provide an ideal way to blend nuts and seeds together with legumes and other ingredients to ensure the body has all the amino acids it needs. The casein found in yogurt is high in amino acids and an ideal addition to smoothies, while nondairy alternatives such as coconut yogurt and almond milk are also good, although less rich, protein sources. Some commercially produced soy milks contain all of the essential amino acids.

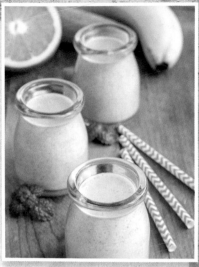

Yogurt provides a creamy base for smoothies, while supplying plenty of protein.

FATS

There are all kinds of fats, including very good ones and very bad ones. Good fats (and oils, which are liquid fats) are essential for good health and should be included in the diet.

Fat is also a secondary source of energy for the body, after carbohydrates and before proteins. When the body runs low on carbohydrates, it can source its energy needs from available fat before drawing on protein (which would break down muscles and other protein structures in the body to provide energy). Fat is crucial for storing fat-soluble vitamins and other nutrients, and it provides cushioning and insulation to the internal organs. And although this may be an uncommon consideration in privileged, well-sheltered, and well-fed societies, fat is a concentrated source of energy. Fat provides about twice as many calories per ounce as carbohydrates and protein do. This has long been of critical importance to indigenous nomadic people dependent on seasonal availability of food, and to those living in very cold climates who have a greater need for energy and fat to both generate and retain warmth in their bodies.

It's widely known that a diet too high in fat will, for most people, result in weight issues and all their attendant problems. It's equally important, however, to understand the relationship between fat and cholesterol, and in turn, "good" (high-density lipoprotein, or HDL) and "bad" (low-density lipoprotein, or LDL) cholesterol.

First, cholesterol itself is not a fat. It is a wax-like substance that is essential for a number of bodily functions. Some cholesterol is made by the body itself, and other cholesterol is found in food. Generally, if a healthy person consumes too much cholesterol, the body will compensate by either producing less cholesterol of its own or excreting the excess. Second, confusion arises because it seems that cholesterol is at once both essential and unhealthy. Not so. In fact, cholesterol only becomes a problem when there is too much in the blood, and when that cholesterol is what is known as LDL cholesterol.

LDL cholesterol is unhealthy because it contributes to the build-up of plaque on the artery walls. Plaque is a thick, hard deposit that clogs and hardens arteries, both narrowing them and making them less flexible, and causing a condition known as atherosclerosis. If a clot then forms and blocks an artery, it is likely to result in a stroke or heart attack. Other diseases are also associated with the buildup of plaque in the arteries, such as peripheral artery disease, which results when narrowing of the arteries reduces the supply of blood to the legs.

On the other hand, HDL cholesterol appears to have a cleansing effect, helping to remove LDL from the arteries and transport it back to the liver where it is broken down and then excreted.

Third, as both a preventative and corrective measure, it makes sense to limit the consumption of saturated fat because our livers appear to make LDL cholesterol from saturated fats. Dietary fats (and oils) are categorized into four different types:

- saturated fats
- monounsaturated fats
- polyunsaturated fats
- trans fats

Saturated fats: These are found mainly in meat and dairy foods, but also in palm oil and coconut oil. Most fruits and vegetables are very low in saturated fats, with some notable exceptions, such as coconut, which is high in saturated fat, and avocados.

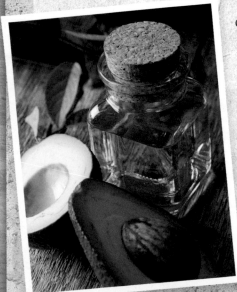

Some saturated fats—not all—contribute to higher levels of "bad" LDL cholesterol, which in turn increases the risk of cardiovascular problems. The link between saturated fat and heart disease is a contentious issue. Some research suggests that when saturated fat is found with calcium in foods like dairy products, the effect of the saturated fat may not be as damaging as once thought.

Avocado oil. Many vegetable and other plants are sources of dietary fats.

Research is also being undertaken to look at the effects of coconut consumption on blood cholesterol levels and plaque formation in the arteries. The research is not yet conclusive, but given that some saturated fats and oils are known to contribute to cholesterol problems, and others seem to be implicated in other serious health disorders, it makes sense to keep consumption of saturated fats to a minimum. Obviously, people with existing heart conditions should avoid them completely. A diet high in fresh fruit and vegetables is less likely to be high in saturated fat, and certain nutrients found in fresh produce may help to counteract the adverse effects of some saturated fats, unless they are cooked in buttery sauces.

Monounsaturated fats: These are high-quality, good fats that are found mainly in oils and fats from plant sources, including olives, avocados, and nuts. Unlike saturated fats, monounsaturated fats help reduce the levels of LDL cholesterol in the blood—although they do so less effectively than polyunsaturated fats—and hence help reduce the risk of heart and cardiovascular diseases.

Olive oil is a source of monounsaturated fats.

Polyunsaturated omega-6 fats: These come mainly from plant seeds, such as sunflower and sesame, and are used to make cooking oils. They are also found in grains, and are effective in reducing all types of cholesterol (both LDL and, less fortunately, HDL) in the blood.

Walnuts

Polyunsaturated omega-3 fats: These are polyunsaturated fats that, in addition to being able to reduce cholesterol levels, are able to thin the blood, reducing its ability to clot. They therefore have an important role in reducing the risk of heart and cardiovascular diseases. Omega-3 fats are found in both seafood and plant foods, with the strongest evidence of benefits to date being associated with seafood. Nonetheless, omega-3 fats can be obtained from plant sources, including canola oil, flaxseed (linseed), chia seeds, and walnuts. Research into the potential benefits of omega-3 fats is continuing, but indications are that they have strong anti-inflammatory effects and positive implications in the treatment and prevention of rheumatoid arthritis, inflammatory bowel disease, stroke, hypertension, and depression. They may also boost immunity and reduce overall inflammation.

Seek out plant-based oils, such as canola, a polyunsaturated omega-3 oil.

Trans fats: These are unsaturated fats that behave like saturated fats and are, therefore, unhealthy. They occur naturally in certain animal foods, including some dairy products as well as beef and lamb, but are not found in fruit, vegetables, or grains—another reason why a diet high in fruit and vegetables is such a healthy option. That said, our bodies have managed the trans fats found in animal foods for centuries without too many problems; the problems are associated more with commercial fats used in food production—for example, liquid vegetable oils that are artificially converted into solids, such as certain margarines. For this reason, it pays to inspect food labels and avoid foods with trans fats as much as possible.

Citrus peel contains high levels of the soluble fiber pectin.

FIBER

Dietary fiber, or roughage, is the indigestible parts of plant food that pass through the digestive tract and bowel and are eventually eliminated. There are three types: soluble, insoluble, and resistant starch.

To boost your fiber intake, use unpeeled apples for both juices and smoothies. The skins are rich in insoluble fiber, while the flesh supplies the soluble kind.

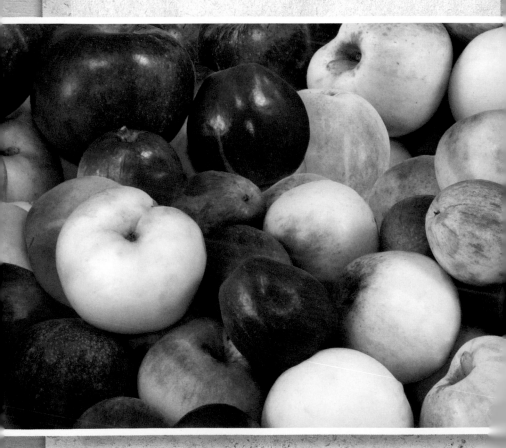

Soluble fiber: This type dissolves in water and forms a gel-like substance. It promotes satiety, contributes to the removal of cholesterol from the body, and helps to control blood sugar levels. Pectin, the fiber in fruit, is a soluble fiber, as is the fiber found in legumes.

Insoluble fiber: This type is the structural component of the plant found in vegetables and fruit peels and, while also promoting satiety, helps speed the passage of food through the bowel. This is important for a number of reasons, not least because it prevents constipation and reduces the length of time that toxic substances are in contact with the membranes of the bowel.

Resistant starch: This type resists digestion and ferments in the large bowel, where it produces acids that offer protection against bowel cancer. Certain grains and cold, cooked potatoes are examples of foods high in resistant starch (warmed potatoes are more digestible but their starch becomes less resistant).

THINK ABOUT IT!
Water is both essential and beneficial in more ways than can be listed here. Suffice to say that our bodies—both the rigid and fluid parts and everything in between—are composed mostly of water, and hence it is needed for our very existence. It is required in some way in every bodily function, as well as the more obvious functions of enabling excretion of waste through the kidneys, transporting nutrients around the body in the blood, helping food to pass through the digestive system, aiding thermoregulation, helping to suppress appetite, moistening our eyes and mouths, and keeping our skin plump and nourished. Without water we could not survive.

ESSENTIAL EQUIPMENT

Juicing equipment can be as simple as an old-fashioned lemon squeezer or as high-tech as a state-of-the art juicing machine. For smoothies, a blender is a must.

A basic handheld lemon squeezer

JUICING NEEDS

Juicing is big business nowadays, and you only need to take a quick look online to see how easy it might be to part with hundreds of dollars buying a state-of-the-art juicer. One of the many refreshing things about juicing, however, is that you can get started with minimal equipment. So, what's best for your needs: the humble citrus juicer, a juicer, or a blender? And what's the difference, anyway?

PRESS, SQUEEZE, AND REAM

The basic juicer is the citrus press, the humble lemon squeezer that you no doubt have hidden away in a kitchen drawer somewhere along with the egg slicer, ice-cream scoop, and a host of other occasional-use gadgets (some more useful than others).

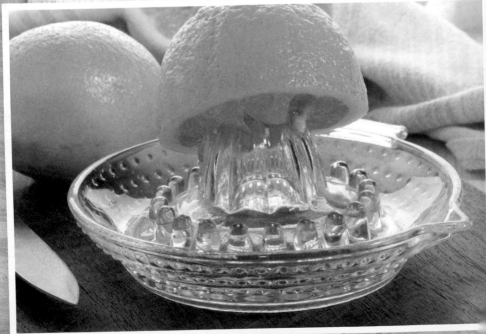

The classic glass citrus press

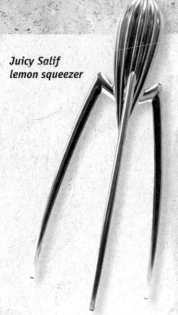

*Juicy Salif
lemon squeezer*

STOP THE PRESS!

In 1990, the citrus juicer emerged from the dark recesses of the kitchen-clutter cabinet and stepped into the limelight (pun intended!) as the now iconic Juicy Salif lemon squeezer. Like a scale model of something from H. G. Wells' sci-fi novel *War of the Worlds*, it is the creation of the design whiz Philippe Starck. Standing at just under a foot tall, the reamer is suspended on three spidery legs and a glass is placed underneath to collect the juice (most of the time). Like much of Starck's work, it is somewhat controversial and is as much a work of art and a dinner-party talking point as a practical kitchen implement. Starck's juicer can be seen in New York City's Museum of Modern Art or in trendy kitchens everywhere—available in aluminum or even gold plate!

Citrus press: The citrus press has the advantage of being cheap and quick to use. You simply slice the fruit in half (horizontally, across its segments) and press the cut end down onto the "reamer," which is itself a half-lemon shape, grooved to increase the pressure on the fruit flesh and to allow the juice to run down into the bowl. In the classic, usually glass, model, the pith and pips are separated from the juice by a simple circle of nodules surrounding the reamer. A flat handle is positioned at ninety degrees to a spout. This is still a great option for that refreshing glass of fresh orange juice.

Lemon squeezer: Even simpler is the true lemon squeezer, a handheld lever device with a bowl on one side and a grooves on the other. You place a half lemon in (or in larger versions, an orange or other citrus fruit), and . . . squeeze.

Citrus reamer: The most simple of all is the citrus reamer, a handled tool with a tapered conical blade and deep straight troughs running the length of the blade. You first half the fruit, pierce the flesh with the tip of the reamer blade, and then grind out the inside with a twisting motion until nearly all of the juice is extracted. This dislodges the seeds and some of the pith, and you will have to strain the juice.

*A simple
wooden
citrus reamer*

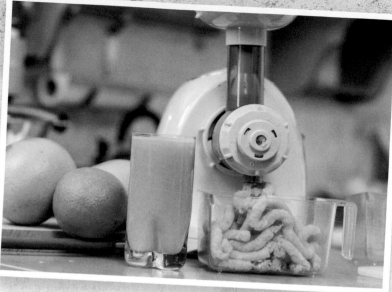

Masticating juicer

THE WHOLE JUICE, AND NOTHING BUT THE JUICE

You can make delicious juices in a blender, but for the true juicing experience, nothing beats a juicer machine. The key difference between blenders and juicers is simply that blenders don't separate the juice from the pulp. If you prefer your health drinks super smooth and easily digestible, with no hint of pith or pip, then you need to consider a juicer, which will separate the juice from the fibers of fruit and vegetables. Prices range from inexpensive to exorbitant but, as in all things in life, you generally get what you pay for. There are two different types of juicers for fruits and vegetables: centrifugal and masticating. A third type, an expeller press juicer, is made for wheatgrass and leafy green vegetables.

Centrifugal juicers: This machine has a perforated metal basket, usually complete with minute "teeth" that grind the fruit or vegetable as the basket spins. The centrifugal force pushes the liquid through the perforations to separate the juice from the pulp.

Masticating juicers: These are more substantial (and considerably more expensive) machines that use a powerful screwlike mechanism to pulverize the food into mush, which is forced down a tapered tube and through

Centrifugal juicer

a wire mesh so that the juice is separated from the pulp. They extract larger amounts of juice than centrifugal models and therefore larger quantities of nutrients. It is argued that their slowly rotating cutters do not expose the juice to oxidization, so that it maintains its nutritional value for longer and doesn't have to be drunk immediately. The quality of a masticating juicer is best gauged by the quantity and dryness of the pulp that is left behind after the juicing process; cheaper juicers leave a higher quantity of damp "mush," whereas a high-end machine will leave bone-dry pulp—and remarkably little of it.

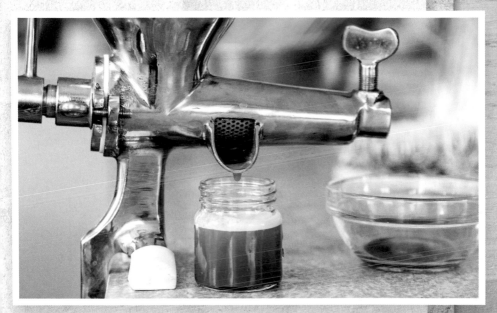

A wheatgrass juice extractor

WHEATGRASS JUICERS

Leafy vegetables and wheatgrass are packed with nutrition, but their "stringiness" means they can only be juiced in specialized juicers—centrifugal juicers simply cannot process them. Fortunately, there are specialized expeller press juicers that are relatively cheap and easy to use. Many models are manually operated with a crank handle and attach to a tabletop using a simple vice to provide stability without bulk. They're light and don't require electricity, so you can take your wheatgrass juicer with you on your travels and need never do without your favorite green drinks. In fact, since such "specialized" machines juice a variety of fruit and vegetables other than wheatgrass, this may be the only juicer you need.

Whichever machine best suits your needs and your budget, check that it dismantles easily so that it can be cleaned quickly and thoroughly. Nothing is more likely to turn you off of juicing than the thought of laboriously scrubbing gunk from the contraption every time you make a drink.

Wheatgrass juice

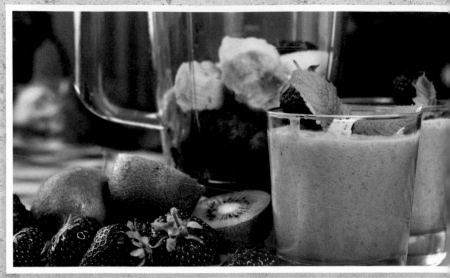

Your blender takes just minutes to turn fresh fruit like strawberries, kiwis, and bananas into healthy and flavorful smoothies.

BLENDERS

Not much equipment is needed for making smoothies. The whole point is that they are quick, easy to make, uncomplicated, not messy—but wonderfully nutritious. Really, the only major piece of equipment for making smoothies is a good-quality blender.

You may or may not need a glass from which to drink the smoothie—in some of the powerful modern blenders, the mixing vessel is also the drinking receptacle, making them super quick and easy to use and to clean up afterward.

There are three main types: jug-style blenders long used for blending milkshakes, smoothies, and other concoctions; the new breed of powerful "nutrient-extracting" upside-down blenders, such as the Nutri Ninja and NutriBullet; and finally, the humble handheld blender. If you are using one of the first two types, clear a space on your kitchen counter—close to a power outlet and ideally the fruit bowl—and keep it there, ready for use whenever a smoothie craving strikes. Don't pack it away where it will fight for space and become less accessible, so that moments of inspiration disappear in a puff of frustration as you fight to retrieve it from the back of the cupboard.

Jug blenders: The powerful (usually more expensive) jug blenders can generally blend most ingredients well, even if they are all loaded into the jug at the same time. Blending times may vary, depending on the level of smoothness desired. You may need several bursts on high power for 15 to 30 seconds. Be aware, however, that even some of the more powerful jug blenders do not have the ability to crush ice. If your blender does not handle ice easily, chilled water or slightly softened frozen fruit, such as berries, might be a better option. You can also use ice that has been crushed beforehand. Powerful blenders are a great choice—not only can they handle tough ingredients, but their ability to finely grind ingredients also enables more nutrients to be released. Don't be tempted to load indiscriminate amounts of nuts, seeds, supplements, and other nonproduce ingredients into the blender just because you can; overloading with some ingredients can have adverse health effects, while pulverizing others can release toxins that cannot be digested.

Making the smoothie: When using a jug-style blender, especially a less powerful one, place ice in the bottom of the jug, followed by the liquid. Add supplements, nuts, seeds, and grains at this point if you are using them, then the soft ingredients, such as spinach, herbs, and soft fruits. Load the heavier ingredients, such as apples and pears, last. Top up with extra fluid if needed.

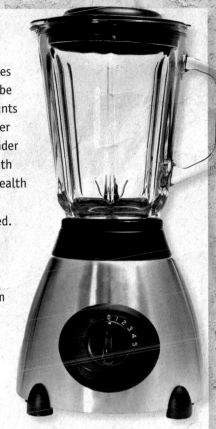

A jug blender

If you have a very powerful blender, mix everything together in one go. If your blender is less powerful, you may need to blend in steps, first blending the ice, liquid, and leafy vegetables, before progressing through the rest.

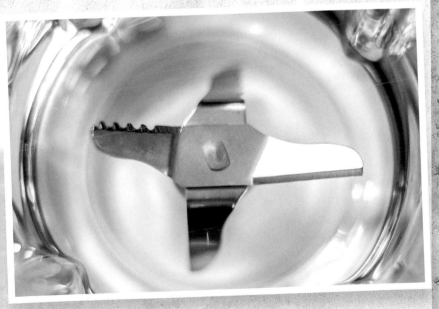

The rotating metal blades at the bottom of the blender mix and puree your ingredients. More powerful models can also crush ice for a frosty-cold smoothie.

Ninjas, NutriBullets, and other "Nutrient-Extracting" blenders: These are the super-powerful upside-down blenders that use a large bottle-like vessel or beaker instead of a jug to hold the ingredients. You fill the vessel with the ingredients before screwing it into a lid that also holds (very securely) the powerful blades. You then insert it upside down (with lid and blades at the bottom) into the machine. The beauty of this design is twofold: First, when blending is complete, you remove the vessel from the machine and take off the lid; you can then drink the smoothie straight from the vessel or tip it into a glass. Second, cleanup is a breeze. The lid is quick and easy to wash, and because the vessel is also used as a drinking cup, there are fewer utensils to wash. There are also claims that the most powerful of these types of blenders are able to extract additional nutrients from fruit and vegetables.

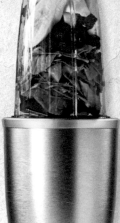

Bullet-style blender

JUICING ACCESSORIES

Many of the accessories you need for juicing will already be in your kitchen, so check your pantry before you make a shopping list. Here are a few handy items to keep with your juicing equipment:

- Scales to weigh solid ingredients
- A measuring cup ensures that you have the correct proportions of liquid ingredients for each recipe.

Scale for dry ingredients

- A vegetable peeler to remove the skin from certain foods—especially many non-organic fruits and root veggies

Peeler

- A small, sharp fruit knife and a larger chopping blade are musts, along with a suitable cutting board.
- Small graters are useful for citrus zest or spices such as nutmeg or stick cinnamon.
- A long-handled spoon or swizzle stick is ideal for combining juices (and the spoon can help you retrieve the maximum amount of those thicker smoothies that tend to stick to the bottom -of the jug).
- A range of glasses to display your wonderful creations to their best advantage.
- Finally, when you really start taking your juicing and smoothie-crafting seriously, you might want to add a few luxury items, such as an apple or pineapple corer.

Grater

These machines also come with extra lids (without blades) that are used to seal the smoothies inside the vessel if they are not consumed right away. This makes it portable, preventing spills and keeping particles in the air from entering, and also suitable for short-term storage in the fridge. Most also have drinking spouts—a practical and fun design that is popular with kids and teenagers.

Making the smoothie: In this type of blender, the ingredients are put into the vessel in the opposite order as in jug blenders, and then it is inverted. First, in go the fruit and vegetables, followed by any nuts, seeds, and supplements, then the liquids, and finally the ice. Then it is just a matter of screwing on the lid, inserting the vessel upside down into the machine, and blending the ingredients.

Handheld immersion blenders: Handheld blenders can be quite useful and have the advantage of being portable, so they can be taken on vacation, to work, and to the gym. Models are available that come with useful accessories, such as a chopping bowl, whisk attachment, beaker, and mini food processor. Although there are powerful ones available, few would be capable of handling tougher ingredients, and so they are limited to making smoothies with softer fruits and vegetables, such as mangoes, berries, and bananas. All in all, handheld blenders can make smoothies, but in a more work-intensive and limited way. If you are serious about smoothies, try to invest in a powerful full-sized machine.

Making the smoothie: Most likely, you will need to cube the fruits and vegetables before blending. Start by putting small amounts of diced ingredients and liquid into a suitable vessel, then begin blending. Add more ingredients and liquid as you go, blending them all together between additions. Some experimentation might be needed.

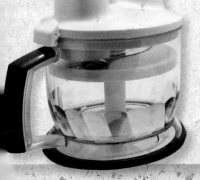

Handheld blender with mini food processor, beaker, and whisk accessories

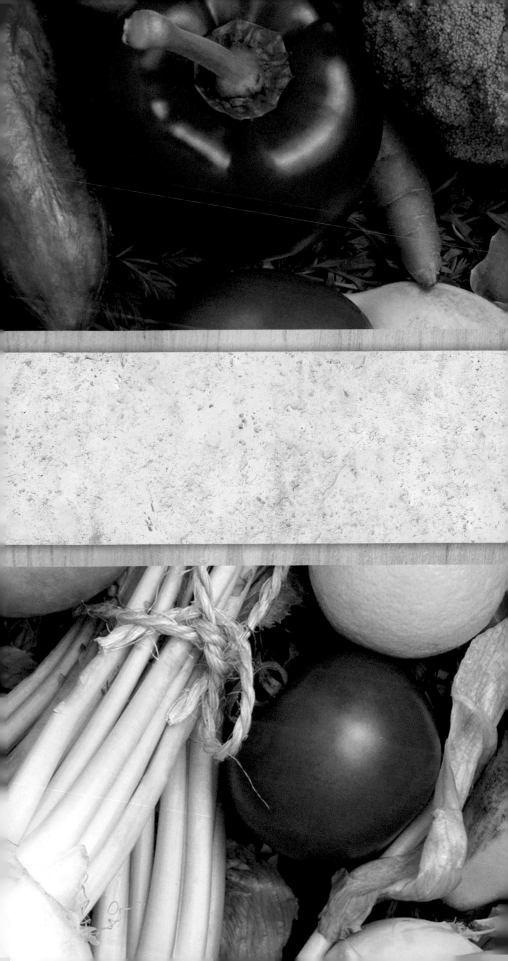

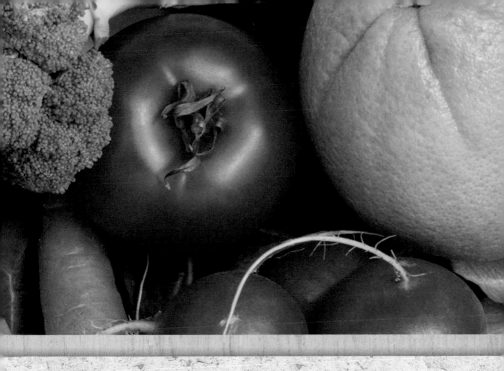

CHAPTER 2
INGREDIENTS
A TO Z

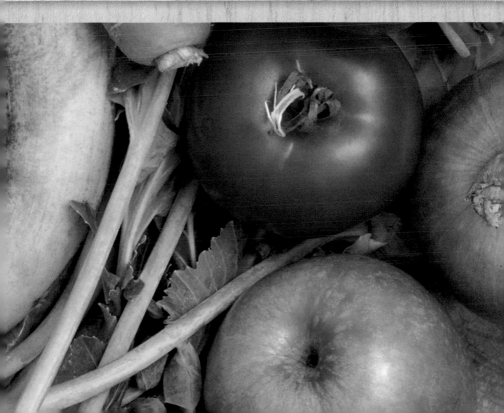

INGREDIENTS A TO Z GALLERY

Let's take some time to get to know the stars of the show: the individual fruits and vegetables that appear in so many wonderful juices, smoothies, and bowls. Each has its own variety of nutritional benefits, and learning a little about those nutrients can go a long way to helping you create a healthy balanced diet.

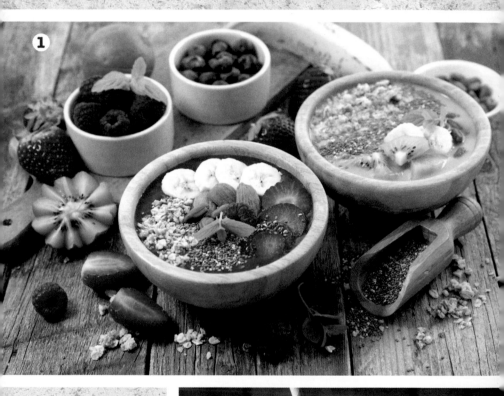

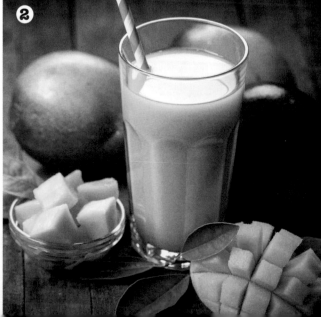

1 Strawberry-banana and kiwi smoothie bowls
2 Mango juice
3 Cucumber smoothie
4 Watermelon and pomegranate smoothie
5 Grapefruit juice
6 Wheatgrass juice

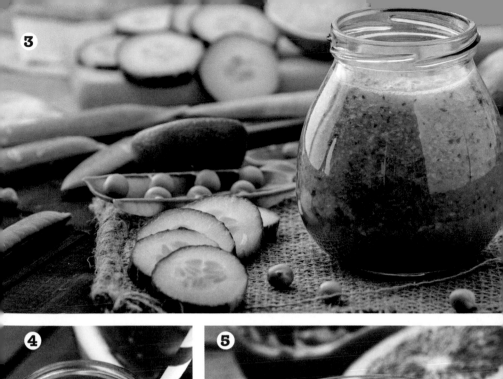

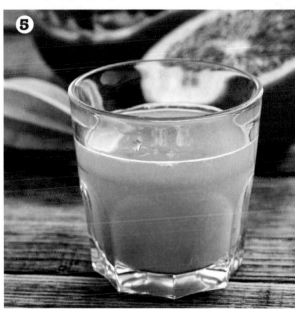

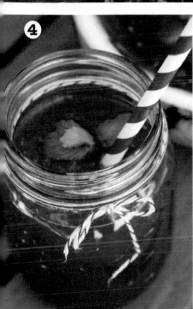

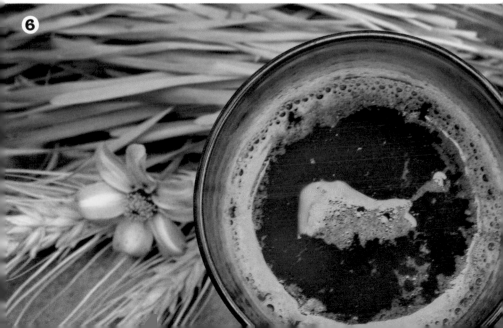

ACAI

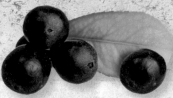

Touted by many people as a "super food," acai just might earn this appellation. It is packed with antioxidants, fiber, and heart-healthy fats.

THE BASICS

Acai is the fruit of the acai palm (*Euterpe oleracea*) and has a large seed and very little flesh. Acai is not a berry, but rather it is a drupe (stone fruit). Its small size and deep blue color most likely account for its association with berries.

It perishes quickly, so it is frozen or freeze-dried immediately after picking. It is then used in a variety of health foods, beverages, and supplements. Like all fruit, acai is nutritious, but many of the more amazing claims regarding its "miracle" properties are yet to be proven. As fresh acai is not generally available, its nutritional quality will vary depending on the quality of the product in which it is contained. Acai has a slightly bitter flavor, so it is generally mixed with fruit juices to improve its taste.

BEST FOR
Antioxidants, for a healthy immune system

CALORIES
80 to 250 per 3.5 ounces

PREPARATION
Add frozen fruit or powdered acai to smoothies and smoothie bowls.

DIY: RECIPES

Acai purée makes a perfect base for a morning smoothie bowl.

Acai Smoothie Bowl

- ½ small banana
- 3.5-ounce (100 g) pack frozen unsweetened acai berry pulp
- ½ cup frozen strawberries
- ¼ cup frozen blueberries
- ¼ cup frozen raspberries
- ½ cup almond milk

In a blender, add banana, acai pulp, strawberries, blueberries, and a splash of milk. Pour mixture into a bowl and top with sliced fruit, nuts, and seeds.

HEALTH BENEFITS

Acai contains antioxidants, which can protect the body's cells from free-radical damage, support cardiovascular health, and help to boost the immune system. Antioxidants are also thought to play a role in slowing down the aging process. Acai has high fiber content, is rich in vitamin E, and contains small amounts of calcium and iron.

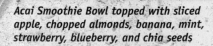

Acai Smoothie Bowl topped with sliced apple, chopped almonds, banana, mint, strawberry, blueberry, and chia seeds

ALFALFA

Long prized as a livestock feed source for its high vitamin, mineral, and protein content, alfalfa is also good for humans and can add a healthy dose of fiber to a savory smoothie.

THE BASICS

Alfalfa *(Medicago sativa)*, a member of the pea (or legume) family, is also called lucerne and buffalo herb. Fresh alfalfa is readily available in supermarkets and health food stores. It is used in salads, sandwiches, and tea, as well as in smoothies.

HEALTH BENEFITS

Although it is thought that alfalfa might assist in the treatment of various health conditions, most of these claims are still subject to further study. Both the seeds and sprouts of this light, crunchy legume are a rich source of beta-carotene, a highly potent antioxidant that the body also converts to vitamin A. Alfalfa contains several other minerals (calcium, iron, magnesium, phosphorus, and potassium) as well as vitamins B1, B3, B12, D, C, E, and K.

BEST FOR
Fiber, which helps lower cholesterol

CALORIES
28 per 3.5 ounces

PREPARATION
Wash and roughly chop, then add to smoothies and smoothie bowls.

An alfalfa in bloom displays the plant's pale purple clover-like flowers.

APPLE

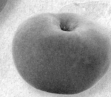
Granny Smith

Perhaps the best known and most popular of all fruits, apples are remarkably nutritious and versatile. Best of all, apples are widely available year-round, and the high number of varieties means there is always a wide selection of varying flavors, from sweet to tart, to choose from.

Golden Russet

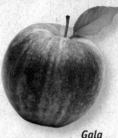
Gala

THE BASICS

An apple is the fruit of the *Malus pumila* tree. There are over 7,500 varieties of apple, and some are particularly good for juicing, including the ubiquitous Cox's Orange Pippin and the Golden Russet. As a rule of thumb, the greener an apple's skin, the sharper its juice will taste, so if you enjoy a tart flavor, opt for Granny Smith apples. For sweeter juice, go for Gala or McIntosh. Whichever variety you choose, select fresh fruit with firm, undamaged skin. Avoid those with waxy skins, as this often disguises a woolly, flavorless fruit. Apples should be washed thoroughly and chopped into quarters. They do not necessarily need to be peeled or cored—apple seeds are a valuable source of potassium.

BEST FOR
Pectin and vitamin C, which lower cholesterol

CALORIES
52 per 3.5 ounces

PREPARATION
Wash and chop into quarters. No need to peel or core.

HEALTH BENEFITS

Apples are full of important nutrients, especially fiber, as well as carbohydrates. They have a low GI (38) and are a source of vitamin C, many of the B-group vitamins, and various minerals, including calcium and potassium.

Apples are full of a fiber called pectin, which is classed as a soluble, fermentable, and viscous fiber, a combination that gives it a huge list of health benefits.

Pectin, a gelling agent, offers particular digestive benefits by speeding the passage of food through the digestive tract, hence reducing the time that the mucous membrane of the colon is exposed to toxic substances in the stool. Additionally, pectin plays a role in reducing cholesterol levels. They are also rich in antioxidants, and it is thought that their polyphenols may provide a protective benefit for our lungs and airways.

DIY: RECIPES

Apple is a versatile fruit that blends well with other veggies and other fruit.

Apple-Carrot Juice

- 1 apple, cored
- 1 carrot
- 1 stalk of celery

Scrub all produce, then put ingredients through a juicer.

Apple-Strawberry Nectar

- 2 cups fresh strawberries
- ¼ cup unsweetened apple juice, or to taste
- 2 tablespoon water, or as needed (optional)

Wash all produce, then put ingredients through a juicer.

Apple-Celery Juice

- 4 green apples, cored
- 6 celery stalks

Scrub all produce, then put ingredients through a juicer.

Waterapple Juice

- 2 apples, cored
- 3 slices of watermelon, rind removed

Scrub all produce, then put ingredients through a juicer.

Apple-Carrot Juice

APRICOT

Hailing from the peach family, apricots are firm, attractive, pinkish orange fruits with velvety skin and a distinctive bittersweet flavor that is something between a peach and a plum.

THE BASICS

Apricots come from one of the many species of *Prunus* that produce flavorsome fruit, including plums, cherries, peaches, and nectarines. These delicious stone fruits—technically drupes—have soft flesh that blends beautifully into smoothies. Their flavor is sweet, but has a distinctive tang. Dried apricots make a tasty snack, and can be added to smoothies if desired.

BEST FOR
Vitamin A and beta-carotene, to promote healthy eyes, skin, hair, and bones

CALORIES
48 per 3.5 ounces

PREPARATION
Wash, remove stone. No need to peel.

HEALTH BENEFITS

Widely recognized as a superfood, apricots are a good source of fiber and an excellent source of vitamin A, which is vital for healthy eyesight and a leading agent in the battle against age-related macular degeneration. Their lovely orange color immediately signals the presence of the antioxidant beta-carotene within. Known to the Greeks as "golden eggs of the sun," apricots are also high in vitamin C and minerals such as calcium, magnesium, silicon, and phosphorus. They are wonderful antioxidant cleansers and are often recommended for respiratory problems. They are not one of the juiciest fruits, so you will need several to produce a reasonable quantity of juice, and they are best mixed with another juice, or diluted with water. Although the stone is edible, it should be removed before juicing.

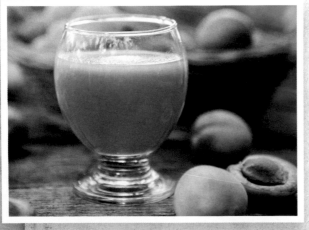

Apricot nectar

AVOCADO

Avocados are a particularly satisfying food that helps to keep hunger at bay for long periods of time. Adding avocados to smoothies can increase the absorption of carotenoids like beta-carotene from other colorful fruits and vegetables.

THE BASICS

Avocados, also known as alligator pears, are the large berries of the avocado tree *(Persea americana)*. The pits, or stones, are the single seed within.

Like apricots and bananas, avocados are not great for juicing. Plus, they tend to receive a lot of bad press for their high fat and calorie content. Nevertheless, they are packed with goodness and can be successfully blended with other juicier fruits and vegetables. The rich, smooth flesh of this subtly flavored fruit lends a seductively creamy texture to green smoothies that works particularly well with cacao and banana.

BEST FOR
Folate, to produce healthy red blood cells

CALORIES
160 per 3.5 ounces

PREPARATION
Wash, cut in half to remove stone, scoop flesh into blender.

HEALTH BENEFITS

Avocados are high in vitamin E, which boosts the immune system, and their cholesterol-lowering properties, along with their folate content, help keep your heart healthy. Folate helps the body produce red blood cells and has several other vital functions. It is particularly important for pregnant women because it reduces the risk of birth defects. Avocados are also an excellent source of potassium, which many health experts claim provides protection against premature aging. As well as improving your complexion, potassium helps combat fatigue and lethargy.

Despite the creamy texture, avocados are also high in fiber. They are also rich in heart-friendly monounsaturated fats. Some research suggests that the monounsaturated fats in avocados may assist in maintaining good cholesterol and blood sugar levels.

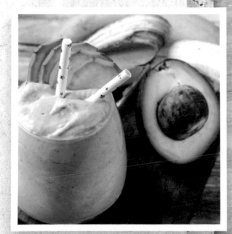

For a postworkout snack, blend avocado and banana with the low-fat milk of your choice and enjoy a potassium-replenishing smoothie.

BANANA

Widely available, bananas are an ideal ingredient in smoothies due to their creamy texture, sweet flavor, high fiber content, and excellent nutritional value.

THE BASICS

Botanically a berry, the banana is the fruit of several species of the tropical tree species *Musa*. Once considered an exotic indulgence, it is now common just about everywhere and comes in many sizes, colors, and degrees of firmness. Most varieties are elongated and

BEST FOR
Vitamin B6 (pyridoxine), which preserves nerves and skin

CALORIES
79 per 3.5 ounces

PREPARATION
Peel and chop into segments.

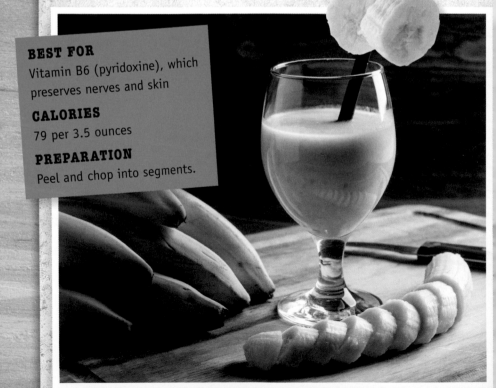

No-Frills Banana Smoothie

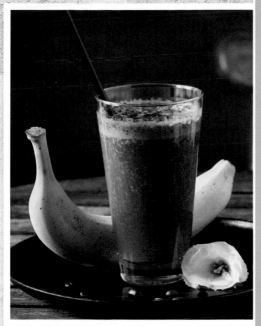

Morning Banana Java

curved, with pale soft flesh covered in green, yellow, red, purple, or brown rind when ripe.

For juicing, use soft bananas, chopped up or mashed, and combined with a juicier fruit that will flush the banana through the juicer. Bananas come into their own in smoothies because they can be blended more successfully and provide a great flavor along with a lovely creamy texture.

HEALTH BENEFITS

Bananas have many claims to fame, but they are perhaps best known for their high levels of potassium, a mineral vital to the functioning of body cells. They are a good source of manganese and magnesium— essential trace minerals involved in the production of cartilage as well as being required for healthy bones and for normal nerve function. They also have small amounts of the other B vitamins and contain vitamin C. They are low in sodium, make a good source of energy-boosting carbohydrates, and have a low GI (52).

Bananas are the best fruit source of vitamin B6, which metabolizes proteins, sugars, and fatty acids. Vitamin B6 also helps with the production of serotonin, the body's natural "happy" chemical that is often prescribed in drug form as an antidepressant. The banana has been described as "a sleeping pill in a peel"—in addition to the soothing serotonin, the magnesium acts as a muscle relaxant.

BEET

These modest round root vegetables have recently found unexpected fame as a fashionable superfood.

THE BASICS

A beet, also known as beetroot, table beet, garden beet, red beet, or golden beet, is the taproot portion of the beet plant *(Beta vulgaris)*. A beet has two edible parts: the root and the leaves.

It has a sweet flavor and comes in a variety of colors ranging from garnet red to white. The beautiful bright red juice gives a colorful lift to other juices, which dilute its strong taste. Beet juice may turn the urine red; this is not unusual, but can sometimes indicate an underlying problem with iron metabolism. Choose small, firm beets and avoid any with wilting foliage.

BEST FOR
Antioxidants, to help prevent cancer and heart disease

CALORIES
44 per 3.5 ounces

PREPARATION
Cut off the tops and wash; scrub the roots, cut into quarters, and use immediately.

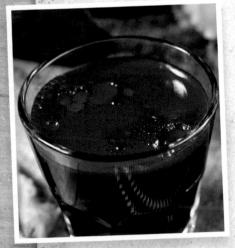

Fresh beet juice (above); beetroot plant (opposite)

HEALTH BENEFITS

The unusual rich red color of a beet comes from phytochemicals known as betalains, which have an antioxidant and anti-inflammatory role. Beet juice has some effect in lowering blood pressure and increasing blood flow to the brain in older people. Surprisingly, it may also make you run a little bit faster!

Nutritionally, beets are a good source of vitamins A and C, iron, beta-carotene, potassium, calcium, folate, and fiber, and they are low in calories. When used raw, beets are very high in folate, which reduces the risk of fetal defects.

The green tops contain certain nutrients in higher concentration than in the roots, with higher levels of phytonutrients and vitamins C and A, so be sure to eat them or throw them in the smoothie, too. They should not be consumed in large quantities, however, because they contain potentially harmful oxalic acid.

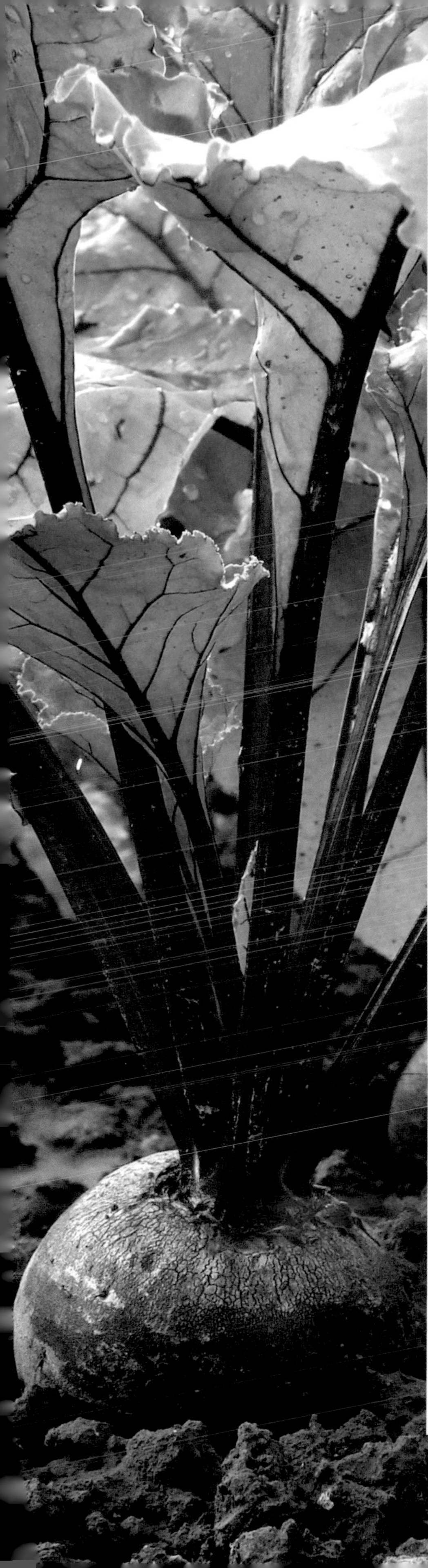

DIY: RECIPES

The red color of beets makes juices and smoothies made from this vivid veggie as pretty as they are healthful.

Beet Base

- 1 small beet
- 2 carrots
- 2 apples
- 1 handful of kale

Wash all produce, then put ingredients through a juicer.

Spicy Sweet Beet Juice

- 1 small beet (reduce to a quarter of a beet if you don't eat raw beets regularly)
- 1 small carrot, peeled
- ¼ yellow bell pepper
- 2 lemon wedges (add some rind if you like a little tartness)
- jalapeño pepper and cilantro to taste
- 2 large romaine lettuce leaves (optional)

Scrub all produce, then put ingredients through a juicer.

Beet, Apple & Blackberry Juice

- 3 small beets
- 2 to 3 apples
- 8 ounces blackberries
- ½ inch ginger

Wash all produce, then put ingredients through a juicer.

Pear, Apple & Beet Juice

- 2 apples, scrubbed
- 1 pear, scrubbed
- 3 medium or 2 large beets
- 1 lemon, peeled
- ½ inch ginger

Scrub all produce, then put ingredients through a juicer.

BLACKBERRY

Low in calories, blackberries have a tart, sweet flavor that enhances juices and smoothies.

Blackberry juice

THE BASICS

Many species in the genus *Rubus* produce tasty blackberries, which grow on thorny brambles that can make gathering them a challenging yet highly rewarding adventure. When buying or picking blackberries, choose ones that are plump, dry, deeply colored, and quite firm to the touch. They are highly perishable, so they should be consumed as soon as possible or refrigerated for up to five days. You can also store them in the freezer for later use.

BEST FOR
Vitamin C, for healthy skin, blood, and bones

CALORIES
43 per 3.5 ounces

PREPARATION
Wash and use immediately.

DIY: RECIPES

Juice blackberries for a wine-colored beverage.

Blackberry-Kiwi Juice

- 1 cup blackberries
- 1 kiwi (2-inch diameter)
- 1 medium pear
- 30 leaves peppermint
- ¼ pineapple, peeled and cored

Wash all produce, then put ingredients through a juicer.

Blackberry Grape Juice

- 2 cups blackberries
- 2 cups black or purple grapes
- 2-inch piece ginger

Wash all produce, then put ingredients through a juicer.

HEALTH BENEFITS

Low-calorie blackberries produce a nutrient-rich mixing juice. High in fiber, they aid digestion and improve cardiovascular health. They also help you to feel satisfied longer, which makes them a great diet food. They also have anthocyanins that help prevent the effects of aging, and gallic acid, an antioxidant used to treat psoriasis and hemorrhoids. They are also a good source of vitamins A and C, which work together as antioxidants to help strengthen the immune system.

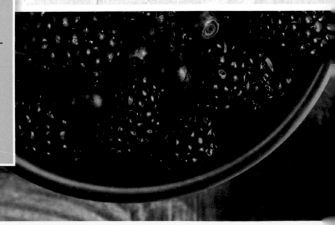

Blackberries and blueberries

BLACKCURRANT

The blackcurrant produces a delightfully piquant juice and is a welcome addition to juice blends and smoothies.

THE BASICS

Blackcurrants are the small fruit that develops along the stems of the shrubby flowering *Ribes nigrum* plant. Fresh blackcurrants are dark purple, almost black, with a glossy skin and a delightfully tangy taste. If not used immediately, store blackcurrants in the refrigerator, where they will keep fresh for several days.

HEALTH BENEFITS

These juicy and acidic berries are rich in vitamin C and iron. Iron is an essential mineral whose main function is to help distribute oxygen from the lungs. When iron is low, oxygen circulates more slowly, often resulting in fatigue, irritability, and headaches. Significant deficiency can lead to anemia. Women are more likely to develop iron deficiency, partly because of the loss of red blood cells during menstruation. Adolescents, both male and female, may also be lacking, due to their rapid growth. Iron absorption can be impaired by the frequent drinking of tea and coffee, so replace at least one of your daily caffeine boosters with another drink—say, a delicious blackcurrant juice.

DIY: RECIPES

Add a handful of blackcurrants and blackberries to grapefruit to sweeten the tart citrus flavor while further boosting your dose of vitamin C.

Citrus Berry Juice

- 2 grapefruits
- 1 handful blackberries
- 1 handful blackcurrants

Wash all produce, then put ingredients through a juicer.

BEST FOR
Vitamin C and iron, to metabolize proteins and promote growth

CALORIES
63 per 3.5 ounces

PREPARATION
Wash and use immediately.

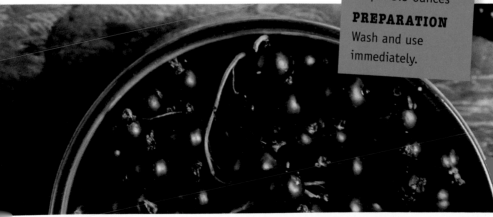

Blackcurrants

BLUEBERRY

Commonly hailed as the ultimate superfood, blueberries are now hugely popular all around the world and are famed for having one of the highest antioxidant capacities among all fruits and vegetables.

THE BASICS

Blueberries *(Vaccinium corymbosum)* have been enjoyed by Native Americans for centuries, and they are one of the few fruits that originated in North America. They have a mild, slightly sweet, slightly tart flavor that is not particularly distinctive but combines well with other fruits. Like all berries, they are highly perishable, and quickly become "squishy" and begin to lose their nutritional value. Fortunately, blueberries can be frozen for three months without damaging their antioxidant properties.

BEST FOR
Antioxidants, for a healthy immune system

CALORIES
57 per 3.5 ounces

PREPARATION
Wash and use immediately.

HEALTH BENEFITS

Blueberries are very rich in vitamin K, which has several important functions, including helping wounds heal properly and building strong bones.

RELATED SPECIES
BILBERRY

A European native, the bilberry *(Vaccinium myrtillus)* is a close cousin of the North American blueberry but has a few notable differences. Both are dark blue, but the slightly smaller bilberry has a smooth, circular outline at one end, while the blueberry shows a rough, star-shaped pattern. Split open, a bilberry reveals red or purple pulp in contrast to the light green of a blueberry. Despite the differences, both berries are highly nutritious, containing diverse anthocyanins, including delphinidin and cyanidin glycosides.

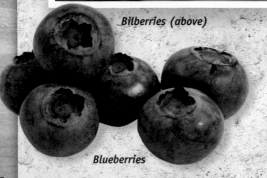

Bilberries (above)

Blueberries

Otherwise, blueberries are thought to be beneficial for everything from promoting a healthy urinary tract to reducing belly fat, preserving eyesight, and combating heart disease.

They are exceptionally high in the phytonutrients called anthocyanins, found in the blue skin of the berry and the source of the blueberry's antioxidant power. The anthocyanin, selenium, and a host of other vitamins and minerals abundant in blueberries may prevent and ease the symptoms of neurotic disorders and promote the health of the central nervous system.

Blueberries are nicknamed brain berries because research in rodents has shown improvements in the rodents' cognitive function when they were fed blueberries. The antioxidants in these berries may also be useful in decreasing the risk of Alzheimer's disease and age-related macular degeneration. So highly regarded are their antioxidant properties that some health experts have suggested that if you are going to make just one change to your diet, make it the addition of blueberries.

DIY: RECIPES

Healthful blueberries are an excellent base for juices, smoothies, and smoothie bowls. Here is a small selection of blended juices.

Blueberry & Ginger Juice

- ¼ pineapple
- 1 cup blueberries
- ¼ to ½ inch ginger

Wash all produce, then put ingredients through a juicer.

Blueberry & Cucumber Juice

- 1 cup blueberries
- 1 cucumber
- ½ lemon, rind removed
- 2 apples

Wash all produce, then put ingredients through a juicer.

Blueberry & Basil Lemonade

- ½ cup fresh lemon juice (about 3 lemons)
- 2 cups fresh blueberries
- ¼ cup fresh torn basil leaves
- 6 tablespoons granulated sugar
- 4 cups water

Pour lemon juice into a pitcher. Add blueberries, basil, and sugar to the pitcher and muddle. Add water and allow to stand for 30 minutes. Pour through a fine mesh sieve into a bowl; discard the solids. Return mixture to the pitcher. Serve chilled over ice.

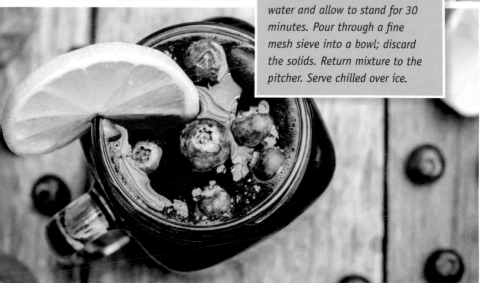

Blueberry & Basil Lemonade

BROCCOLI

Broccoli is blessed with numerous health-enhancing qualities, making it one of the most powerful superfoods.

THE BASICS

A member of the powerhouse Brassicaceae, this cruciferous vegetable is the flowering head of *Brassica oleracea* var. *italica*. The list of broccoli's virtues is almost endless, but sadly it can turn a bit bitter when juiced, so it works best when mixed with sweeter vegetables such as carrots or beets. Choose firm, unbruised dark green heads with no yellowing.

Despite its name, broccoli rabe is actually a different species, *Brassica rapa*. Broccoli rabe presents small green florets atop its long, leafy stalks. It is a good source of vitamins A and C, among other nutrients. Like broccoli, it is thought to have anti-cancer properties.

BEST FOR
A wide array of essential vitamins and minerals, for all-around health

CALORIES
34 per 3.5 ounces

PREPARATION
Rinse and cut into smaller pieces, including the stalk and fresh leaves.

HEALTH BENEFITS

Broccoli is an important source of the detoxifying phytonutrients that are thought to help protect us from cancers of the breast, colon, and prostate. It is also rich in many antioxidant vitamins and minerals, containing more than the daily recommended intake of the vitamins C and K in a single portion, as well as useful amounts of vitamin A and folate, which is known to reduce fetal abnormalities when taken before conception and during pregnancy.

It is also full of iron, chlorophyll, and sulfur compounds. Sulfur is an important mineral often omitted from nutrition tables—probably because it is widely available in foods. Present in every cell in the human

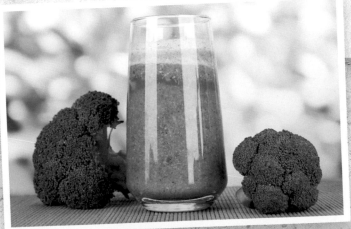

Juiced broccoli

CRUCIFEROUS VEGETABLES

Cruciferous vegetables are members of the Brassicaceae (or Cruciferae), a family of plants known as the mustards, the crucifers, or the cabbages. One of the species in this family, *Brassica oleracea*, is divided into seven groups of cultivars:

- **Acephala Group:** *kale and collard greens*
- **Alboglabra Group:** *kai-lan (Chinese broccoli)*
- **Botrytis Group:** *cauliflower, Romanesco broccoli, and broccoflower*
- **Capitata Group:** *cabbage*
- **Gemmifera Group:** *brussels sprouts*
- **Gongylodes Group:** *kohlrabi*
- **Italica Group:** *broccoli*

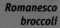

Romanesco broccoli

Crucifers may be the superstars of the veggie universe—no other family is as high in vitamin A carotenoids, vitamin C, folic acid, and fiber.

body, it has important roles in insulin function, metabolizing protein, and fighting bacteria. It is also known as the beauty mineral because it helps promote smooth skin, glossy hair, and hard nails. Broccoli contains an enzyme, myrosinase, that converts some sulfur compounds into other compounds called isothiocyanates, which have anti-cancer properties. It also contains a specific trio of phytonutrients that work together to assist in detoxification and the elimination of contaminants. Animal proteins are considered the best dietary sources of sulfur. Vegans and vegetarians may therefore be at greater risk of a deficiency, and so sulfur-rich vegetables have a special role in their diets. Because broccoli is low in calories and high in bulk and fiber, it is also an ideal inclusion in any weight-management plan.

Another reason to choose broccoli is that it is a great source of calcium for maintaining healthy bones, and like many vegetables is very low in calories.

White, purple, and green cauliflower

RELATED SPECIES
CAULIFLOWER

Lacking carotenoids and chlorophyll, white cauliflower is the least nutrient-dense of the crucifers. Nonetheless, it is an excellent source of the B vitamins and vitamin C and is rich in the minerals potassium, calcium, magnesium, manganese, copper, iron, molybdenum, phosphorus, and boron. To up its nutritional value, try one of the colored varieties.

Cauliflower doesn't yield the tastiest juice, but mixed with more flavorful veggies, like carrots and green apples, it makes a healthful drink. It can also add body to smoothie bowls.

CABBAGE

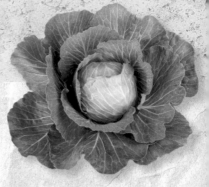

The smell of overcooked cabbage may have put you off it for life, but think again! It turns out that eating your greens really is a good idea, as the cabbage family is now known to be full of valuable hidden health benefits.

THE BASICS

Members of the Brassicaceae, cabbages (*Brassica oleracea* var. *capitsta*) are biennial plants grown for their dense-leaved heads. Cabbages can be dark green, light green, or red, with red varieties having the highest amount of the beneficial nutrients. People often dislike cooked cabbage because of its unappealing smell, but raw cabbage has a subtle, fresh scent and a light flavor. In smoothies, it works best when combined with other vegetables and fruit. Choose firm, tightly packed heads with no yellowing.

HEALTH BENEFITS

When eaten raw, cabbage contains a number of antioxidants, such as polyphenols and glucosinolates, which play an important part in helping to prevent cancer and lower cholesterol.

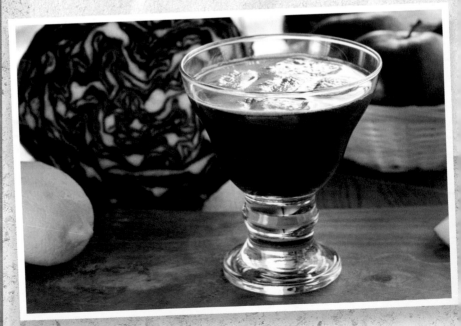

Red cabbage juice is a deep red to purple.

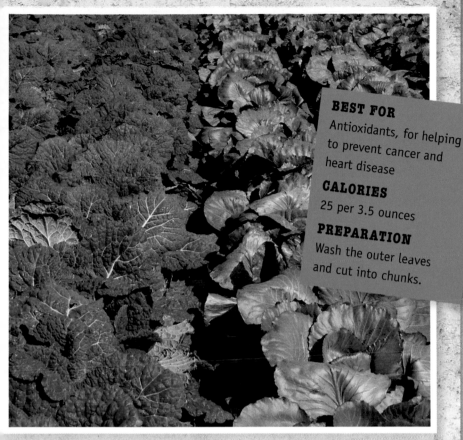

A field of cabbages. Both green and red varieties can be successfully juiced.

Cabbage is a rich source of vitamin C, and it also has useful amounts of vitamin K and folate. It also contains high levels of sulfur together with a number of other minerals. The health benefits of sulfur are gradually attaining increased recognition, and it is thought that cabbage's sulfur-containing compounds called sulphurophanes may play a critical role in detoxification and the treatment of inflammatory conditions. Cabbage is also full of antioxidants that assist in lowering cholesterol and might help prevent certain cancers. Many naturopaths also recommend cabbage to alleviate depression and to help constipation and other digestive issues.

RELATED SPECIES
BRUSSELS SPROUTS

In the Gemmifera Group of *Brassica oleracea*, brussels sprouts look like miniature cabbages and have a very similar nutritional content, although they come from a different plant and grow on upright stalks. At just 43 calories per 3.5 ounces, they have a light, nutty taste when juiced.

Brussels sprouts. Toss whole sprouts in the juicer for best results.

CARROT

The natural sugars in this root veggie lend it a sweet flavor. Enjoy it straight from the juicer or incorporate it into delectable blends.

THE BASICS

Carrots are the root of the *Daucus carota sativus* plant. They make plentiful quantities of sweet, mild-tasting juice that can be drunk on its own or used as a base for mixing with fruits and other vegetables. Look for firm roots that are brightly colored; small roots taste sweeter than older woody ones.

HEALTH BENEFITS

Carrots are low in calories and full of vitamins and minerals. Their fabulous orange color is a clue to the powerful presence of beta-carotene. These days, though, carrots range in color from deep blues and purples to orange and red to yellow and cream. The phytonutrient plant pigment beta-carotene is responsible for their delightful red-orange-yellow colors, while the blue-purple varieties contain another pigment, anthocyanin.

Both beta-carotene and anthocyanin are powerful antioxidants. Beta-carotene assists in the prevention of age-related macular degeneration, for example. A natural antioxidant that helps protect the body from various cancers and can lessen the signs of aging, it converts to vitamin A once in the body. A regular supply of this vitamin is essential for maintaining healthy functioning of the eyes and other parts of the nervous system, as well as keeping the immune system in good working order, and carrots are one of the very best sources. They also contain many other carotenoids like lutein, also vitally important for protecting against macular degeneration. They are high in fiber, and their slightly sweet taste enhances the flavor of less palatable vegetables.

BEST FOR
Beta-carotene, for eye health

CALORIES
41 per 3.5 ounces

PREPARATION
Cut off any green foliage, scrub roots, and cut into chunks.

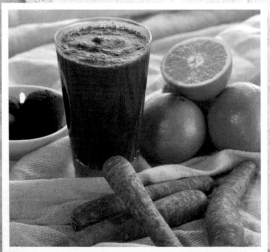

Carrot, Beet & Orange Juice (left); carrots growing in the field (opposite)

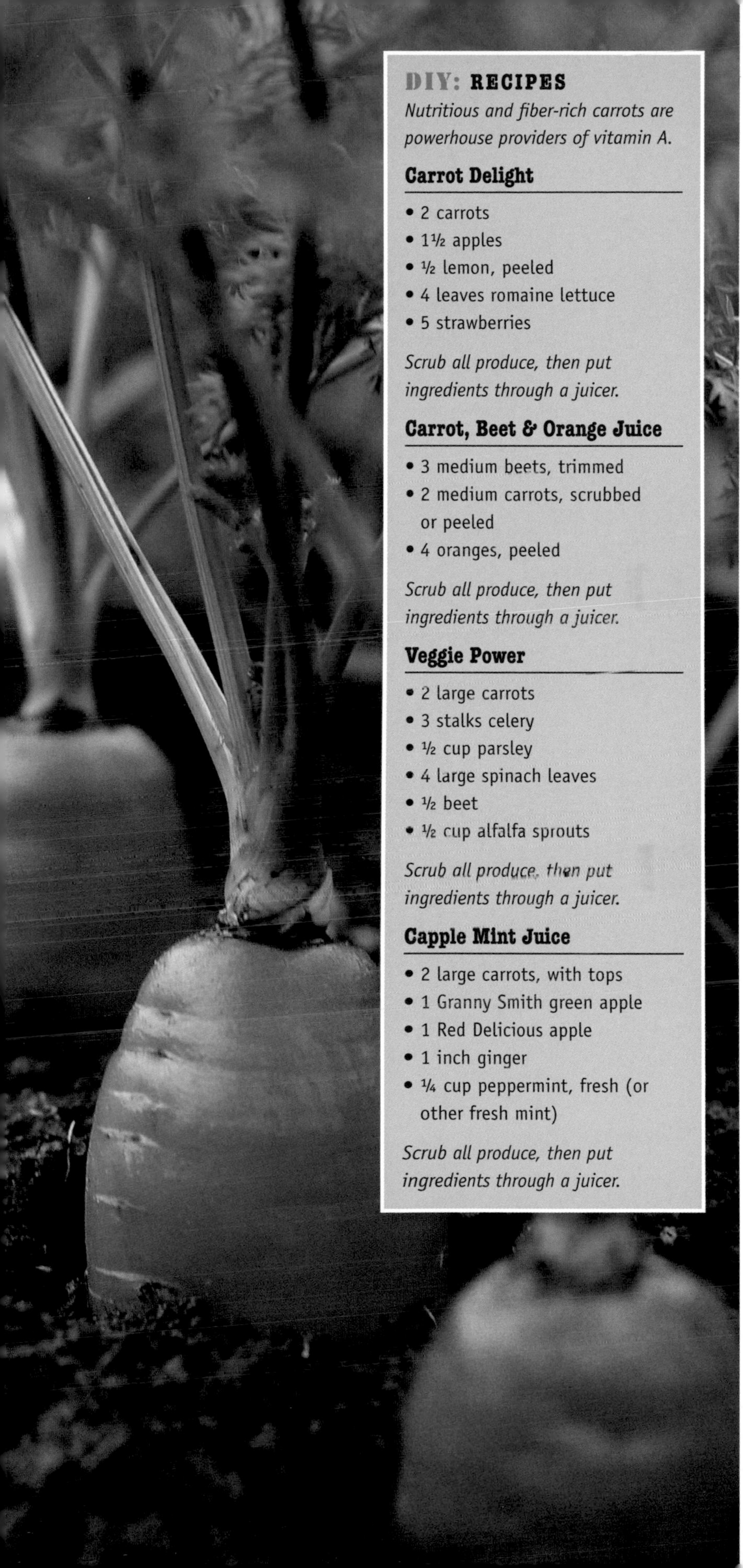

DIY: RECIPES

Nutritious and fiber-rich carrots are powerhouse providers of vitamin A.

Carrot Delight

- 2 carrots
- 1½ apples
- ½ lemon, peeled
- 4 leaves romaine lettuce
- 5 strawberries

Scrub all produce, then put ingredients through a juicer.

Carrot, Beet & Orange Juice

- 3 medium beets, trimmed
- 2 medium carrots, scrubbed or peeled
- 4 oranges, peeled

Scrub all produce, then put ingredients through a juicer.

Veggie Power

- 2 large carrots
- 3 stalks celery
- ½ cup parsley
- 4 large spinach leaves
- ½ beet
- ½ cup alfalfa sprouts

Scrub all produce, then put ingredients through a juicer.

Capple Mint Juice

- 2 large carrots, with tops
- 1 Granny Smith green apple
- 1 Red Delicious apple
- 1 inch ginger
- ¼ cup peppermint, fresh (or other fresh mint)

Scrub all produce, then put ingredients through a juicer.

CELERY

Celery has a lovely fresh, slightly peppery taste that helps to lift the flavor of vegetable smoothies but also combines beautifully with fruits like pears and apples to produce light, refreshing beverages.

THE BASICS

Celery *(Apium graveolens)* has a long history as a cultivated vegetable, grown in the Mediterranean since antiquity. Celery's crisp, ridged, upright stalks are topped by foliage that looks rather like flat-leaf parsley, though the two plants come from different families. Celery has a strong, distinctive taste and is best mixed with other vegetables when juiced. Choose heads with bright, fresh-looking leaves and firm stems.

HEALTH BENEFITS

Celery is a good source of vitamin K, which helps maintain bone density, and the leaves contain vitamin A, for healthy eyes and skin. The antioxidant action of its vitamins is supported by a number of

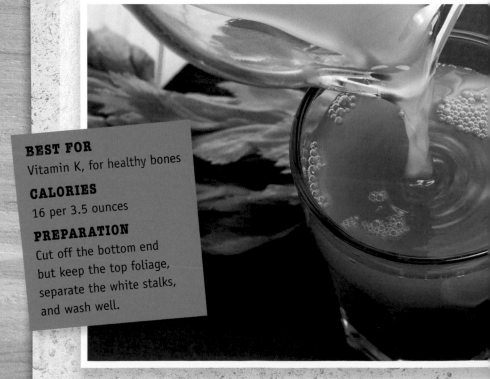

BEST FOR
Vitamin K, for healthy bones

CALORIES
16 per 3.5 ounces

PREPARATION
Cut off the bottom end but keep the top foliage, separate the white stalks, and wash well.

other phytonutrients that have recently been identified and also have an anti-inflammatory role. It is especially rich in potassium and is also a source of vitamin C and folate, as well as phosphorus and sodium. Some studies have found that compounds in celery known as phthalides are capable of reducing high blood pressure, but it is not yet clear whether the consumption of everyday amounts of celery would deliver sufficient phthalides to be effective. It does seem likely that future research will establish clear links between cardiovascular health and the phthalides found in celery.

Celery has traditionally been eaten as an aid to digestion and is particularly low in calories, making it popular for people on a weight-loss diet. Pregnant women should avoid celery, and it can cause an allergic reaction with anaphylactic shock in some individuals.

DIY: RECIPES

Celery's salty taste is a great counterpoint for tomato-based blended juices.

Celery Juice with Carrots & Apple

- 3 carrots
- ½ cucumber
- 2 apples
- 2 celery sticks

Scrub all produce, then put ingredients through a juicer.

Savory Celery Juice

- 2 tomatoes
- 6 stalks celery
- 1 broccoli stem and crown
- 1 red bell pepper
- 1 lemon
- ½ bunch green kale
- ½ bunch curly parsley
- ½ bunch cilantro
- ½ cup fresh basil
- 1 small clove garlic

Wash all produce, then put ingredients through a juicer.

Vegetable Cocktail

- ¾ pound fresh tomatoes
- 2 tablespoons chopped celery
- ⅛ large onion, peeled
- ⅛ green bell pepper
- ⅛ medium beet
- ¼ carrot
- ⅛ clove garlic, peeled
- ½ teaspoon sugar
- ⅛ teaspoon black pepper
- ⅛ teaspoon prepared horseradish
- ¾ teaspoon lemon juice
- 1 cup and 3 tablespoons water, or as needed
- ⅛ teaspoon Worcestershire sauce, or to taste
- 2½ teaspoons brown sugar
- ½ teaspoon salt, or to taste

Wash all produce, then put ingredients through a juicer.

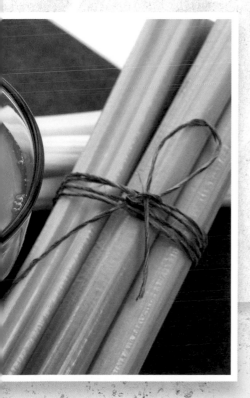

Fresh celery juice

CHERRY

Juicing these cheery little summer fruits may be time-consuming, but the effort is worth it—their sweet-tart flavor brightens many blended juices and smoothies.

THE BASICS

The cherries you find at the supermarket or roadside stand are most likely one of a limited number of varieties, of which *Prunus avium* (the wild, or sweet cherry) and *P. cerasus* (the sour, or tart cherry) are the most popular. These delicious little fruits are a type of drupe (stone fruit). The darker-skinned sour varieties are thought to have greater health benefits, though all are low-calorie and nutritious.

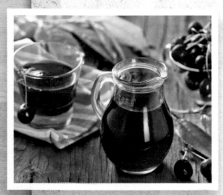

Cherry juice

HEALTH BENEFITS

Rather fiddly to prepare, this delicious fruit has so many health-boosting benefits that it's well worth the effort. Cherries are one of the few known food sources of melatonin, a naturally occurring hormone that helps to regulate the body's sleep patterns. They are also a fantastic source of vitamins C and A. Cherries also have an important role in the production of collagen, the protein that holds our body together and supports the skin.

Anthocyanins, which are also a powerful antioxidant, give cherries their deep red-purple color. These pigments have been shown to have anti-inflammatory properties, and may assist in the treatment of arthritis. Indeed, folk medicine has traditionally used cherries in the management of osteoarthritis, rheumatoid arthritis, and gout. The antioxidants in cherries might also have anti-aging properties—from the brain cells right down to the skin.

These fabulous little fruits also contain quercetin, which is said to prevent damaging lesions from forming in the colon. As if all of this wasn't enough, cherries are low in sugar compared to most other fruits, which makes them an ideal choice for people who want to lose weight.

BEST FOR
Vitamin A (retinol), for healthy eyes, hair, teeth, and skin

CALORIES
50 per 3.5 ounces

PREPARATION
Wash, cut in half to remove stone. No need to peel.

COLLARD GREENS

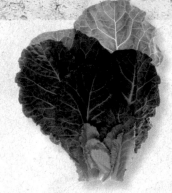

This soul food staple easily makes the leap from side dish to juice glass, lending its healthy goodness to green cleanses and smoothies.

THE BASICS

The collard plant (*Brassica oleracea* var. *acephala*) is a member of the nutritious Brassicaceae, closely related to kale and kin to cabbage and broccoli. It is cultivated for its large, dark-green, edible leaves.

HEALTH BENEFITS

Collards are low in calories, and the leaves are rich in vitamin C, beta-carotene, lutein, and vitamin K, as well as many of the B-group vitamins, including folate. Collard greens also contain good amounts of soluble fiber, which can decrease cholesterol absorption, help to prevent constipation, and assist with overall bowel function. Certain sulfur compounds found in collard greens may help protect against some cancers. The leaves and stems are both good sources of various minerals including iron, calcium, and copper.

BEST FOR
Vitamin K, for bones and teeth

CALORIES
31.5 per 3.5 ounces

PREPARATION
Discard any discolored leaves and wash.

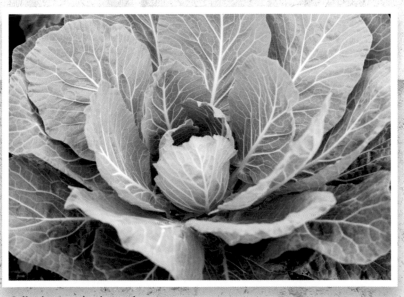

Collard greens in the garden

CRANBERRY

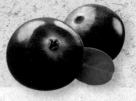

A fruit native to the Americas and cousin to the similarly super blueberries, these glossy, scarlet berries produce a tart juice that mixes especially well with orange or apple.

THE BASICS

Cranberries are the fruit of evergreen bushes in the genus *Vaccinium*. They are hard, sour, and bitter, so in most cases, you will want to blend them with a sweeter fruit, such as apple, orange, or pineapple. Choose fresh, plump, bright red fruit, which will keep in the fridge for several weeks. You can freeze fresh cranberries, and they will keep up to nine months; use them directly in recipes without thawing.

BEST FOR
Manganese, to neutralize free radicals and maintain healthy nerves

CALORIES
46 per 3.5 ounces

PREPARATION
Wash. No need to peel.

HEALTH BENEFITS

Cranberries are another fruit rich in antioxidants, particularly anthocyanins, the pigments that give them their deep, rich red and blue colors. Cranberries are also a good source of vitamin C, copper, and fiber, among other nutrients, yet it's actually their amazing cocktail of phytonutrients that makes them stand out from the crowd.

Cranberries have been associated with promotion of a healthy urinary tract, and recent tests indicate that they may similarly protect the stomach lining, but the findings are not yet conclusive. Other health benefits attributed to cranberries include anti-inflammatory and anti-cancer properties. The latter are now thought to extend to cancers of the breast, colon, lung, and prostate.

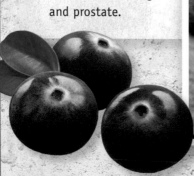

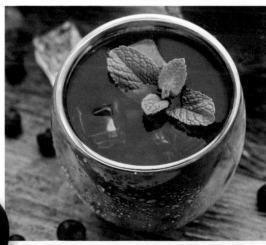

Minty Cranapple (above); ripe cranberries (opposite)

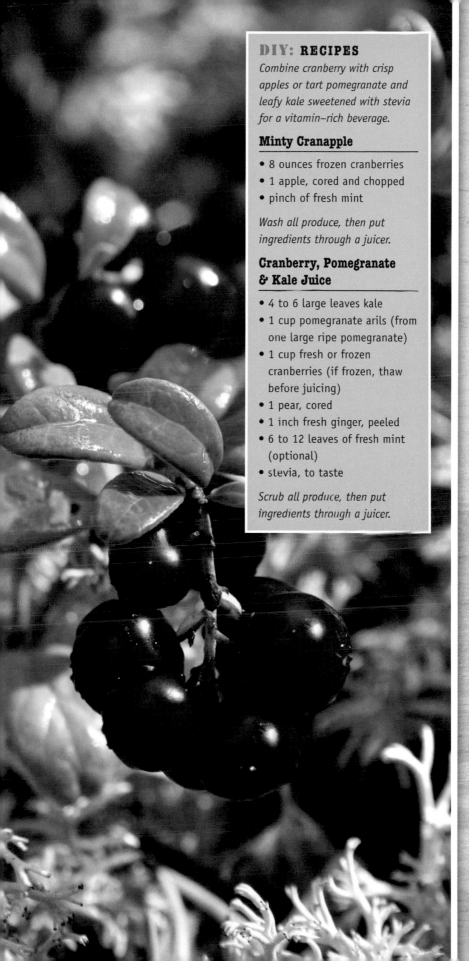

DIY: RECIPES

Combine cranberry with crisp apples or tart pomegranate and leafy kale sweetened with stevia for a vitamin–rich beverage.

Minty Cranapple

- 8 ounces frozen cranberries
- 1 apple, cored and chopped
- pinch of fresh mint

Wash all produce, then put ingredients through a juicer.

Cranberry, Pomegranate & Kale Juice

- 4 to 6 large leaves kale
- 1 cup pomegranate arils (from one large ripe pomegranate)
- 1 cup fresh or frozen cranberries (if frozen, thaw before juicing)
- 1 pear, cored
- 1 inch fresh ginger, peeled
- 6 to 12 leaves of fresh mint (optional)
- stevia, to taste

Scrub all produce, then put ingredients through a juicer.

CUCUMBER

With a nearly 95 percent water content, this summertime veggie will help you stay hydrated and as cool as a . . . well . . . cucumber.

THE BASICS

A member of the cucurbit family, which also includes zucchini, melons, and squash, cucumbers *(Cucumis sativus)* have a fairly tough green skin which hides the pale, watery flesh. Cucumber has a crisp, refreshing flavor that works well on its own but also combines well with other fruits and vegetables. Look for vivid color and firm texture when buying. Avoid anything yellowing or flabby.

BEST FOR
Potassium, to aid cleansing

CALORIES
16 per 3.5 ounces

PREPARATION
Wash but don't peel, and cut into chunks.

HEALTH BENEFITS

Given their high moisture content, it will be no surprise that cucumbers are very low in calories, making them a good inclusion for those wanting to manage their weight. The skin is edible and should not be removed when juicing; eating cucumbers with the skin provides several beneficial nutrients, including dietary fiber, vitamins K and C, and some useful minerals. As well as being a source of antioxidants, cucumber is also thought to have an anti-inflammatory effect, and there is some evidence that its phytonutrients, known as lignans, may play a part in reducing the risk of cancers of the breast, ovaries, womb, and prostate.

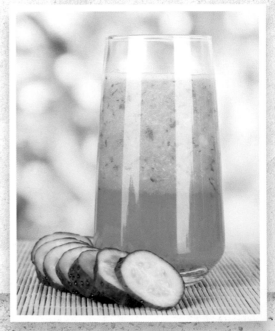

Fresh cucumber juice

DATE

Dates provide a delicious sweetness when blended into a smoothie, and also loads of fiber.

THE BASICS
Dates are the fruit of the date palm tree *(Phoenix dactylifera)*. They add a delectable sweetness to smoothies and smoothie bowls; however, because they are high in calories and fructose, they should be used in moderation. Most varieties, except for the Medjool date, are available only in dried form.

HEALTH BENEFITS
Dates are highly nutritious. They are an excellent source of iron and potassium and contain loads of fiber. They also provide vitamins A and K, as well as the B-group vitamins. Dates are rich in antioxidants such as beta-carotene; tannins, which are anti-inflammatory and anti-infective; and lutein and zeaxanthin, which are thought to protect against age-related macular degeneration.

BEST FOR
Iron, for healthy red blood cells

CALORIES
277 per 3.5 ounces

PREPARATION
Wash and chop into small pieces.

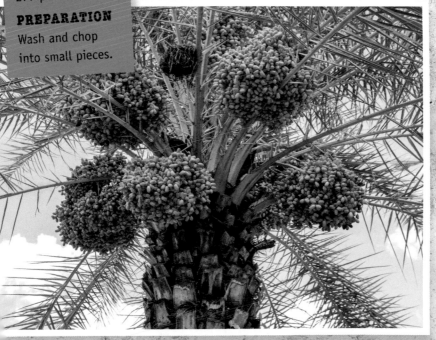

Clusters of yellow dates ripen on a date palm.

FENNEL

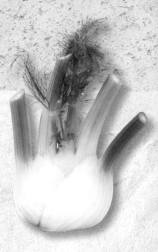

Originally a Mediterranean plant, fennel smells and tastes of aniseed and is powerfully reminiscent of warm summer evenings in France or Greece.

THE BASICS

Topped by a spray of feathery fronds, the fennel bulb sits prettily above the ground. It is not a true bulb at all, and its bulbous shape is formed from the swollen bases of its leaf stems. Originally from the Mediterranean, fennel *(Foeniculum vulgare)* is known in Italy as *finocchio,* which, rather sweetly, rhymes with Pinocchio.

It has a sweet yet pungent flavor and a light anise or licorice scent. The smell comes from its essential oils, which have some antifungal and antibacterial effects, so that it is used traditionally as an aid to digestion. It was also one of the herbs in a medicinal mixture that later became the notorious alcoholic drink absinthe.

The anise-licorice taste can be quite strong and the juice is best mixed with other juices. It blends especially well with apples and oranges and forms a particularly intriguing flavor when paired with cilantro. When buying, choose fresh-looking white bulbs.

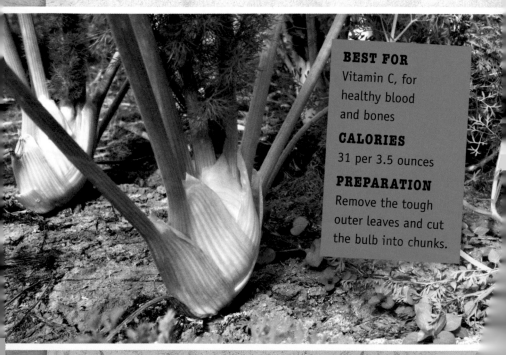

BEST FOR
Vitamin C, for healthy blood and bones

CALORIES
31 per 3.5 ounces

PREPARATION
Remove the tough outer leaves and cut the bulb into chunks.

Fennel plants in a garden show their bulbous stem base and feathery leaves.

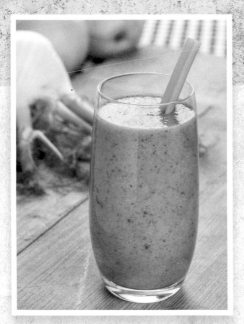

Fennel Fest

HEALTH BENEFITS

The bulb and its fronds contain useful amounts of antioxidant vitamin C, one of the essential vitamins that keep the body in a good state of repair, as well as some vitamin A, folate, and potassium. Teas made from the seeds and roots are sometimes used to suppress appetite as well as relieve flatulence.

DIY: RECIPES

The light aniseed flavor of fennel works well in both sweet and savory juices and smoothies.

Fennel Fest

- 2 large apples
- ½ lime, peeled
- 2 cucumbers
- 4 stalks celery
- 1 to 2 large handfuls fennel
- 1-inch piece ginger

Scrub all produce, then put ingredients through a juicer.

Fenneltastic

- 2 small fennel bulbs
- 3 small apples
- 1 lemon, whole
- 8 leaves kale
- ¼ medium-sized green cabbage

Wash all produce, then put ingredients through a juicer.

Orange Fennel Juice

- 1 wedge purple cabbage
- 4 kale leaves
- 1 large cucumber
- ½ fennel bulb
- 2 oranges
- 1 apple

Scrub all produce, then put ingredients through a juicer.

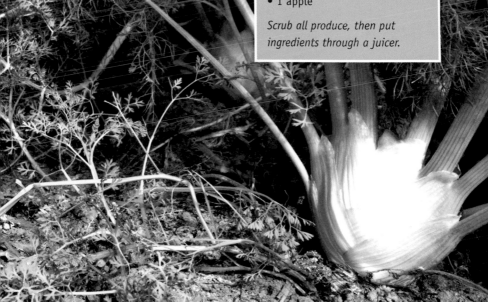

GINGER

Ginger has an intriguing sweet, peppery, sharp taste that can be enjoyed on its own or added to any beverage for a bit of zing.

THE BASICS

In powdered or grated form, the root of the ginger plant has long been used as a culinary spice and in various tea infusions. It lends itself to both sweet and savory combinations, mixing beautifully with cacao for a sweet treat and just as well with garlic and chili pepper.

HEALTH BENEFITS

It is claimed that ginger is a stimulant that relieves flatulence, clears the nasal passages, strengthens digestion, and eases nausea and vomiting. It is also commonly used to prevent motion sickness.

ADDING AN HERBAL FLOURISH

In the past, herbs were used only to enhance the flavor of other foods, but we now know they are also very high in antioxidants—in fact, adding a handful of fresh herbs to a smoothie can enhance its antioxidant capacity by 200 percent! The list of available herbs and their health and culinary benefits is endless. Nearly all are suitable for juices and smoothies, but here are the most popular. They are each used dry, fresh, or in infusions, and are all low in calories.

- **Basil:** This fragrant herb is an excellent source of vitamins C, K, and A, as well as many minerals. Its antioxidants include rosmarinic and caffeic acids, as well as beta-carotene. It has a sweet yet peppery flavor.

- **Chamomile:** This daisylike flower has long been used for its calming effect, as well as to help ease digestive conditions and insomnia. It has an unusual subtle yet earthy flavor. It should be cooled before being added to smoothies.

- **Cilantro:** This green leafy herb has a uniquely fresh, sweet, yet piquant flavor and can be used as an ingredient or garnish. It is rich in antioxidants, including beta-carotene and vitamin C. It contains many B-group vitamins, including folate, as well as vitamins K and A.

- **Garlic:** This pungent bulb has long been used in the preparation of both food and herbal medicines and is commonly referred to as "nature's penicillin." It is high in sulfur-containing compounds that are thought to boost immunity and also have antibacterial and antifungal properties. Consuming garlic has been associated with a reduction in total cholesterol, LDL cholesterol,

Gingerol, one of the many phytonutrients in ginger, is thought to have anti-inflammatory effects, and research has shown positive effects of ginger consumption on reducing osteoarthritic pain.

Ginger is low in calories and provides modest amounts of essential vitamins like vitamin C and B6, and minerals including manganese, magnesium, and potassium.

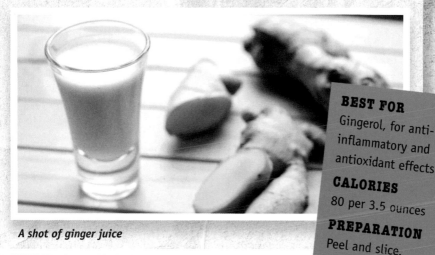

A shot of ginger juice

BEST FOR
Gingerol, for anti-inflammatory and antioxidant effects

CALORIES
80 per 3.5 ounces

PREPARATION
Peel and slice.

and triglycerides. An intake between one half and one clove of garlic per day can reduce cholesterol levels by nine percent. It seems that garlic can lower blood pressure and may also thin the blood and reduce clotting.

- **Lemongrass:** It has a spicy citrus flavor and tastes surprisingly good in smoothies. It is a source of essential vitamins, such as A and C and many B-group vitamins. It also provides essential minerals.

- **Mint:** This family comprises many varieties, of which peppermint is perhaps the most well known. Its cool, sweet, and refreshing flavor works equally well with both savory and sweet. It is an excellent source of vitamins A and C, and

also includes many B-group vitamins. Exceptionally rich in iron and manganese, it is also a very good source of copper, calcium, and magnesium. Mint is high in antioxidants.

- **Rosemary:** This evergreen herb has a warm, bitter, and astringent taste, and it can add a lot of flavor to blended juices and smoothies. It is high in antioxidants and contains vitamins like A, C, B6, thiamin, and folate, as well as several essential minerals.

- **Thyme:** A bit of thyme will add depth to a smoothie. This herb has a woody, slightly minty flavor and can help liven up a green smoothie. It's also good for you. Thyme contains thymol which has been shown to have antifungal properties.

GOJI

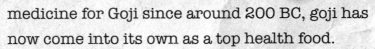

A staple in Chinese medicine for Goji since around 200 BC, goji has now come into its own as a top health food.

THE BASICS

Goji, also called wolfberry or goji berry, is the small oblong fruit of two species of boxthorn in the nightshade family: *Lycium barbarum* and *L. chinense*. It is a tender red berry with a distinctive sweet-and-sour taste. Their unusual flavor adds an interesting touch to smoothie combinations. Dried goji berries are more readily available than fresh.

BEST FOR
Iron, for healthy red blood cells

CALORIES
320 per 3.5 ounces

PREPARATION
Wash dried berries.

HEALTH BENEFITS

Goji berries are highly nutritious and contain surprisingly high levels of protein and iron, together with a wide range of other vitamins and minerals. They also have antioxidant properties and have long been used in traditional Chinese medicine to treat various conditions including kidney disorders, diabetes, and high cholesterol. At this stage, the medical research into the touted health benefits is inconclusive, and it is likely that some of the more miraculous claims are overstated. Still, these delicious little berries are undoubtedly nutritious and a good source of fiber.

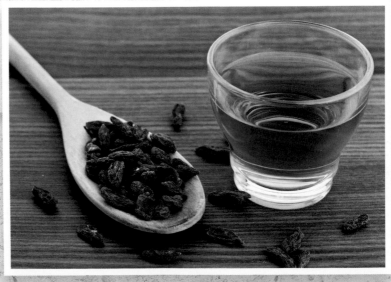

Water infused with dried goji. Add this infusion to juice blends and smoothies.

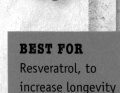

GRAPE

Ideal for juicing, freshly ripened grapes are bursting with goodness, and their health benefits have been appreciated for centuries, if not millennia.

THE BASICS

Botanically a berry, grapes *(Vitis vinifera)* are among the world's oldest and most widely cultivated fruits. Cultivated plants can yield green, red, or purple-black fruits.

Deliciously flavorful, grapes are a natural way to sweeten smoothies, but because a high portion of their calories is derived from sugars, they should be used in moderation.

HEALTH BENEFITS

Every year the list of health benefits from their consumption grows longer. The fruit of the grapevine is a rich source of phytonutrients with antioxidant properties. One of these, resveratrol, is found in the skin of red grapes and is thought to have cardiovascular benefits and has been shown to increase our chances of aging healthily. It may also prevent the development of certain cancers and liver disorders. Grapes also contain the antioxidants lutein and zeaxanthin, which are important for eye health, as well as myricetin and quercetin, which help the body to prevent free radicals from forming.

Grapes have a high water content and are useful for hydration. They are also high in potassium and dietary fiber and contain small amounts of other vitamins and minerals.

BEST FOR
Resveratrol, to increase longevity

CALORIES
67 per 3.5 ounces

PREPARATION
Wash, remove stalks. No need to remove pips.

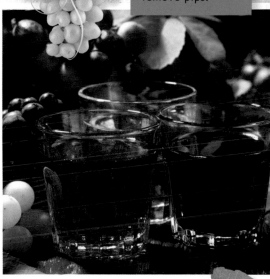

Red, green, and purple grape juice

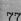

GRAPEFRUIT

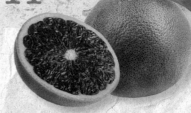

The grapefruit's Latin name, *Citrus paradisi*, reflects its origins on the paradise island of Barbados in the eighteenth century, where the fruit grew wild and hung from the trees in clusters like overgrown grapes.

THE BASICS

Whether or not the fruit is "a taste of paradise" is open to debate—it is way too tangy for some palates. Grapefruit's juiciness and fresh, uplifting flavor combines well in smoothies with other citrus fruits and melons, and with herbs such as mint. Use the full fruit (except the peel and seeds) in order to retain the benefits of extra fiber and bulk as well as nutrition in the pith and pulp. The pith can add a bitter but not unpleasant flavor, and zest from the peel can be used as a nutritious garnish that also provides freshness, color, and zing.

BEST FOR
Pectin, to improve circulatory or digestive problems

CALORIES
40 per 3.5 ounces

PREPARATION
Peel and break into segments.

HEALTH BENEFITS

There is no doubt, however, that grapefruit is an excellent source of vitamin C, and red varieties are so rich in vitamin A that they are ranked among those fruits with the highest antioxidant activity. Both the ruby and pink varieties contain lycopene, a phytonutrient thought to offer some protection against prostate cancer. It has long had a reputation as a "slimming food," with the half-a-grapefruit-for-breakfast regimen, a popular dieting practice that dates back to the 1960s. Grapefruit, like all citrus fruits, contains soluble fiber, which can help stabilize blood sugar levels and stave off hunger—both useful for weight management.

Recent studies also suggest that grapefruits may be particularly effective in combating lung and colon cancers and can significantly

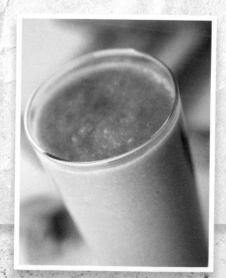

Grapefruit, Carrot & Ginger Juice

lower cholesterol. Again, although both red and yellow grapefruits positively influence cholesterol levels, it is worth noting that red grapefruit is more than twice as effective. So, if you're already healthy and want to stay that way, grapefruits are indeed a heavenly fruit. The controversy arises because certain compounds in grapefruit are known to increase circulating levels of a number of prescription drugs, including statins, and the risk of toxicity associated with such drugs may actually increase when grapefruit is consumed. Therefore, if you're taking any kind of prescription drugs, check with your healthcare practitioner before adding grapefruit juice to your diet.

DIY: RECIPES

Grapefruit is a perfect base for healthful morning juices.

Ruby Red

- 2 pink grapefruits
- 2 stalks celery
- ½ beet

Scrub all produce, then put ingredients through a juicer.

Grapefruit, Carrot & Ginger Juice

- 2 chopped grapefruits, peel and pith removed
- 5 carrots, chopped
- 1 inch fresh ginger, peeled and chopped

Scrub all produce, then put ingredients through a juicer.

Grapefruit, Apple & Beet Juice

- 3 beets, thoroughly washed and peeled
- 1 whole grapefruit, peeled
- 1 organic Fuji apple
- 3 to 4 organic carrots

Scrub all produce, then put ingredients through a juicer.

Grapefruit, Lemon & Pineapple

- 1 grapefruit, peeled, halved, cut into wedges, seeds removed
- ½ ripe pineapple, peeled, cut lengthwise into quarters
- 1 lemon, peeled, halved, cut into wedges, seeds removed

Scrub all produce, then put ingredients through a juicer.

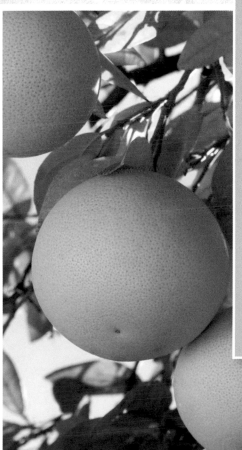

Grapefruits ripening on tree

GREEN TEA

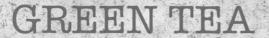

Long prized in China and Japan, green tea has become one of the go-to beverages for the health conscious throughout the world.

THE BASICS

Green tea is harvested from the leaves and buds of *Camellia sinensis,* an evergreen shrub or small tree. Known as the small leaf variety, it grows best in the cool, high mountains of central China and Japan. The green tea leaf is the same as a black tea leaf that hasn't yet been oxidized.

Green tea is the favorite drink of the people of Okinawa in Japan, which also happens to have the world's highest percentage of centenarians; there may well be a link between these two observations.

When used in smoothies, green tea is first brewed, strained, and cooled before it is added to the blend. The tea should be quite strong, but should not be left to brew too long, as it will become bitter.

The brew has no calories and is a terrific way to add nutritious fluids, particularly if a lighter, more

BEST FOR
Antioxidants, for cardiovascular health

CALORIES
Fewer than 1 per 3.5 ounces

PREPARATION
Brew, strain, and cool tea leaves.

refreshing and hydrating beverage is desired. Green tea has a subtle flavor that works well with herbs like mint but also combines well with almost all fruits and vegetables. For convenience, green tea can be prepared in advance and frozen into ice cubes, ready to add to smoothies when needed.

HEALTH BENEFITS

Green tea offers many health benefits and has been proven to help prevent heart disease by decreasing inflammation. Phytonutrients in green tea might protect against certain cancers. It is renowned for its antioxidant properties, which stem from its flavonols called catechins. It is likely these are responsible for most of its healthy benefits.

MATCHA

Both matcha and green tea are derived from *Camellia sinensis*. While green tea is sold as loose dried leaves or in tea bags, matcha is green tea leaves that have been ground into a fine powder. When you drink matcha brews, you ingest the entire leaf, which means you absorb more of its health benefits. Like green tea, matcha is packed with antioxidants and is rich in fiber, chlorophyllm, and vitamins and minerals, including vitamin C, zinc selenium, and chromium. It is also said to help boost metabolism and burn calories. You can add matcha to juices and smoothies.

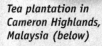

Matcha powder

Tea plantation in Cameron Highlands, Malaysia (below)

KALE

This leafy green vegetable has not had a glamorous past but its reputation has undergone a transformation since it was identified as one of the new superfoods.

THE BASICS

A member of the cabbage family, kale *(Brassica oleracea* var. *acephala)* is so nutritious and easy to grow that farmers have traditionally fed it to cattle during the winter. Now embraced as a health food, humans have come to love its strong, peppery flavor. It does tends toward the bitter, however, so it tastes best when blended with other vegetables and fruits. This, together with washing, will help minimize the pungent and sometimes mildly unpleasant odor that kale is known to emit.

HEALTH BENEFITS

Packed full of all the healthy nutrients associated with the cabbage family, including beta-carotene, lutein, and zeaxanthin, it provides more than the recommended daily intake of vitamins A, C, and K in a single serving and is an important source of calcium and iron. Together, its powerful phytonutrients help prevent cancer and promote healthy eyes, skin, and bones. A winter crop, the leaves should be bought when fresh, crisp, and strongly colored, with no yellowing or wilting. Use without delay, as their nutrient value deteriorates rapidly after harvest. The juice can taste bitter and is best used in small quantities and mixed with other vegetable juices.

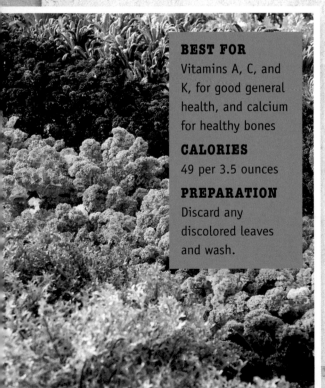

BEST FOR
Vitamins A, C, and K, for good general health, and calcium for healthy bones

CALORIES
49 per 3.5 ounces

PREPARATION
Discard any discolored leaves and wash.

Rows of purple and green kale growing in a garden

DIY: **RECIPES**

Juicing with kale is a smart way to boost your intake of essential nutrients. Its blends well other veggies and with fruit, which can tame its bitterness.

Hail King Kale

- 3 leaves green kale
- 2 apples
- 2 slices watermelon
- ¼ lemon, peeled

Scrub all produce, then put ingredients through a juicer.

Red Kale

- 8 kale leaves
- 1 ruby grapefruit
- 2 oranges

Wash all produce, then put ingredients through a juicer.

Tomato-Kale with Celery, Horseradish & Soy Juice

- 1 tablespoon prepared horseradish
- 1 tablespoon soy sauce
- ½ cup plus 2 tablespoons fresh tomato juice (from about 2 pints grape or cherry tomatoes)
- ¼ cup fresh kale juice (from about ½ pound kale)
- 2 tablespoons fresh celery juice (from 4 stalks celery)
- 2 tablespoons juice from 2 lemons
- dash hot sauce

Mix horseradish and soy sauce in a glass. Add tomato juice and stir well until horseradish is well distributed. Add kale juice, celery juice, lemon juice, and hot sauce. Stir well. Serve with celery stalk garnish, over ice if desired.

Ultimate Green Dream

- 2 green apples
- 2 celery stalks
- ½ cucumber
- 3 leaves kale
- ¼ lemon, peeled
- ½-inch piece fresh ginger

Scrub all produce, then put ingredients through a juicer.

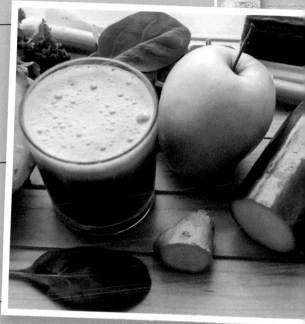

Ultimate Green Dream

Celery Kale Juice

- 3 apples
- 16 to 20 stalks celery
- 2 handfuls kale
- ½-inch piece fresh ginger
- 1 lemon

Scrub all produce, then put ingredients through a juicer.

Parsnip, Apple, Mint, Lime & Kale Melange

- 1 cup freshly squeezed kale juice, from about 1½ pounds kale
- ½ cup parsnip juice, from about 4 peeled parsnips
- ½ cup fresh apple juice, from 4 large (or up to 8 small) green apples
- 4 teaspoons juice from 1 lime (more or less to taste)
- ¼ cup mint juice, from about 2 large bunches

Scrub all produce, then put ingredients through a juicer. Garnish with mint and lime wedge.

KIWIFRUIT

A furry-skinned berry about the same size as a hen's egg, kiwifruits possess delicious emerald flesh. Kids often enjoy them in a similar way to a boiled-egg breakfast—slicing off the top and scooping out the delicious emerald flesh with a teaspoon.

BEST FOR
Magnesium, to regulate blood pressure and build strong bones

CALORIES
61 per 3.5 ounces

PREPARATION
Peel, and chop to fit into feeder tube.

THE BASICS

Kiwifruit (often just called kiwi) is the berry of several species of woody vines in the genus *Actinidia*—the most common is the species *A. deliciosa*. Also known as the Chinese gooseberry, this fruit originated in China but was later cultivated in New Zealand, where it was affectionately given the name of the national bird, the kiwi.

Kiwifruit is similar in size and shape to an egg, although covered in a thin, brown, fuzzy peel that conceals the luscious bright green or gold flesh and tiny black seeds within. The flesh has a slightly wet texture, a little like partially-set jelly, and has a deliciously sweet, uplifting flavor that tastes something like a blend of banana and pineapple. The peel has a mild earthy flavor. When juiced, a kiwi produces a thick, green juice that is delicious by itself but is wonderful when mixed with fruits such as pineapple or melon. Be sure to select firm fruit with unwrinkled skin. You can ripen hard fruit at room temperature, but be sure to store the kiwifruits away from other fruits—hormones released by them will cause other fruit to ripen too quickly.

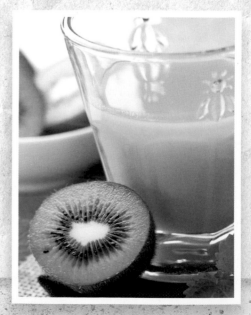

Kiwifruit juice

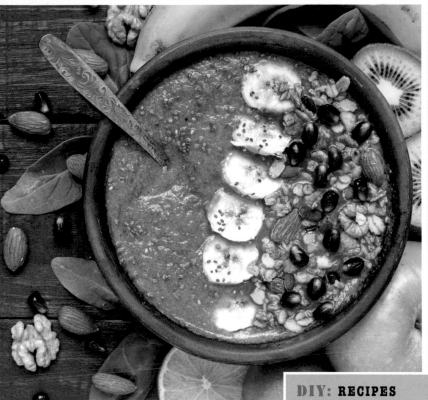

Green Kiwi Breakfast Bowl

HEALTH BENEFITS

Positively bursting with vitamin C, kiwis
are also an excellent source of magnesium,
which offers multiple health benefits that
include aiding the transmission of nerve
impulses, regulating body temperature,
detoxifying the blood, boosting energy
production, and promoting the formation of
healthy bones and teeth. Magnesium also
aids the treatment of migraines, insomnia,
and symptoms of depression. It is used to
help combat such psychiatric problems as
anxiety and panic attacks.

Both the peel and seeds contain dietary fiber, while the seeds
provide small amounts of ALA, the plant source of omega-3 fatty acids.
Gold kiwifruit contains high amounts of lutein and zeaxanthin, which
can help protect against macular degeneration. Furthermore, studies
in Norway have shown that eating two to three kiwifruits per day can
help thin the blood and reduce the risk of blood clots. The kiwifruit is
also thought to assist in treating a host of other disorders, including
mood imbalances, respiratory problems, and diabetes; research is not
yet conclusive, but indications are very positive.

DIY: RECIPES

*Kiwi not only adds bright color to
a breakfast bowl, it's also packed
with nutrients and fiber.*

Green Kiwi Breakfast Bowl

- 2 kiwis
- 1 handful spinach
- ½ frozen banana
- ½ regular banana
- ¾ cup almond milk
- squeeze of lime

*Layer ingredients in blender. Blend
until smooth. Top with sliced
bananas and other toppings, such
as granola, pomegranate, and
pumpkin and chia seeds.*

LEEK

Prized for their medicinal properties for centuries, leeks can also be appreciated for their delicate onion-like flavor.

THE BASICS

Although leeks *(Allium ampeloprasum)* are members of the onion family, they do not form an obvious bulb but are grown for their thick white stems, which make them look rather like large scallions. Curiously, the seedlings are planted in trenches and covered with soil to prevent the stems from turning green. Although leeks taste quite bland when cooked, their juice can be surprisingly strong and is best added to other juices. When buying, look for firm stems and avoid produce with yellowing tops.

BEST FOR
Antioxidants, for cardiovascular health

CALORIES
61 per 3.5 ounces

PREPARATION
Remove the stem end and tough outer leaves, wash well to remove grit between the leaf layers, and cut into chunks.

HEALTH BENEFITS

Like onions and garlic, leeks contain a number of significant antioxidants that are known to promote a healthy cardiovascular system, although these tend to be found in smaller quantities in leeks than onions. They are good sources of folate and vitamin A, and contain useful amounts of vitamins K and C, as well as a high level of iron, with other minerals. Like so many vegetables, they are also low in calories.

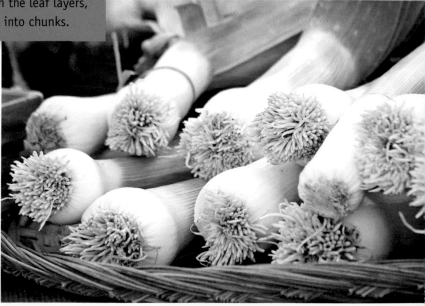

Use the stalk, bulb, and leaves to prepare leek juice.

LEGUMES

Known as legumes, the Fabaceae (or Leguminosae) is a family of plants that houses its fruit inside a pod.

THE BASICS

The Fabaceae includes all types of beans (such as French beans, kidney beans, soy beans, mung beans, and cannellini beans), peas (including green peas and chickpeas), lentils, and, surprisingly, peanuts.

A few legumes can easily be slipped into a fruit-based smoothie to boost the protein and fiber content without affecting flavor. Cannellini beans (also known as white beans or white kidney beans) add a delicious creaminess that blends well with banana without altering taste. Green peas have a light, slightly nutty flavor that will be imperceptible when mixed with more strongly flavored fruits and vegetables, but conversely complements certain flavors such as avocado very nicely. Some peas and beans also work as juicing veggies.

HEALTH BENEFITS

They are highly nutritious, providing both low GI carbohydrates and protein, together with a host of vitamins and minerals like calcium, potassium, iron, B-group vitamins, and vitamin C. Their high levels of protein make them especially important in vegetarian and vegan diets.

DIY: RECIPES

White beans will lend a creamy texture and a protein boost to this blend of melon and mangoes.

Beany Melon-Mango Smoothie

- 2 cups cooked white beans
- ½ medium cantaloupe, skinned and chopped into small cubes
- 2 medium mangoes, skinned and chopped into small cubes
- 2 ice cubes
- ½ to 1 cup water, if needed

Add (in this order) melon, mango, beans, and ice. Blend until smooth, adding water if necessary.

BEST FOR
Protein, for every part of the body to develop, grow, and function properly

CALORIES
125 to 360 per 3.5 ounces

PREPARATION
Soak and rinse dried beans; rinse canned beans.

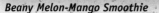

Beany Melon-Mango Smoothie

LEMON

Even diluted, the tart taste of lemon shines through and brightens any beverage you add it to.

THE BASICS

Lemons *(Citrus limon)* originated in Asia and were brought by the troops of Alexander the Great to Greece where, even then, they were used for medicinal purposes. More recently, they were distributed to sailors in the British navy to combat the debilitating effects of scurvy. Today, they are still employed for medicinal purposes in cold remedies, are used in kitchens throughout the world to bring out the flavor of other foods, and are squeezed in water to cleanse the palate (and the fingers!) between meals.

Most lemon varieties have a sour taste that can be far too bitter for the average palate, and they should always be diluted. To sweeten lemon juice, add a small amount of raw honey; combine it with sweeter citrus juices, such as orange; or mix it with water. The Meyer lemon is thought to be a cross between a lemon and an orange or mandarin and has a naturally sweet flavor. Remove the skin to avoid contaminating the juice with the wax that is often used to prolong the shelf life of lemons and other fruits, but preserve as much of the flavonoid-rich pith as you can.

BEST FOR
Vitamin C, for healthy skin, bones, teeth, and hair

CALORIES
29 per 3.5 ounces

PREPARATION
Peel, and divide into segments.

Fresh-squeezed lemon juice

HEALTH BENEFITS

They are rich in flavonoids, which recent studies suggest may have antihistamine, antimicrobial, and even memory-enhancing and mood-elevating properties. Although approximately half the size of the average orange, they contain twice the amount of vitamin C and also contain small amounts of various minerals, including calcium, phosphorus, iron, and potassium. Lemons can assist in weight management because they are low in calories, high in fiber, and also have a low GI. The citric acid in lemon juice slows the rate of digestion and when added to a food or meal can reduce its GI score.

LETTUCE

A popular salad vegetable, lettuce comes in a number of varieties and colors from light green leaves to dark green leaves tinged with purple and also a bewildering array of shapes and textures.

THE BASICS

Lettuce *(Lactuca sativa)* is certainly a variable veggie. As a general rule, varieties with firmer heads—such as Iceberg—are easier to juice, but the darker-leafed varieties tend to be more nutritious. The leaves can taste bitter when juiced, so mix them with other fruit and vegetable juices. Avoid buying lettuces with limp or discolored leaves.

HEALTH BENEFITS

Lettuce is well known for being low in calories and frequently forms an important part of a weight-reduction diet. Like all green leafy vegetables, lettuce is also full of healthy nutrients. It supplies vitamins A and K, with useful amounts of vitamin C and folate, as well as chlorophyll, iron, potassium, silicon, and a substance known as lactucarium, which is, among other things, a natural sedative. It is also a good source of manganese, and zeaxanthin (which helps protect the eyes), and it is a great source of beta-carotene. The amount of beta-carotene increases with the amount of color in the lettuce, with red-leaf lettuce like Lollo Rossa being the richest source.

BEST FOR
Vitamin A, for healthy eyes

CALORIES
15 per 3.5 ounces

PREPARATION
Wash and juice whole leaves or cut firmer varieties into chunks.

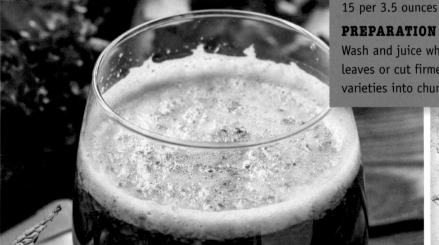

Choose red- or violet-leaf lettuces, such as Lollo Rossa, for the most nutritious juice.

LIME

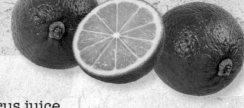

Among the most popular of the citrus juice fruits, the lime has a pleasantly tart-sour flavor.

THE BASICS

More than a dozen fruits go by the name *lime,* but three species are the most widely produced. The green fruit that supermarkets label as "lime" is most likely *Citrus × latifolia* (or Persian lime). The other two most common species are key lime *(C. × aurantifolia)* and Kaffir lime *(C. hystrix)*. Like lemon juice, lime juice can be overwhelmingly sour on its own, so be sure to dilute it with sweeter juices, or dilute it with water and sweeten it with a bit of honey.

The smallest of the citrus fruits, limes are also the most perishable, so be sure to select an unblemished specimen that feels heavy for its size, with a rich green color. Limes can be kept out at room temperature where they will stay fresh for up to one week. Lime juice can bestored for later use. Pour freshly squeezed lime juice in ice cube trays until frozen, then store them in plastic bags in the freezer.

BEST FOR
Vitamin C, for healthy skin, bones, teeth, and hair

CALORIES
28 per 3.5 ounces

PREPARATION
Peel and divide into segments.

HEALTH BENEFITS

Emerald-green limes are an excellent source of vitamin C and, like lemons, were eaten to prevent the degenerative disease scurvy that was so prevalent among sailors in the 17th and 18th centuries. One of the most important antioxidants in food, vitamin C neutralizes damaging free radicals. Limes also contain flavonoids that may have anti-cancer properties. They also possess antibiotic properties and have been used in Africa to protect against cholera.

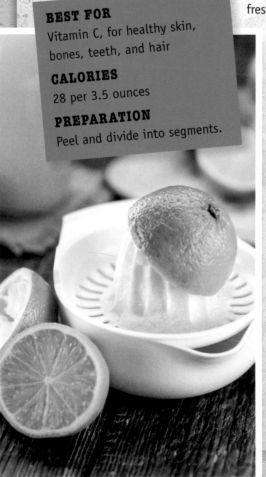

Fresh-squeezed lime juice

MACA

In recent years, maca has seen a rise in popularity, and it is now mainly grown for the nutritional value of its root.

THE BASICS

A cousin of the radish, maca (*Lepidium meyenii*) looks something like a small parsnip or turnip and has a nutty, slightly sweet flavor. It is best added to smoothies in liquid or powdered form; a teaspoon, which has only about 10 calories, is sufficient. Higher quantities are not generally recommended—maca is known to have certain nontoxic side effects that may nonetheless disturb other processes within the body. Many health practitioners recommend that it be taken in cycles of week on/week off, rather than continually. This can both prevent the body from becoming immune to its benefits and provide a way to assess the body's response to it.

HEALTH BENEFITS

Maca has a high number of nutrients, including B-group vitamins, vitamin C, zinc, calcium, and fatty acids, and hence it supports general good health. There are numerous other claims regarding the health benefits of maca but as yet there is insufficient evidence to confirm them conclusively—although they do sound promising. Supposedly, maca can boost energy, boost sex drive, increase fertility in men and women, relieve migraines, relieve stress, improve memory, and boost immunity, among other things.

BEST FOR
A variety of amino acids, to balance hormones

CALORIES
210 per 3.5 ounces (limit serving to 1 teaspoon)

PREPARATION
Add powdered or liquid maca to a smoothie or smoothie bowl.

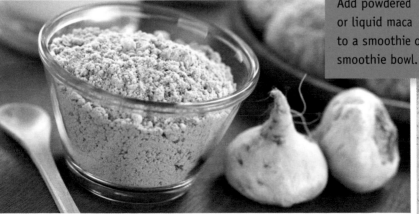

Maca root is sold in powdered form to use in juices and smoothies.

MANGO

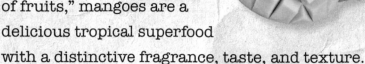

Often hailed as "the king of fruits," mangoes are a delicious tropical superfood with a distinctive fragrance, taste, and texture.

THE BASICS

The mango is the fruit of the tropical tree *(Mangifera indica)*. The orange flesh of this delicious drupe (stone fruit) has a soft, juicy texture, appealing aroma, and deliciously sweet taste. Mangoes blend beautifully with bananas, berries, and other fruits and can also add a sweet touch to more savory blends. They are fiber-rich, and hence good for digestion and also for promoting satiety.

Mangoes are best to juice when they reach the peak of ripeness and are just starting to give slightly to the touch. Mangoes do not last well in the refrigerator and are best left out at room temperature, where they will keep for three or four days.

HEALTH BENEFITS

Mangoes are particularly rich in the antioxidant vitamin C and are a good source of vitamins A, E, potassium, iron, and copper. They also contain high levels of antioxidants like beta-carotene.

Recent research suggests that the polyphenolic antioxidant compounds found in mangoes are especially effective in helping to protect against colon, breast, and prostate cancers. They are rich in vitamins and minerals, including vitamin A for healthy skin and B6 for protecting gray matter. They are an excellent source of vitamin C, potassium, and niacin.

BEST FOR
Carotenes, to boost the immune system

CALORIES
70 per 3.5 ounces

PREPARATION
Slice in half or quarters, remove the stone, and scoop the flesh out of the skin.

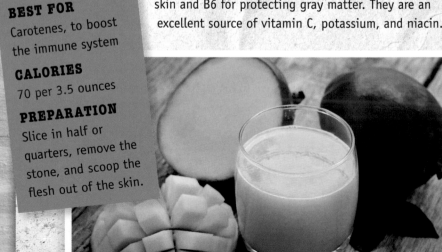

Fresh mango juice (above); mangoes growing in the tree (opposite)

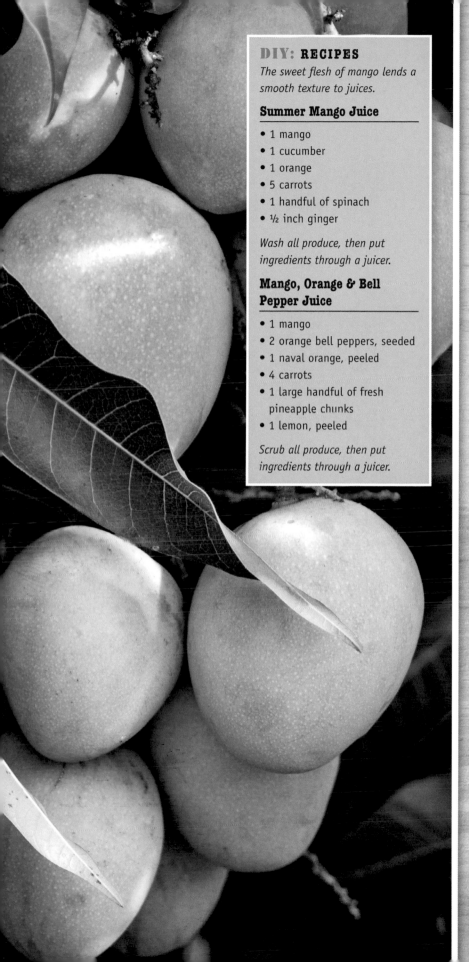

DIY: RECIPES

The sweet flesh of mango lends a smooth texture to juices.

Summer Mango Juice

- 1 mango
- 1 cucumber
- 1 orange
- 5 carrots
- 1 handful of spinach
- ½ inch ginger

Wash all produce, then put ingredients through a juicer.

Mango, Orange & Bell Pepper Juice

- 1 mango
- 2 orange bell peppers, seeded
- 1 naval orange, peeled
- 4 carrots
- 1 large handful of fresh pineapple chunks
- 1 lemon, peeled

Scrub all produce, then put ingredients through a juicer.

MELON

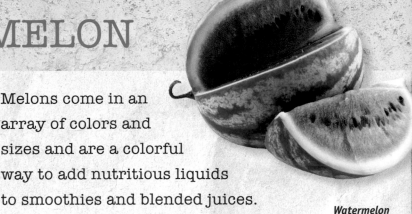

Melons come in an array of colors and sizes and are a colorful way to add nutritious liquids to smoothies and blended juices.

Watermelon

THE BASICS

Melons are part of the Cucurbitaceae (the gourd family), whose members are also called cucurbits. This plant family consists of about 965 species in around 95 genera. Three of the most popular melons for juicing and smoothies are watermelon, cantaloupe (rock melon), and honeydew. All three have a high water content (upwards of 90 percent) and are low in calories. The plentiful seeds are edible, but are usually scooped out prior to eating.

HEALTH BENEFITS

Nutritionally, melons are excellent sources of vitamin A and other antioxidants, and also contain moderate amounts of B-group vitamins and some minerals, particularly copper and potassium.

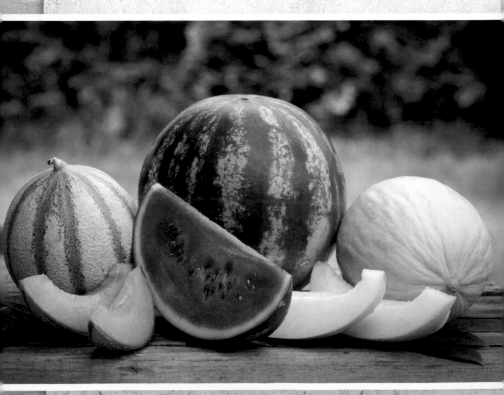

Cantaloupe, watermelon, and honeydew

WATERMELON

Watermelon *(Citrullus lanatus)* grows as a trailing flowering vine that produces large fruit with a thick green rind. It has a light, sweet taste and aroma. The flesh is pink and crisp, but quickly becomes watery. Notably, watermelon is a good source of lycopene—a carotenoid phytonutrient that's especially good for the heart and a powerful antioxidant that is thought to be even more effective than beta-carotene at combating free radicals in the body.

This quintessential summer fruit has attracted a good deal of scientific interest in recent years because of its lycopene content. It's worth noting that lycopene, beta-carotene, and other antioxidants are highest in ripe watermelon—when its flesh is almost red. The seeds in watermelon are a good source of iron, zinc, vitamin E, and essential fatty acids. The rind, too, is full of nutrients but can alter the flavor significantly. You might want to add a little honey if you decide to juice a significant portion of rind.

BEST FOR
Lycopene, for cardiovascular health

CALORIES
32 per 3.5 ounces

PREPARATION
Slice into quarters, remove the pips if preferred, and cut away the flesh in chunks.

DIY: RECIPES
Nothing evokes summer like the refreshingly sweet flavor of colorful watermelon.

Watermelon-Orange Juice
- 4 to 5 cups chopped watermelon cubes, deseeded
- 1 medium or large orange, juiced, or ¾ to 1 cup orange juice
- organic, unrefined cane sugar
- a few fresh mint leaves for garnishing
- 4 to 5 fresh mint leaves (optional)
- ice cubes (optional)

Peel and chop the orange and extract the juice, using a juicer. Blend the watermelon, mint leaves, and sugar in a blender. Pour the watermelon juice in a jar or bowl. Add the orange juice to the watermelon juice. Stir well and serve immediately, with or without ice cubes, garnished with mint leaves.

Watermelon-Lime Juice
- 3 cups diced watermelon, deseeded
- 1 lime, peeled

Scrub all produce, then put ingredients through a juicer.

Watermelon, Blueberry & Swiss Chard Juice
- 2½ cups watermelon deseeded
- 1 cup blueberries
- 6 to 8 leaves Swiss chard

Wash all produce, then put ingredients through a juicer.

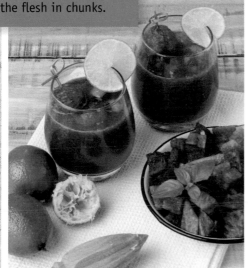

Watermelon-Lime Juice

MUSKMELON

Muskmelons, such as cantaloupe and honeydew, produce wonderfully refreshing juice that can be absorbed very quickly by the digestive system and is great for mixing with a host of other fruits. Muskmelons are a good source of folic acid, which preserves the nervous system.

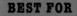
Cantaloupe

Cantaloupe: The cantaloupe (also called muskmelon, mushmelon, rock melon, and sweet melon) is a variety of the *Cucumis melo* species. The North American cantaloupe, *C. melo* var. *reticulatus,* has a reticulated skin covering that looks like netting. This round melon has firm flesh.

BEST FOR
Lycopene, for cardiovascular health

CALORIES
28 per 3.5 ounces

PREPARATION
Slice into quarters, remove the pips if preferred, and cut away the flesh in chunks.

RELATED SPECIES
OTHER MUSKMELONS

Cantaloupe and honeydew are commonly available, but just about any muskmelon will add flavor and color to juice blends, smoothies, and bowls. Here are just a few:

- **Casaba:** This easy-to-identify melon has an ovoid to round shape with a thick, hard rind that displays shallow furrows running from end to end and a golden yellow color with hints of green. The pale-green to white flesh is mildly sweet, with hints of pear and cucumber.

- **Crenshaw:** A mix between the casaba and the Persian, this melon (also known as the Cranshaw) has a rich yellow skin that is often tinged with green. Its golden flesh has a spicy-sweet flavor.

- **Galia:** This intensely sweet melon is a cross between cantaloupe and honeydew. It resembles a yellow version of the former on the outside and the latter on the inside.

- **Hami:** Also known as the snow melon, this is an oblong fruit with yellow skin and green streaks throughout. The juicy orange flesh is reminiscent of very sweet cantaloupe, with a firmer texture.

- **Korean:** This little "single-serving" melon has a large seed cavity filled with edible seeds and juicy white flesh that seems to blend cantaloupe, pear, and banana flavors.

- **Santa Claus:** Also known as the Christmas melon, the Santa Claus looks like a small, bumpy, football-shaped watermelon. Its succulent flesh is pale green to white and has a mildly sweet flavor.

with a sweet taste and slightly musky aroma. The flesh ranges in color from soft peach tones to orange; the texture is quite soft compared to other melons, but can be crisp when unripe. The European cantaloupe, *C. melo* var. *cantalupensis*, looks quite different from its New World cousin, with a lightly ribbed gray-green skin that covers a sweet and flavorful flesh.

Honeydew: Another variety of the *Cucumis melo* species, the honeydew melon (also known as a honeymelon), is classified with the Inodorus group, which also includes Crenshaw, casaba, winter, and other mixed melons. It has a round to slightly oval shape, with a smooth skin that ranges in color from greenish to yellow. When ripe, its pale green, juicy flesh bursts with floral sweetness reminiscent of honey.

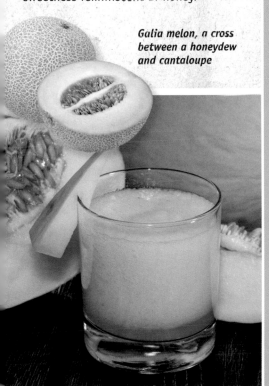

Galia melon, a cross between a honeydew and cantaloupe

Fresh-made honeydew juice

DIY: RECIPES

Whether you choose cantaloupe, honeydew, or any other yellow melon, the result will be rich, flavorful, and refreshing.

Melon & Orange

- ½ muskmelon, without rind
- 1 carrot
- 4 oranges, peeled

Scrub all produce, then put ingredients through a juicer.

Apple, Cantaloupe & Honeydew

- 2 apples
- ½ cantaloupe
- ½ honeydew
- 6 to 8 kale leaves
- 6 to 8 Swiss chard leaves

Wash all produce, then put ingredients through a juicer.

Rock 'n' Roll Melon Juice

- ½ cantaloupe
- 4 to 6 leaves rainbow chard
- 1 apple
- 1 handful fresh mint leaves

Scrub all produce, then put ingredients through a juicer.

Heaven's Honeydew

- 1 handful spinach with stems
- ¼ honeydew, rind removed
- 1 cucumber
- ½ lemon, peeled

Peel the lemon or scrub thoroughly. Wash and chop the ingredients to fit through your juicer.

Substitutions:
- Spinach: *kale, dandelion leaves, lettuce, watercress, choy sum*
- Honeydew: *cantaloupe, pineapple, apple*
- Cucumber: *celery, zucchini, celeriac root*
- Lemon: *lime, grapefruit, orange*

NECTARINE

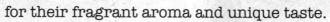

A close relative of the peach but lacking the velvety skin, nectarines are popular worldwide for their fragrant aroma and unique taste.

THE BASICS

Like the peach, nectarines *(Prunus persica)* originated in China, and then spread to central Asia and Europe via the Silk Road. The flesh is juicy and, depending upon the variety, yellow or pale cream in color with a single stone in the center. The seed is very hard and inedible. Nectarines are classified into free-stone variety or clinging variety depending on whether the seed is free or firmly attached to the pulp.

HEALTH BENEFITS

As well as being a source of antioxidants, such as vitamin C and vitamin A, nectarines are a good source of some B vitamins, including niacin, pantothenic acid, thiamin, and pyridoxine. They also contain important minerals, including iron, potassium, and phosphorus. Iron is required for red blood cell formation; potassium helps regulate heart rate and blood pressure; and phosphorus helps to preserve the nervous system.

BEST FOR
Vitamin B3 (niacin), to lower cholesterol

CALORIES
44 per 3.5 ounces

PREPARATION
Wash, slice to remove the stone. No need to remove skin.

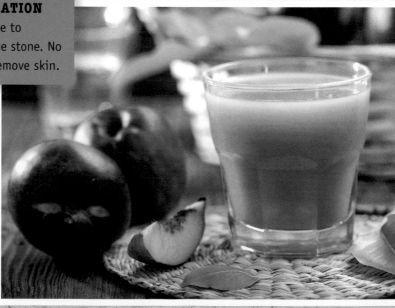

Unfiltered nectarine yields a sweet juice with a natural cloudiness.

ONION

Onions may not be the first veggie you think of when you reach for your juicer, but adding this pungent bulb to juice blends can add a layer of complexity.

THE BASICS

The onion *(Allium cepa)* is a culinary staple that has been in cultivation for at least 7,000 years. Onions come in a variety of sizes and colors and the underground bulb is made up of modified leaves, rather than being a foodstore for the plant, so it is very low in calories.

Common onions vary in color depending on variety. Yellow or brown onions are noted for their full flavor, and cultivars like Vidalia, Walla Walla, Cévennes, and Bermuda are bred for sweetness. Yellow onions, which caramelize to a rich, dark brown, and white onions, which have a golden color, are particularly sweet when sautéed; both of these varieties are better suited for cooking than juicing. Red onions add color to a dish, and their savory-sweet flavor makes them the best juicing onion. Beneath the skin, the flesh of the bulb is pale-colored. Choose bulbs that are firm and unbruised.

HEALTH BENEFITS

Although it is a useful source of vitamin C, it lacks the healthy complement of other vitamins found in the leafy green vegetables. It does, however, contain powerful phytonutrients that more than make up for this. Onions are high in polyphenols and flavonoids, together with other beneficial compounds, which are thought to have a role in protecting the body from cancer, as well as lowering blood sugar levels and helping to reduce the risk of heart disease and stroke. Yet you would probably need to eat onions on a regular, daily basis in order to receive their full benefit.

BEST FOR
Polyphenols, for prevention of cancer and heart disease

CALORIES
40 per 3.5 ounces

PREPARATION
Remove the papery skin and cut into quarters.

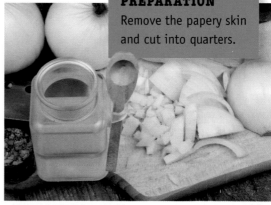

Just a dash of onion juice can add tons of flavor to juice blends and smoothies.

ORANGE

They may be commonplace, but oranges are still a treasure trove in terms of health benefits and their status in the world of juicing, where they provide the base juice for so many wonderful drinks.

THE BASICS

Once regarded as a luxury item available only to the mega-rich, oranges first became more widely available in the seventeenth century with the establishment of trade routes to India. Often called sweet orange to distinguish it from the bitter orange *(Citrus × aurantium)*, the orange is the fruit of the citrus tree *C. × sinensis*. Aromatic, delicious, and refreshing, fresh orange juice is the classic breakfast drink that provides the perfect start to a day.

HEALTH BENEFITS

Packed with goodness, at the expense of just a few calories, a single orange can provide your full day's quota of antioxidant vitamin C. It's worth noting

BEST FOR
Vitamin C, for healthy bones, teeth, skin, and hair

CALORIES
46 per 3.5 ounces

PREPARATION
Peel and quarter.

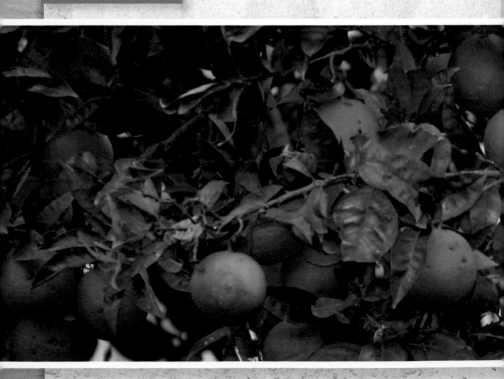

that juicing—rather than squeezing—is more beneficial healthwise because it includes the pith that contains the super-antioxidant bioflavonoids that help the body process that precious vitamin C. Foods high in vitamin C help your body to absorb iron, so it's always a good idea to blend them with iron-rich green leafy vegetables.

Note, too, that the seeds are a good source of calcium, magnesium, and potassium, so for the greatest benefit, simply peel the orange and juice the flesh, pith, and pips. This ensures that the fiber is retained, along with the white pith, a source of antioxidants. The fiber in the pith contains pectin, a type of soluble fiber that is also a natural gelling substance used to set jam. Pectin helps to protect the bowel from disease and also helps to reduce cholesterol levels. And even the peel is good for you, containing phytonutrients (called terpenes), which have antioxidant power.

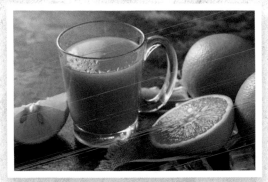

A classic breakfast juice, OJ also mixes well with both sweet and savory blends and smoothies (above); ready-to-pick oranges on the tree (below)

DIY: RECIPES

Orange juice is a classic morning beverage, rich in vitamin C. You can juice this fruit in a simple citrus press, squeezer, or reamer, or run it through a juicing machine.

Minty Orange Juice

- 2 oranges, peeled
- ½ pink grapefruit, peeled
- 2 carrots
- 2 celery stalks
- ⅓ bunch mint

Scrub all produce, then put ingredients through a juicer.

Citrus Cucumber Reviver

- ½ cucumber
- 2 oranges, peeled
- 1 lemon, peeled

Scrub all produce, then put ingredients through a juicer.

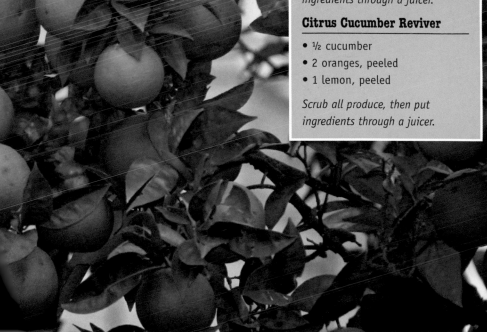

PAPAYA

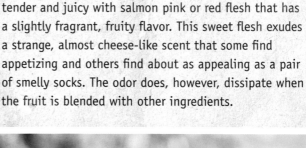

A native of the
tropics, papayas
have a sweet, almost
melon-like flavor that enhances blended juices,
summer smoothies, and smoothie bowls.

THE BASICS

Papaya is the fruit of a small tropical tree, *Carica papaya*. The pear-shaped fruit is quite large, growing up to 20 inches in length and 12 inches in diameter. There are two commonly grown varieties: a sweet papaya with red or orange flesh (sometimes called red papaya) and a yellow one (yellow papaw). A green papaya can be either the red or yellow variety that has been picked while still green. In US supermarkets, you will likely find the large-fruited, red-fleshed Maradol, Sunrise, and Caribbean Red cultivars, which tend to be delightfully tender and juicy with salmon pink or red flesh that has a slightly fragrant, fruity flavor. This sweet flesh exudes a strange, almost cheese-like scent that some find appetizing and others find about as appealing as a pair of smelly socks. The odor does, however, dissipate when the fruit is blended with other ingredients.

BEST FOR
Papain, for healthy digestion

CALORIES
25 per 3.5 ounces

PREPARATION
Slice into quarters, remove the pips, and cut away the flesh in chunks.

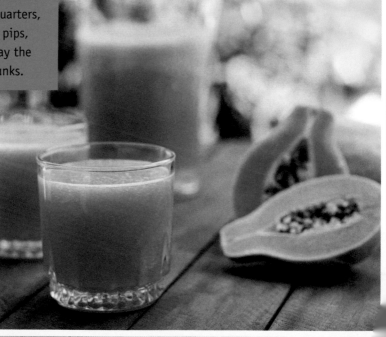

Fresh-made papaya juice

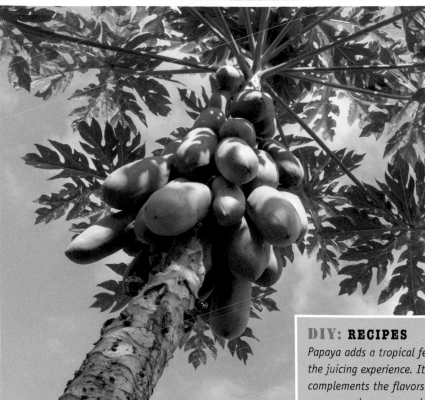

Papaya fruit ripening on the tree

HEALTH BENEFITS

Papaya is perhaps best known as an aid to digestion. It contains a particular enzyme (papain) that helps to digest protein and may also help ease some disorders related to incomplete digestion. It is itself easily digested and high in fiber, which further enhances its digestive properties. Papaya is a rich source of the antioxidants beta-carotene and vitamin C, and a good source of vitamin A and many of the B-group vitamins. It also provides moderate amounts of potassium, calcium, and iron. Interestingly, papaya seeds (which are edible but have a bitter taste) have long been used in folk medicine for their purported anti-inflammatory, antiparasitic, and analgesic properties, but these are yet to be scientifically proven.

DIY: RECIPES

Papaya adds a tropical feel to the juicing experience. It nicely complements the flavors of mango and orange, and these three fruits can be mixed in any combination and blended to your desired consistency.

Pabamao Smoothie

- ½ cup papaya, diced, peeled and seeded
- 1 small banana, peeled and sliced
- ½ cup mango, peeled and cut into chunks
- ¼ cup freshly squeezed orange juice

Place all the ingredients in a blender. Blend until smooth, adding ice if desired.

Lime, Papaya & Mango

- 1 mango
- ½ standard papaya
- 1 cup orange juice
- 1 cup mango juice
- 1 tablespoon lime juice (the juice of ½ small lime)

Scrub all produce, then put ingredients through a juicer.

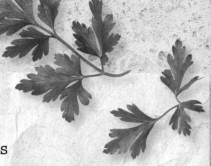

PARSLEY

Once upon a time, parsley was just a pretty garnish that no one ever ate. Times have changed and it has grown up to become an important source of phytonutrients, many of which are particularly helpful to elderly people.

THE BASICS

Garden parsley *(Petroselinum crispum)* is a bright green herb that has two common varieties: curly leaf and flat leaf (also known as Italian parsley). Flat-leaf parsley has a stronger flavor than the curly-leaf variety, and both types are best drunk in combination with other juices, where they contribute a high dose of nutrients and a lovely shot of color. Look for fresh bunches and avoid any with wilting stems or yellowing leaves. For the ultimate in freshness, try growing your own in a pot by the back door or on a kitchen windowsill.

BEST FOR
Vitamin K, for healthy bones

CALORIES
36 per 3.5 ounces

PREPARATION
Wash and juice in handfuls.

HEALTH BENEFITS

Both the flat- and curly-leaf varieties can work as a diuretic to flush unwanted water and salt from the body and may, theoretically, assist in the treatment of kidney disorders, high blood pressure, and water retention—although the amounts needed may well exceed the usual intake. With a high content of zeaxanthin for maintaining the aging retina in good health, it is also full of antioxidants (such as beta-carotene and vitamins A and C) and some B-group vitamins like folate. It is particularly rich in vitamin K, which helps keep bones healthy and is thought to limit the damage to the brain caused by Alzheimer's disease, and is a good source of various minerals, including potassium, calcium, iron, and magnesium. To absorb the iron from parsley, it is important that you combine it with a food containing vitamin C. Parsley also has hardly any calories

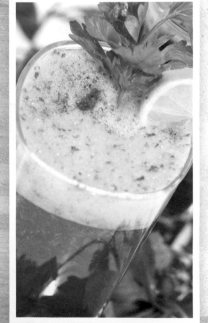

Parsley juice

PARSNIP

Try not to think of the parsnip as merely a pale carrot. This root veggie is packed with minerals and other nutrients, and its juice makes a rich and creamy base for smoothies.

THE BASICS

With a higher sugar content (and calorie count) than carrots, parsnips *(Pastinaca sativa)* make a fabulous thick, sweet juice which is best mixed in small quantities with other juices. A winter crop, they come into their own when other vegetables are out of season. Look for firm roots that are not too big.

HEALTH BENEFITS

Parsnips may not have the healthy color of their carrot cousins, but don't let their looks deceive you. Never mind the lack of vitamin A and beta-carotene in these white root vegetables: they have a plentiful supply of other antioxidants which are thought to protect against cancer, particularly of the colon, and are a good source of vitamins C and K and of folate. They also contain useful amounts of the various minerals that keep the body in good health, such as copper, manganese, and calcium. To retain as many of these vitamins and minerals as possible, leave the skin on the roots but scrub well before juicing to remove any dirt.

DIY: RECIPES

Parsnips, like most other root veggies, yield a thick juice.

Parsnapple

- 3 parsnips
- 3 apples
- ½ lime
- 3 sprigs fresh mint

Wash all produce, then put ingredients through a juicer.

Citrus Frootjuice

- 1 parsnip
- 2 grapefruit
- 2-inch slice sweet potato
- 1 stalk celery

Scrub all produce, then put ingredients through a juicer.

BEST FOR
Potassium, for heart health

CALORIES
75 per 3.5 ounces

PREPARATION
Scrub the roots and cut into chunks.

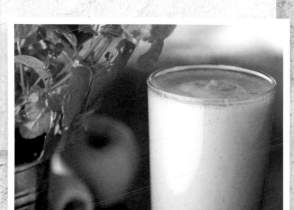

Parsnapple. Juicing parsnips results in a satisfyingly thick and filling beverage.

PEACH

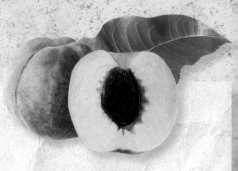

Ripe peaches, dripping with juice, evoke the taste of summer, and a glass of this sweet nectar is sublime on its own or added to smoothies and bowls.

THE BASICS

The fuzzy peach is the fruit of the flowering *Prunus persica* tree. The fruit, technically a drupe, or stone fruit, has yellow or whitish flesh, a delicately sweet-acrid aroma, and velvety skin. In some cultivars, especially the heirloom varieties, the flesh bruises easily. The red-brown, oval-shaped stone is actually a single large seed and is surrounded by a wood-like husk.

It is not surprising that the peach is full of goodness when sipped as a deliciously refreshing juice or smoothie. Very ripe peaches can also be pulped and blended with water (or coconut water) to produce a delicious, nutritious nectar that is perfect for fruit smoothies, either on its own or blended with other fruits. Peaches combine particularly well with pineapple, but are also delicious when mixed with a host of other fruits, including grapes, cherries, and plums. Not for nothing, they are called the "nectar of the gods."

HEALTH BENEFITS

The sweet, juicy flesh of peaches hosts a spectacular array of nutrients. Despite their sweetness, peaches are low in calories (less than 12 calories per ounce). They contain health-boosting flavonoids that combat free radicals and may play an important role in forestalling many signs of aging and protecting against cancer and heart disease. Peaches are high in antioxidants, including vitamins A and C, beta-carotene, and lutein. It is widely believed that foods high in antioxidants may reduce the risk of cancer and degenerative diseases such as Alzheimer's disease, as well as assist in the treatment and prevention of other disorders. Peaches, especially the yellow variety, also contain useful amounts of minerals like potassium, considered helpful in the treatment of high blood pressure, as well as iron, fluoride, copper, and manganese.

Like other stone fruits, peaches yield a sweet, cloudy nectar (opposite).

BEST FOR
Flavonoids, to delay the aging process

CALORIES
45 per 3.5 ounces

PREPARATION
Slice in half, remove stone, then chop to feed into juicer.

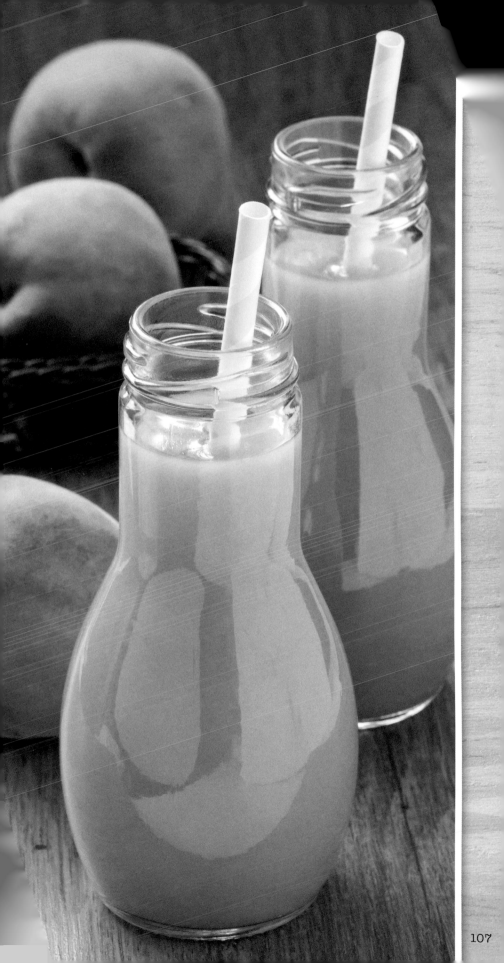

PEAR

The teardrop-shaped pear has a sweet taste and grainy texture that juices well and also adds rich flavor to a smoothie or any blended beverage.

THE BASICS

Close cousins of the apple, pears have a high water and fiber content and are very low-calorie, providing around 100 calories. There are more than 5,000 varieties of pear out there, but they are broadly divided into just two categories: Asian pears *(Pyrus pyrifolia)*, which tend to be firm and crisp (and stay that way); and European pears *(P. communis)*, which tend to become softer as they ripen, making them ideal for juicing. European pears are what we typically think of when we picture this fruit: smooth, mottled skin with gentle bumps and a bottom-heavy shape. Asian pears look more like apples, round and a uniformly yellowish tan. Both Asian and European pears are suitable for smoothies, adding a pleasant, light, sweet taste.

HEALTH BENEFITS

Although low in calories, pears are packed with the usual suspects in the world of fruity nutrients, such as dietary fiber, antioxidants, vitamins, and minerals. Pears are a good source of copper, iron, potassium, and magnesium, as well as antioxidant vitamin C

BEST FOR
Copper, to help your body process iron and protect the nervous system

CALORIES
60 per 3.5 ounces

PREPARATION
Wash, and chop to fit into juicer.

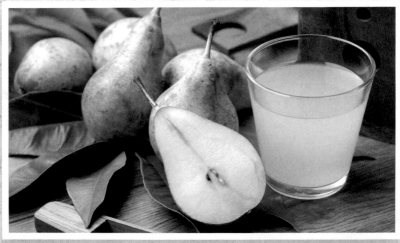

Pear nectar made from European pears. European pears, such as Boscs, Anjous, and Bartletts, have the classic teardrop pear shape.

and a heap of B complex vitamins. Pears are thought to have a special role to play in the fight against colon cancer, helping to cleanse the colon of carcinogenic toxins. They are very high in dietary fiber, as well as sorbitol, which together provide laxative benefits. Pears appear in a range of traditional medicines designed to treat such chronic disorders as colitis, arthritis, and gout. They are also known as one of the least allergenic fruits and are therefore often recommended for inclusion in low-allergen diets. Pear juice oxidizes very rapidly, so to obtain the maximum health benefits, be sure to drink the juice as soon as it is made.

DIY: RECIPES

The sweet flavor of pear makes it suitable for both morning juices and afternoon smoothies.

Pear Pineapple Nectar

- 2 pears
- ¼ large pineapple
- ½ inch ginger

Scrub all produce, then put ingredients through a juicer.

Rupert the Pear

- 3 parsnips
- 3 pears
- 1 lime

Scrub all produce, then put ingredients through a juicer.

Wash all produce, then put ingredients through a juicer.

Spiced Pear Smoothie

- 1 cup vanilla almond milk
- ½ cup sliced pear
- 1 frozen banana
- ½ teaspoon grated ginger
- ¼ teaspoon cinnamon
- 1 teaspoon ground flaxseed

Place all the ingredients in a blender. Blend until smooth.

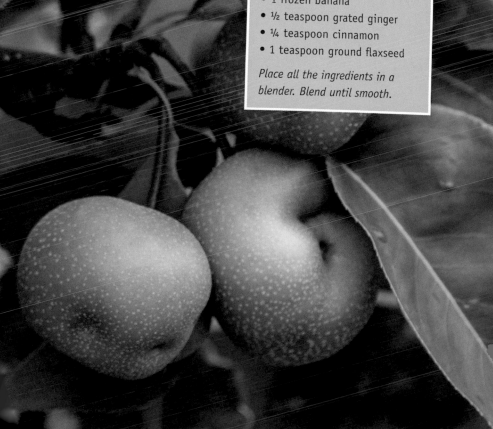

Golden Asian pears. Asian pears are rounder than their European cousins.

PEPPER

Heat up your juices, smoothies, and bowls with brightly colored and flavorful peppers, all fruits of the Capsicum annuum plant.

THE BASICS

There are several varieties of peppers, ranging from the large, mild bell peppers to the hot little chili peppers, which have an intense heat that most people can tolerate in small doses only.

HEALTH BENEFITS

Peppers contain the chemical capsaicin. Preliminary research suggests that capsaicin might offer, among other benefits, antibacterial and anticarcinogenic properties, and might assist in lowering LDL cholesterol.

BEST FOR
Vitamin C, for healthy blood and bones

CALORIES
20 per 3.5 ounces

PREPARATION
Wash and cut open lengthwise, removing the stem, pips, and pith.

BELL PEPPER

Originating in Central America, where it was discovered by European explorers in the fifteenth century, the bell pepper has a cheerfully tropical appearance. The gloriously bright colors of ripe bell peppers—red, orange, and yellow—send a clear signal that they are full of beta-carotene. The juice combines well with tomato juice. Buy peppers when they look shiny and unwrinkled, and choose the red, orange, and yellow fruits for higher levels of beta-carotene and vitamin C.

Bell peppers are crunchy and quite sweet to the taste, yet low in calories. Green peppers are the unripe form, tasting slightly bitter when compared with the brightly colored ripe fruits and containing much lower levels of beneficial nutrients.

Bell peppers range in color from red to orange to yellow to green.

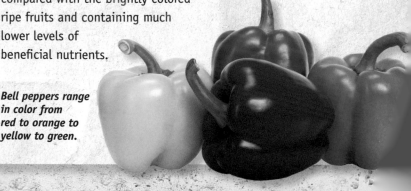

CHILI PEPPER

There are scores of chili peppers available, prized for both the flavor and heat that they bring to food and beverages. They contain high concentrations of nutrients, but can be consumed only in very small quantities due to their hot flavor. A high level of capsaicin is responsible for this heat, but also imbues these peppers with pain-relieving capabilities. It is thought that, when ingested, capsaicin is able to interrupt the transmission of pain messages to the brain, thereby diverting or otherwise reducing the pain experience. Chili peppers are a rich source of vitamin C and beta-carotene as well as other antioxidants. They are a good source of B-group vitamins and also contain various minerals. Here are just a few that you can use to spice up your juices and smoothies.

Jalapeño: These moderately hot peppers are smooth, green, shiny, and plump. They pack a mild punch, with a green, grassy flavor under the heat.

Serrano: Slim green serranos have a taste similar to jalapeños—an herby, even grass-like flavor, but with a tad more heat.

Cayenne: These thin red peppers have a deceptively mild aroma that masks a fiery taste. They pack a spicy punch in any savory smoothie.

Habanero and Scotch bonnet: These squat little peppers are some of the hottest chilis out there, with a scorching level of heat. They look nearly identical, both starting out bright green before turning sunny yellow, then brilliant orange, and finally deep red when ripe.

THINK ABOUT IT!

Peppers vary in heat from just about nothing to scorching. Scoville heat units (SHU) measure this heat and are a good guide to help you choose the level you are comfortable with. Remember, the higher the number, the hotter the pepper.

SHU	PEPPER VARIETY
800,000 to 3,200,000	• Pepper X • Carolina Reaper • Dragon's Breath
350,000 to 800,000	• Red Savina • Chocolate habanero
100,000 to 350,000	• Habanero • Scotch bonnet
10,000 to 100,000	• Malagueta • Cayenne • Serrano • Chipotle • Chile de arbol
1,000 to 10,000	• Guajillo • Poblano • Jalapeño • Ancho
100 to 1,000	• Banana pepper • Cubanelle
0 to 100	• Bell pepper • Pimiento

PINEAPPLE

Perhaps the most distinctive of all fruits, the exotic pineapple originated in the South American tropics and was brought to Europe by Christopher Columbus in 1493.

THE BASICS

The exotic appearance of tropical fruit has strong associations with celebrations and beachside holidays in the sun—and these alone are capable of conjuring up happy thoughts that in turn can be beneficial to health. Holidays and celebrations aside, the pineapple *(Ananas comosus)* is in fact a compound fruit, meaning that it is not one but rather a number of smaller fruits fused together around the very fibrous core. They are relatively fiddly to prepare but the nutritional benefits and the distinctive, delightfully refreshing taste are more than worth the effort. While the pineapple core is less sweet than the flesh and so fibrous that it can be impossible to eat (unless puréed), it does contain bromelain and also offers digestive benefits. It is therefore worth including at least some of the core in smoothie blends.

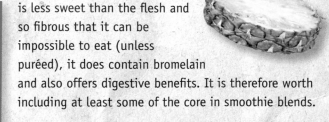

BEST FOR
Bromelain, to aid the digestive system

CALORIES
50 per 3.5 ounces

PREPARATION
Slice off the crown and base, then place the fruit on its base to carefully remove the skin. Cut into chunks to feed into the juicer.

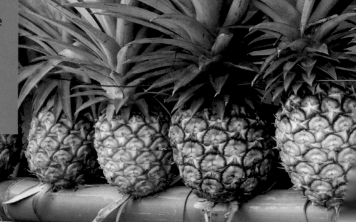

Fresh pineapples for sale in a Thai marketplace

HEALTH BENEFITS

Today, pineapple is hugely popular all around the world and is renowned for its manifold health benefits. It is an excellent source of vitamin C, and also contains modest quantities of a wide range of other nutrients. It is hailed as being especially good for the digestive system due to the presence of potent bromelain, an enzyme that breaks down protein and aids digestion. Bromelain also has anti-inflammatory, anti-clotting, and anti-cancer properties.

It is also used to help alleviate chest conditions such as bronchitis and pneumonia. Pineapples are high in thiamin, vitamin B6, and copper, and are an excellent source of vitamin C.

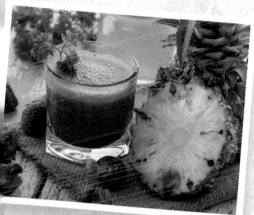

Pink Pineapple Juice

DIY: RECIPES

Pineapples call to mind tropic beaches and summer sunshine. Juice these sweet fruits to make delicious drinks to get that feeling all year round.

Pink Pineapple Juice

- ½ pineapple
- 2 handfuls of strawberries

Wash all produce, then put ingredients through a juicer.

Black & Blue Pineapple

- 1 cup blackberries
- 3 sprigs fresh parsley
- 2 spears pineapple
- ½ cup blueberries
- ½ cup raspberries

Wash all produce, then put ingredients through a juicer.

Aniseed Pineapple Juice

- ½ pineapple
- 1½ handfuls blackcurrants
- ½ fennel bulb

Wash all produce, then put ingredients through a juicer.

Pineapple, Blueberry & Ginger Juice

- ¼ pineapple
- 1 cup blueberries
- ½ inch ginger

Wash all produce, then put ingredients through a juicer.

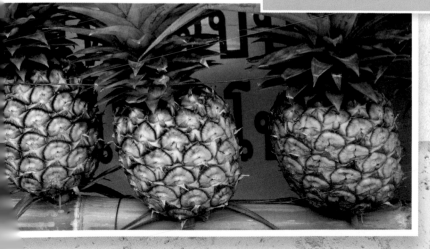

PLUM

Wonderfully delicious and juicy, plums yield a healthful juice that keeps your digestive tract functioning well.

THE BASICS

A plum is a fruit of a flowering, medium-sized tree in the subgenus *Prunus* of the genus *Prunus* (which includes cherries, peaches, nectarines, apricots, and almonds). Fleshy and succulent, plums are small, attractive fruits that originated in China and range in color from yellow to deep purple. The juicy flesh, which ranges from sweet to tart, encases a hard, inedible stone that needs to be removed before juicing.

HEALTH BENEFITS

Plums are perhaps most renowned for aiding digestion and helping to relieve constipation. Besides their gentle laxative effect, thanks largely to the presence of sorbitol, plums are a good source of flavonoid polyphenolic antioxidants, which devour the oxygen-derived free radicals

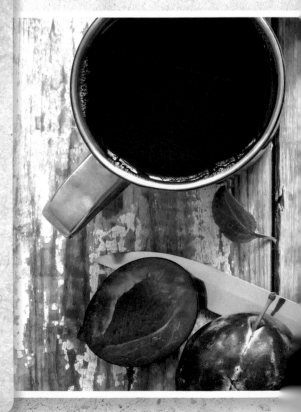

 RELATED SPECIES
PLUM HYBRIDS

Crossbreeding tart, juicy plums and sweet, fleshy apricots now gives us three tasty hybrids:

• *Plumcot:* This a 50-50 hybrid of the plum and the apricot. There are many varieties of plumcot, depending on the kinds of plums and apricots used. It is also goes by the name "apriplum."

• *Pluot:* The pluot is a plum-apricot hybrid, genetically one-fourth apricot and three-fourths plum. A pluot looks and tastes like a plum, but without the bitter skin.

• *Apriums:* An aprium is one-fourth plum and three-fourths apricot. It looks like an apricot, but has firmer, juicier plum-like flesh.

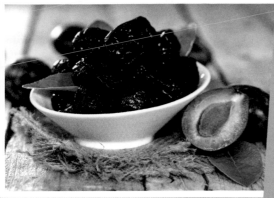

Prunes, otherwise known as dried plums

THE DREADED PRUNE
The prune is made from a prune–plum variety that has a very high sugar content, which allows it to be dried without fermenting while still containing the pit. With its association with constipation (which it helps relieve), it sometimes gets a bad rap—so much so that these days, they are often called "dried plums." Whatever you call it, this chewy, nearly black fruit makes a healthy and flavorful addition to blended juices and smoothies.

that are thought to cause a number of illnesses. They are also a good source of potassium, which helps control the heart rate and blood pressure; vitamin A, which is essential for healthy eyesight; and vitamin K, which is beneficial for bone strength and is thought to help reduce the occurrence of Alzheimer's. Do not peel the fruit, as the skin contains antioxidant pigments and is a good source of fiber.

BEST FOR
Beta-carotene to boost the immune system

CALORIES
46 per 3.5 ounces

PREPARATION
Wash, and slice to remove stone. No need to peel.

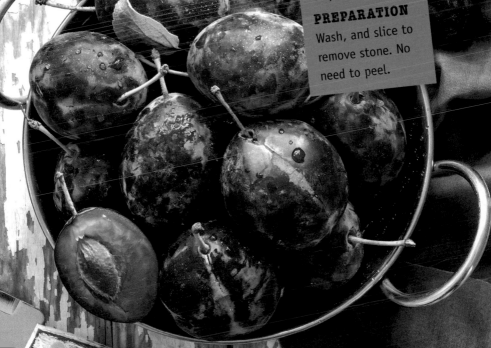

Plums often have a white or silvery coating on them, called wax bloom.

POMEGRANATE

The crimson-red juice of this ancient and exotic fruit is hailed as a heart protector.

THE BASICS

The pomegranate (*Punica granatum*) is a deciduous shrub or small tree that bears deep red fruit. A pomegranate fruit is actually a berry, and its husk has two parts: an outer, hard pericarp and an inner, spongy mesocarp. Within the inner wall are seeds individually encased in a crimson sac that contains the tasty juice. Its flavor varies depending on pomegranate variety and how ripe it is, ranging from a bit sour like a ripe cherry to quite sharp, reminiscent of a fresh cranberry. One of the best ways to remove the seeds from a pomegranate is to cut it in half and hit the backs with the side of a wooden spoon over a bowl.

HEALTH BENEFITS

Pomegranate seeds (arils) are rich in polyphenols, a powerful group of antioxidants that may offer significant health benefits, particularly relating to cardiovascular and prostate health. Research has shown that drinking a daily glass of pomegranate juice (made by blending the fruit's seeds) can reduce the risk of cardiovascular disease by helping to clear clogged arteries. It may even reverse the progression of the disease. This pomegranate potion also has strong anti-inflammatory effects that result in improved blood flow and delayed oxidation of LDL cholesterol in patients with heart disease and arthritis. Pomegranates are a nutrition powerhouse and a good source of vitamin C, potassium, B-group vitamins such as folate, vitamin K, and dietary fiber.

BEST FOR
Polyphenols, antioxidants that support cardiovascular and immune systems

CALORIES
67 per 3.5 ounces

PREPARATION
Remove seeds to extract the juice.

Ripening pomegranate fruit (opposite)

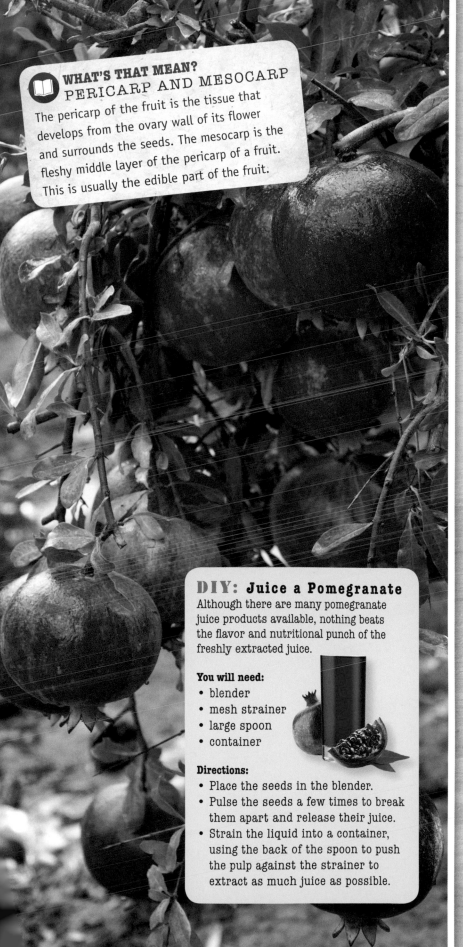

WHAT'S THAT MEAN?
PERICARP AND MESOCARP

The pericarp of the fruit is the tissue that develops from the ovary wall of its flower and surrounds the seeds. The mesocarp is the fleshy middle layer of the pericarp of a fruit. This is usually the edible part of the fruit.

DIY: Juice a Pomegranate

Although there are many pomegranate juice products available, nothing beats the flavor and nutritional punch of the freshly extracted juice.

You will need:
- blender
- mesh strainer
- large spoon
- container

Directions:
- Place the seeds in the blender.
- Pulse the seeds a few times to break them apart and release their juice.
- Strain the liquid into a container, using the back of the spoon to push the pulp against the strainer to extract as much juice as possible.

RASPBERRY

Raspberries are delicately fragrant, pink fruits that, like their cousin the blackberry, grow on sprawling thorny brambles.

THE BASICS

A member of the rose family, the raspberry is the fruit of a multitude of species in the genus *Rubus*, which also includes blackberries. The most common raspberries are the red *(R. idaeus)* and the black *(R. occidentalis)*. Pretty and fragrant, raspberries have an interesting structure. As with blackberries, each raspberry is a collection of small drupes or drupelets (small stone fruits), gathered around a hollow center. Each drupelet has its own tiny seed surrounded

DIY: RECIPES

These late-summer berries brighten any juice blend, whether you combine them with other berries or use them to sweeten a green juice.

Berry Blast

• 2 pounds raspberries
• 1 pound cranberries
• 2 oranges, peeled

Wash the cranberries and raspberries. Remove the stems and any other debris from the cranberries. Juice the berries first, and save the pulp or other fruit toppings. Next, juice up the oranges. Mix the two together and serve over crushed ice.

Raspberry Sensation

• 2 large handfuls raspberries
• 1 apple
• ½ pineapple

Wash all produce, then put ingredients through a juicer.

Raspberry, Carrot, Pear & Cucumber Juice

• 4 or 5 carrots
• 1 pear (green Anjou)
• 2 large handfuls raspberries
• 1 cucumber

Wash all produce, then put ingredients through a juicer.

Berry Blitz

• 2 large handfuls red and black raspberries
• 1 handful blackcurrants
• 1 handful blueberries

Wash all produce, then put ingredients through a juicer.

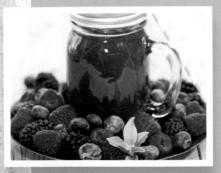

Berry Blitz

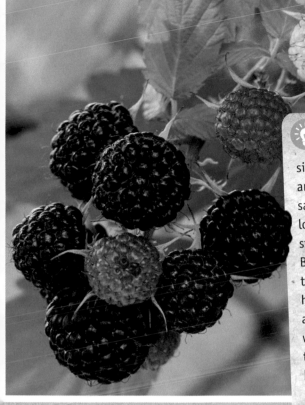

Ripening black raspberries

THINK ABOUT IT!
They may look very similar, but black raspberries and blackberries are not the same fruit. To tell them apart, look at the core, where the stem attaches to the berry. Black raspberries are hollow in the center, while blackberries have a white core. Blackberries are usually larger and shinier, with bigger "cells" that lack the minute hairs that cover black raspberries. As for flavor, black raspberries are sweeter than tart blackberries.

by the berry pulp. Raspberries are ideal for freezing, and there's no need to defrost them before juicing. You can use them in place of ice cubes when making smoothies.

HEALTH BENEFITS

For such a little fruit, raspberries are packed with nutrients. Their health benefits are as multitudinous as their seeds, and they are credited with strengthening the immune system, protecting against heart disease and liver fibrosis, and promoting wound healing. They are low in calories, high in fiber, and high in antioxidants, including tannin and anthocyanin (which gives them their color).

Raspberries are also a good source of the anticarcinogen ellagic acid. All this goodness stems from a plethora of anti-inflammatory and antioxidant phytonutrients and a multitude of minerals, including zinc to help maintain the body's acid/alkaline balance and magnesium, which is vital for a healthy heart. Raspberries are especially rich in manganese, which is important for strong bones. With all these fabulous health benefits, it's great to know that raspberries freeze well and can be enjoyed at any time of the year.

BEST FOR
Vitamin K, which helps prevent postmenopausal bone loss

CALORIES
53 per 3.5 ounces

PREPARATION
Wash carefully before hulling.

SPINACH

One of the great leafy greens, spinach is very low in calories, high in fiber, and exceptionally high in a spectacular array of vitamins, minerals, and other nutrients.

THE BASICS

Spinach (*Spinacia oleracea*) is a flowering plant harvested for its abundant tasty leaves, which yield a bright green juice. Drink it alone, or add to blended recipes—a little goes a long way to up the nutrient value of less powerful juices. Choose fresh young leaves, as these have a better flavor, and use them promptly to avoid loss of vitamins.

HEALTH BENEFITS

One of the invaluable leafy green vegetables, spinach has endless nutritional virtues, not least that it has very few calories. It is well known for its high iron content, but is also a rich source of vitamins A and C, lutein, beta-carotene, and zeaxanthin. Its antioxidant beta-carotene and vitamin C help prevent cancer and reduce the risk of heart disease, and plentiful amounts of vitamin A will keep the skin and eyes in good condition. Zeaxanthin is thought to help prevent macular disease in the elderly, and substantial amounts of vitamin K keep bones strong as well as limiting damage to the brain's neurons in people suffering from Alzheimer's disease. Potassium, manganese, magnesium, copper, and zinc are also found in its leaves. Fresh, young spinach leaves are best in smoothies. The leaves, while high in fiber, are also soft, and have a delicate flavor.

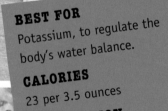

BEST FOR
Potassium, to regulate the body's water balance.

CALORIES
23 per 3.5 ounces

PREPARATION
Wash leaves and use whole.

Spinach in the garden

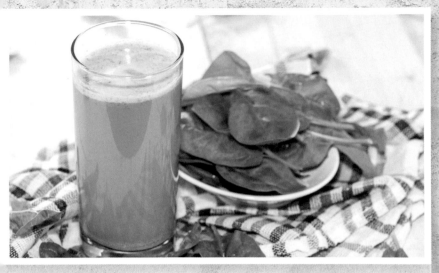

Fresh spinach juice

DIY: RECIPES

Spinach is a true superfood with a distinctive peppery taste, and makes a very appealing and highly nutritious green juice.

Spinach & Apple Juice

- 1½ cups spinach
- ½ grapefruit, peeled, with pith removed
- 2 green apples, cut into eighths
- 1-inch piece peeled fresh ginger
- 2 large stalks celery
- ice (optional)

Wash all produce, then put ingredients through a juicer.

Spinach Lemonade

- ½ chopped lemon
- 2 cups baby spinach
- 1 chopped cucumber
- 2 sweet apples, cored and chopped

Wash all produce, then put ingredients through a juicer.

Spinach, Blueberry, Apple & Lemon

- 1 small handful spinach
- 1 pint of blueberries (10 ounces)
- 1 Granny Smith apple, cored and cut into quarters
- 1 lemon, peeled

Wash all produce, then put ingredients through a juicer.

Healthy Juice

- 2 heads broccoli
- 4 cups spinach, chard, or kale (or a mixture)
- 1 green bell pepper
- 2 Granny Smith apples
- 1 lime, peeled

Wash all produce, then put ingredients through a juicer.

Spicy Spinach, Carrot, Pineapple & Cilantro

- 1 big handful spinach (about 3 ounces)
- 2 medium carrots
- ¼ pineapple
- 1 small bunch cilantro
- 1 lime
- 1 drop liquid cayenne

Wash all produce, then put ingredients through a juicer.

Spinach Cucumber

- 2 cups packed spinach (4 ounces)
- 1 cucumber
- 1 celery stalk

Wash all produce, then put ingredients through a juicer.

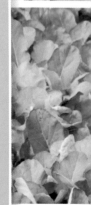

SQUASH

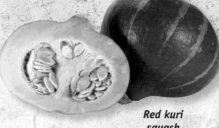

Red kuri squash

Squash traces its origins back more than 10,000 years to Mesoamerican settlements. There are many kinds to choose from that will add taste and texture to smoothies.

THE BASICS

Squash is classified into two varieties. Summer squash, most of which are *Cucurbita pepo* cultivars, includes round squash, straightneck squash, and green and yellow zucchini. Winter squash, which is a range of *Cucurbita* species, includes acorn, butternut, buttercup, and Hubbard squash, as well as pumpkin.

BEST FOR
Vitamin A, for eyes
CALORIES
15 to 40 per 3.5 ounces
PREPARATION
Remove skin, slice into quarters, remove the pips, and cut away the flesh in chunks.

HEALTH BENEFITS

Squash is an excellent source of vitamins A and C and also provides B complex vitamins, fiber—including pectin—anti-inflammatory omega-3 fatty acids, folate, magnesium, potassium, iron, and copper. Its antioxidant compounds help to support the body's immune system.

SUMMER SQUASH

Summer squash is so called because it is harvested earlier than winter squash, while it is immature with thin skin. These delicate, sweet-flavored veggies can be eaten raw and blended into smoothies.

Round squash: Also called avocado squash or round zucchini, round squash is a pale green globe with darker green mottling and dense flesh.

Straightneck squash: Also known as yellow summer squash, straightneck looks like a tapering zucchini and has a creamy-yellow, tender flesh with a nutty flavor.

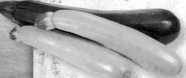

Zucchini: Zucchini can be green or golden yellow. They are cucumber-shaped squashes with smooth, thin skin; the yellow ones are slightly more tender. The flesh is firm, crisp, and sweet.

WINTER SQUASH

These squashes are harvested when mature, resulting in a thick-skinned vegetable that is more nutritious than their summer cousins. You can use them raw or parboiled in smoothies.

Acorn squash
squash

Acorn squash: Shaped like its name, the orange flesh of this squat squash has a subtle nutty flavor. The rind is a dull deep green with small orange splotches.

Buttercup squash: This round, green, and compact squash has orange flesh that smells like cucumber.

Buttercup
squash

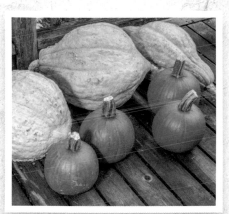

Sugar pumpkins and blue Hubbards

Hubbard squash:
The flesh of this large teardrop-shaped squash is sweet and delicious, with hints of pumpkin. You will see three major varieties: golden Hubbard squash has a bright orange skin; blue Hubbard has bumpy blue-gray skin; and hokkaido, or red kuri squash, looks like a miniature pumpkin with red-orange, ridgeless skin.

Pumpkin: Pumpkin grows as a fibrous flowering vine. The large (sometimes enormous) fruit has a ridged, orange or yellow smooth shell and dense flesh that contains a pulpy mass of seeds. Its rich, hearty flavor can be enjoyed raw or parboiled before being added to juice blends and smoothies. Pumpkins are full of nutrients, including twice the recommended intake of antioxidant vitamin A, and they are also a good source of fiber, vitamin C, riboflavin, potassium, copper, and manganese.

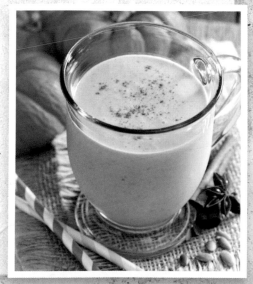

Pumpkins and other squashes
are the perfect base for autumn
smoothies flavored with warm
spices, such as cinnamon.

STRAWBERRY

Low in calories but extremely high in vitamin C, strawberries are synonymous with summertime.

THE BASICS

The garden strawberry is a hybrid species of the genus *Fragaria*. This little berry is pinkish red in color and boasts the unusual feature of having seeds outside rather than inside its flesh. This gives it a peculiar, yet attractive, tailored appearance. The flavor is sweet but slightly tart, and combines very well in smoothies with other berries and fruits, lending their lovely pink color as well as (when fresh from the field at least) lots of wholesome vitamins and minerals. Like all berries, they are highly perishable, but if frozen when fresh, they can

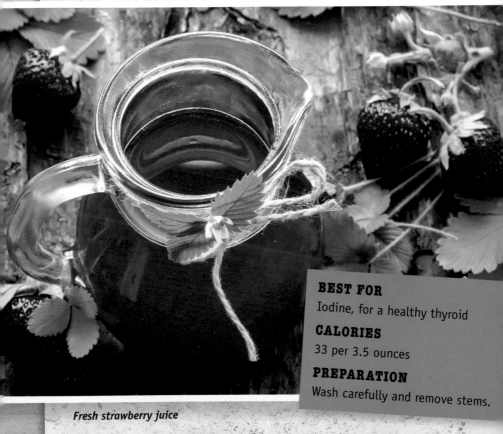

BEST FOR
Iodine, for a healthy thyroid

CALORIES
33 per 3.5 ounces

PREPARATION
Wash carefully and remove stems.

Fresh strawberry juice

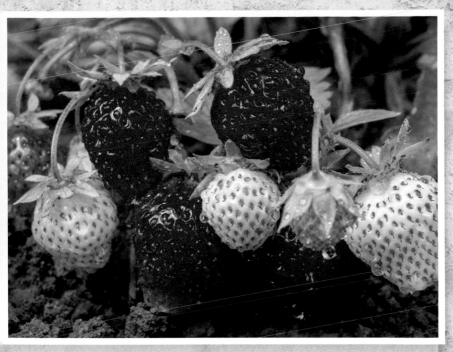

Strawberries ripen from a pale green to vibrant red.

be added to smoothies later in the form of ice blocks without any compromise to their nutritional value. Sadly, strawberries do not keep well but they can be frozen if you cut away the leaves from the base and wash (and dry) them beforehand. Upon thawing, they often become soft or even mushy, but there's no need to defrost them before juicing. Just toss them into your juicer, or add them to smoothies.

HEALTH BENEFITS

Strawberries are packed with vitamin C and other antioxidants, including anthocyanins (the pigment that is responsible for their color), ellagic acid, vitamins A and E, beta-carotene, lutein, and zeaxanthin.

Recent research suggests that strawberries can help maintain healthy blood sugar levels, and they famously promote a healthy heart thanks to their outstanding antioxidant and anti-inflammatory content. A good source of vitamin B, potassium, and magnesium, strawberries make an excellent cleansing juice. But, let's face it, nobody needs an excuse to consume strawberries—their delicious summertime flavor is reason enough.

DIY: RECIPES

Sweet-tart strawberries add a fresh taste to summer juices.

Fresh Strawberries with Ginger, Cucumber, Spinach & Apple

- 10 to 12 strawberries
- 1 inch fresh ginger
- 1 small cucumber
- 3 handfuls fresh spinach (about 4 cups)
- 3 apples
- ½ lemon

Wash all produce, then put ingredients through a juicer.

Strawberry Lime

- 3 cups fresh organic strawberries, stems removed and halved
- 1 apple
- 1 lime

Scrub all produce, then put ingredients through a juicer.

SWISS CHARD

Swiss chard is up there with spinach as one of the great green-leafers that offer a host of health benefits.

THE BASICS

A Mediterranean favorite, Swiss chard is a subspecies of *Beta vulgaris* (the beet). The leaf blade can be green or reddish in color; the leaf stalks are usually white, yellow, or red. A small handful in a smoothie blended together with other greens or perhaps some sweeter fruits and berries packs a nutritional punch. Rainbow Swiss chard is a variety that features brightly colored stems.

BEST FOR
Thiamin, to boost the immune system

CALORIES
18 per 3.5 ounces

PREPARATION
Wash leaves and use whole.

HEALTH BENEFITS

Swiss chard is low in calories; high in fiber; high in antioxidants, including vitamins C and A, beta-carotene, and lutein; high in many B-group vitamins; and a good source of iron, magnesium, manganese, copper, and potassium. It is no surprise that Swiss chard is touted as one of the most health-boosting vegetables.

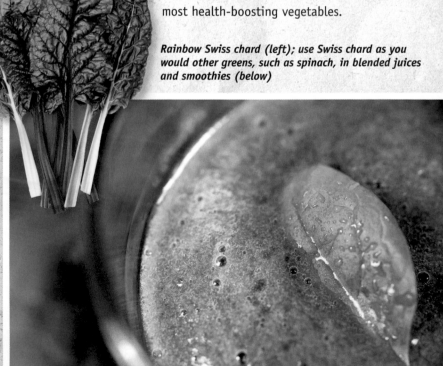

Rainbow Swiss chard (left); use Swiss chard as you would other greens, such as spinach, in blended juices and smoothies (below)

TANGERINE

The fresh sweet flavor of the fragrant tangerine enlivens juices or smoothies.

THE BASICS

A number of smaller citrus fruits are orange in color but are unrelated to the larger fruit and have a more intense flavor; among the intense are satsumas and tangerines. The tangerine *(Citrus tangerina)* is a hybrid of the mandarin orange *(C. reticulata)*. It shares many of the mandarin's traits: it is smaller and squatter than common oranges and its taste is sweeter and stronger. A ripe tangerine should be firm to slightly soft, and feel heavy for its size. Tangerines also divide more easily than oranges into 8 to 10 juicy segments. They will store in the refrigerator for a week or so, but enjoy them as early as possible to gain the maximum nutritional benefits.

DIY: RECIPES

Tangerine combines well with carrots and apples to give you an alternative "orange" juice.

Tangerine, Apple & Carrot

- 1 Minneola tangerine
- 8 large carrots
- 1 Braeburn apple

Scrub all produce, then put ingredients through a juicer.

HEALTH BENEFITS

Like oranges, tangerines are low in calories and high in vitamin C, and they are an even more valuable source of antioxidants such as carotenes and vitamin A. Tangerines are a good source of potassium, as well as some important minerals such as copper and magnesium. Like other citrus fruits, they are believed to help protect against a range of cancers, including stomach, mouth, larynx, and pharynx cancers. Some studies indicate benefits for heart disease and strokes, as well as numerous other debilitating conditions such as arthritis, Alzheimer's disease, cataracts, and gallstones.

BEST FOR
Thiamin, to boost the immune system

CALORIES
53 per 3.5 ounces

PREPARATION
Peel, and divide into segments.

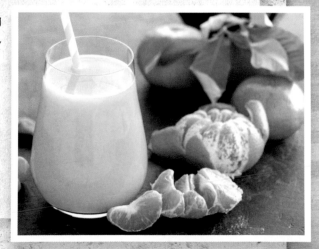

Tangerine juice has a sweeter flavor than orange.

TOMATO

Often thought to be a vegetable, the tomato is actually a fruit that boasts an enormous number of health-promoting properties.

THE BASICS

The tomato *(Solanum lycopersicum)* is now an everyday staple that was originally a native of Central America. Part of the nightshade family, it is a distant cousin of the potato and bell pepper.

Tomatoes are flavorful and juicy, and their thick juice blends well in smoothies with other fruits and vegetables, particularly celery and peppers. Their high water content makes tomatoes an ideal base for a number of smoothies—but they also work exceptionally well as almost the only ingredient, perhaps accompanied by a few healthy herbs and spices. Choose smooth, firm fruits that are a strong, uniform color.

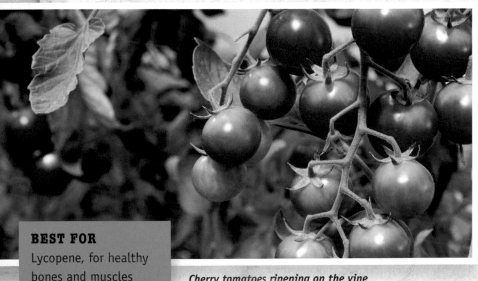

Cherry tomatoes ripening on the vine

BEST FOR
Lycopene, for healthy bones and muscles

CALORIES
18 per 3.5 ounces

PREPARATION
Remove the stem and rinse. Cut into halves or quarters to fit into the juicer feed tube.

HEALTH BENEFITS
The brilliant red color indicates the presence of the important antioxidant lycopene (also found in yellow and orange-colored tomatoes), which has an important role to play in reducing the risk of heart disease, and is also thought to help prevent cancers of the prostate, lung, stomach and breast, and

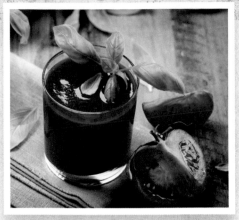

A touch of basil adds a pungent kick to a simple glass of freshly made tomato juice.

protect bones from osteoporosis. Other antioxidants found in tomatoes include beta-carotene and zeaxanthin. These powerful molecules neutralize free radicals in the body. Tomatoes are also rich in potassium and provide vitamins C, A, and K, all of which are vital for keeping the body functioning well.

Liquid Bruschetta

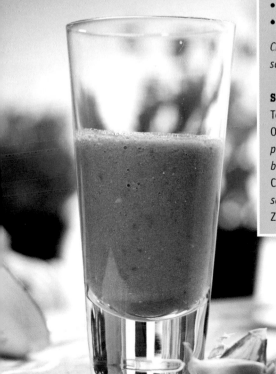

WATERCRESS

Watercress is not just for tea sandwiches. Take this green veggie out from the slices of bread, and add it to flavorful juices and smoothies that burst with nutrient-rich goodness.

THE BASICS

Watercress *(Nasturtium officinale)* is an aquatic plant species that, despite its name, is not related to the flower, but instead to other piquant-tasting members of the Brassicaceae (the cabbages), including garden cress, mustard, radish, and wasabi.

BEST FOR
Sulfur, to promote healthy skin and hair

CALORIES
11 per 3.5 ounces

PREPARATION
Remove roots, wash leaves well, and use while fresh.

This small-leaved plant is usually grown in beds of running water and has a peppery taste and an abundance of health benefits. Because it tastes so strong, it is best added to other juices, where it contributes greatly to the flavor and healthiness. Fresh watercress is a deep green color; avoid leaves that are wilting or yellow.

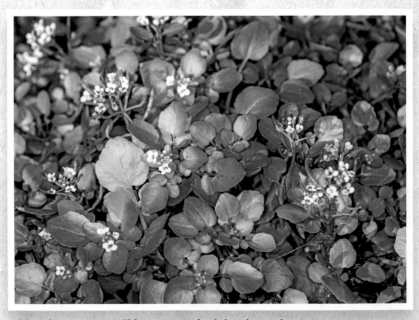

Blooming watercress. This green veggie thrives in running water.

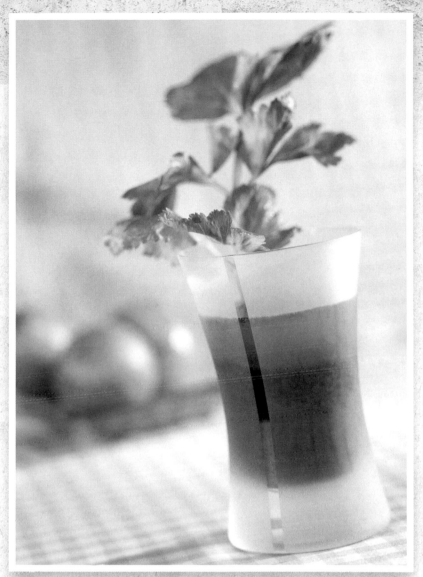

A shot of green juice gets a nutrient boost from watercress.

HEALTH BENEFITS

According to some research, watercress is the most nutrient dense of all foods. It shares many of the virtues of broccoli and brussels sprouts, being low in calories but rich in antioxidant phytochemicals, vitamins, and minerals. It has been eaten by humans for millennia, but has only recently been recognized as one of the superfoods.

Of particular note is its exceptionally high levels of vitamin K, which has an established role in the treatment and prevention of degenerative conditions such as Alzheimer's disease. Watercress contains high levels of antioxidants, including beta-carotene, lutein, zeaxanthin, and vitamins A, C, and E, which together assist in the prevention of cancer and inflammatory diseases and are important for eye health. It is also a good source of B-group vitamins, potassium, and various other minerals, including calcium and iron, for healthy bones and blood.

WHEATGRASS

This brilliantly colored emerald-green juice is certainly a boost to the spirits, and its consumption has grown apace in recent years.

THE BASICS

Derived from the common wheat plant (*Triticum aestivum*), wheatgrass has been touted as a cure-all for a multitude of conditions. You can grow your own—by all accounts, it's a lot of fun for the entire family—or, if you don't have room to grow it or to store a wheatgrass juicer, you can buy it in ounce-size quantities to add to smoothies or juices. Before you turn up your nose at using something that isn't totally fresh, these actually work very well and keep all of the nutritional benefits of freshly juiced wheatgrass.

A few individuals may suffer from an allergic reaction in the form of facial swelling, throat tightening, or difficulty breathing soon after drinking wheatgrass juice; these symptoms should be treated as a medical emergency.

BEST FOR
Essential vitamins, for healthy eyes, skin, and bones

CALORIES
28 per 3.5 ounces

PREPARATION
Wash and juice the stalks.

HEALTH BENEFITS

The nutritional content of wheatgrass is similar to leafy green vegetables, which play an important role in a healthy diet. It contains plenty of vitamin E, and smaller amounts of vitamins A, C, and K, all of which are essential for maintaining the body in good health. It is also a good source of iron.

Wheatgrass is available as fresh produce, tablets, fresh juice, frozen juice, and powder.

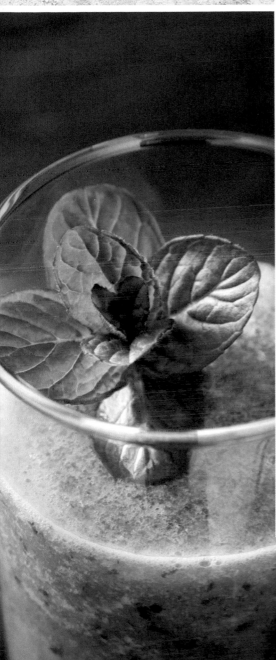

Minty Applegrass

DIY: RECIPES

Not everyone enjoys the taste of wheatgrass (some liken it to lawn clippings). Blending it with more flavorful ingredients, such as apples, allows you to reap the benefits without holding your nose.

Simple Applegrass

- 1 ounce wheatgrass juice
- 2 medium apples

Scrub the apples, then put ingredients through a juicer.

Apple Wheatgrass

- 1 to 2 apples
- ¼ cup water (optional)
- 2- to 3-inch round wheatgrass

Scrub the apples, then put ingredients through a juicer.

Minty Applegrass

- 2 apples
- 1 small handful fresh mint
- 1 ounce wheatgrass juice

Scrub the apples, then put ingredients through a juicer.

Apple Carrot Delight

- 3 carrots
- 2 apples
- 1 ounce wheatgrass juice
- 1-inch piece ginger (optional)

Scrub all produce, then put ingredients through a juicer.

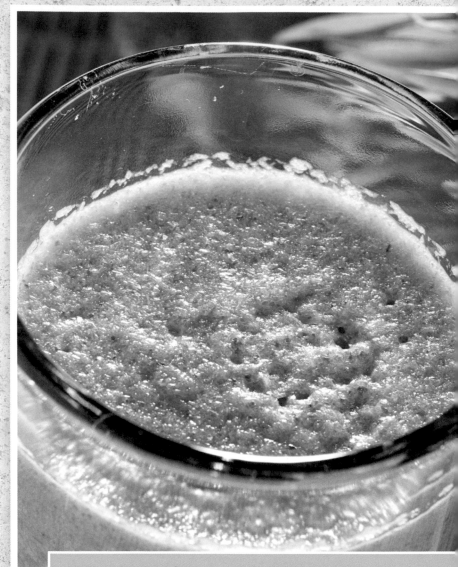

Get Your Greens Juice

- 3 celery stalks
- 4 large spinach leaves
- ½ cup parsley
- 2- to 3-inch round wheatgrass
- ¼ cup water (optional)

Wash greens thoroughly, cut up celery, and juice. Dilute with water if desired.

Green Grass

- 1 ounce wheatgrass
- 2 stalks celery
- 1 handful parsley

Wash all produce, then put ingredients through a juicer.

The Sunblast

- 1 ounce fresh organic wheatgrass juice
- 6 ounces fresh carrot juice

Mix juices together and drink while fresh.

Fresh Juicy Cleanser

- 1 ounce wheatgrass
- 2 carrots
- 2 apples
- 1 celery stalk
- 1 thin slice beet
- ¼ medium cucumber
- ½ inch ginger

Scrub all produce, then put ingredients through a juicer.

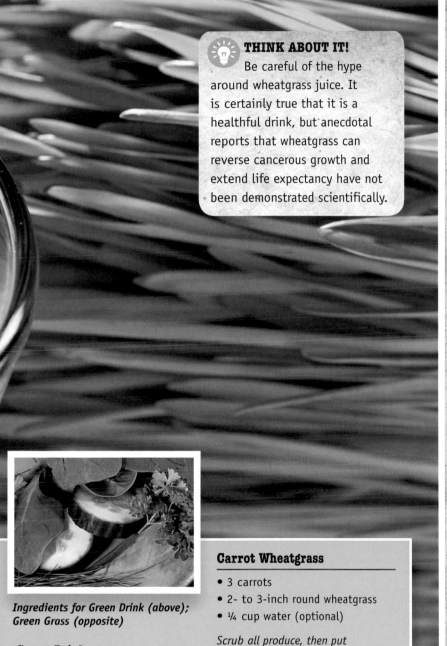

THINK ABOUT IT!
Be careful of the hype around wheatgrass juice. It is certainly true that it is a healthful drink, but anecdotal reports that wheatgrass can reverse cancerous growth and extend life expectancy have not been demonstrated scientifically.

Ingredients for Green Drink (above); Green Grass (opposite)

Green Drink

- 3 stalks celery
- 2 medium cucumbers
- 5 fresh spinach leaves
- ½ cup fresh parsley
- 2 ounces fresh wheatgrass
- water, as needed

Cut celery and cucumber into chunks small enough to fit through your juicer. Juice them, and then dilute with pure springwater for texture and taste.

Carrot Wheatgrass

- 3 carrots
- 2- to 3-inch round wheatgrass
- ¼ cup water (optional)

Scrub all produce, then put ingredients through a juicer.

Carrot Special

- 3 carrots
- ½ beet
- 2 celery sticks
- ½ lemon
- 1 ounce wheatgrass juice
- 1 small handful parsley and/or mint

Scrub all produce, then put ingredients through a juicer.

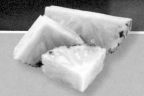

Pineapple Wheatgrass

- 1 cup roughly chopped wheatgrass
- 6½ cups roughly chopped pineapple
- 6 to 8 sprigs mint
- 1 cup crushed ice

After thoroughly scrubbing the pineapple, blend all ingredients until smooth.

Pineapple & Papaya Grass

- 2 cups fresh pineapple
- 1 papaya
- 2- to 3-inch round wheatgrass

Scrub all produce, then put ingredients through a juicer.

Tropical Wheatgrass

- 2 kiwi
- 1 guava or papaya
- 1 cup pineapple
- 5 strawberries
- 3- to 4-inch round wheatgrass

Wash all produce, then put ingredients through a juicer.

Minty Madam

- 1 handful mint leaves
- 1 ounce fresh wheatgrass juicer

Wash all produce, then put ingredients through a juicer.

Ginger Grass

- 1 inch fresh ginger
- 1 ounce wheatgrass juice
- ½ lemon
- 2½ cups water

Wash all produce, then put ingredients through a juicer.

Ginger Wheatgrass Juice

- 1 bunch wheatgrass (about a handful)
- 1 lemon
- 3 large apples
- 3 carrots
- 2-inch piece ginger

Put all ingredients through a juicer. If using a juice press, blend ingredients in a blender with a few inches of water. Send the mixture through the juice press. Serve and enjoy! Refrigerate any leftover ginger lemonade.

Wheatgrass Reviver

- 1 ounce wheatgrass juice
- ½ watermelon (enough for 1 glass)

After thoroughly scrubbing the watermelon, put ingredients through a juicer. This combo is a great, refreshing summer combination that disguises the taste of wheatgrass.

Lemon Grass

- 6 ounces lemonade
- 2 ounces fresh organic wheatgrass juice

Scrub all produce, then put ingredients through a juicer.

Green Orange

- 3 oranges
- 1 tablespoon grated ginger
- 1 ounce wheatgrass juice

After thoroughly scrubbing the oranges, put ingredients through a juicer. Garnish with mint leaves.

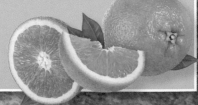

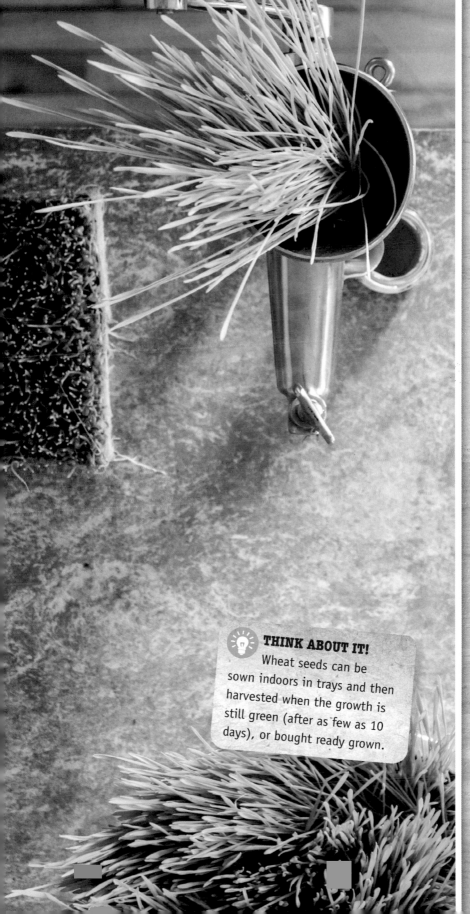

THINK ABOUT IT!
Wheat seeds can be sown indoors in trays and then harvested when the growth is still green (after as few as 10 days), or bought ready grown.

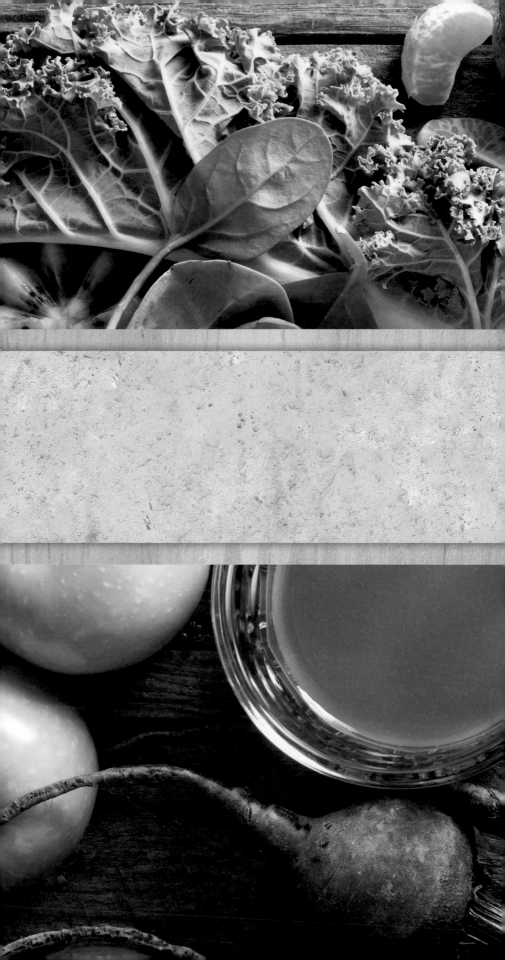

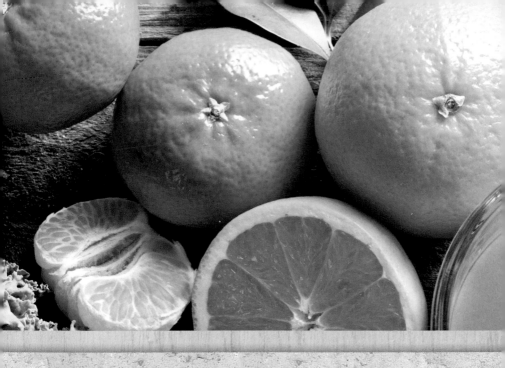

CHAPTER 3
HIGH-ENERGY JUICES

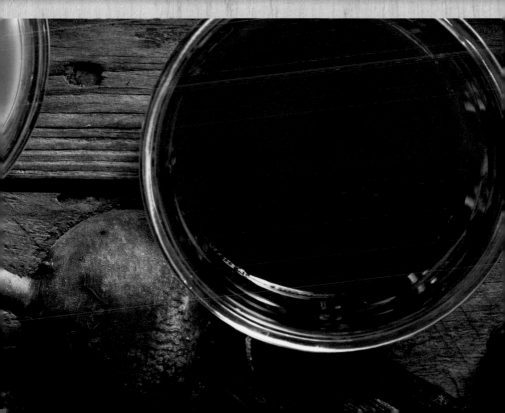

HIGH-ENERGY JUICES

Fresh fruit and vegetable juices are a natural in the ongoing search for maximum physical fitness, both in the gym and out. This is true among serious marathoners, weekend athletes, and anyone just going about their day. The following recipes have been created to give you that morning surge before you head off to work or go to the gym, and you can drink them either before or after a workout. There are also juices to keep you going morning, noon, and night.

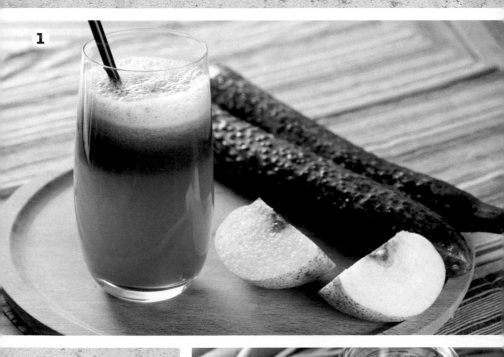

1. Lemon, Pear, Celery & Cucumber Blend
2. Sunburst Juice
3. The Morning Drive
4. Coconut Splash
5. Morning Boost Juice
6. Sunset Blend

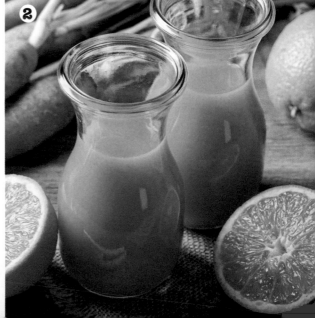

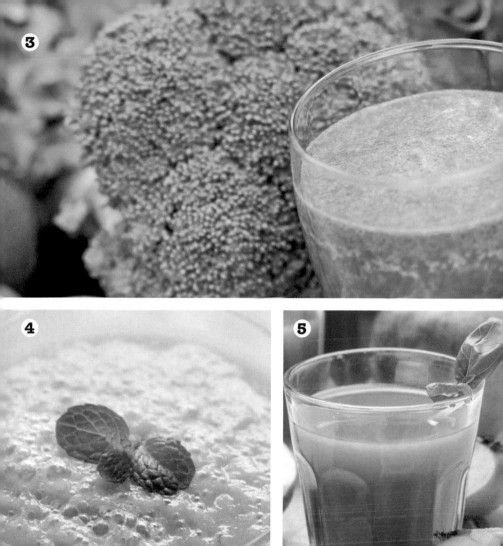

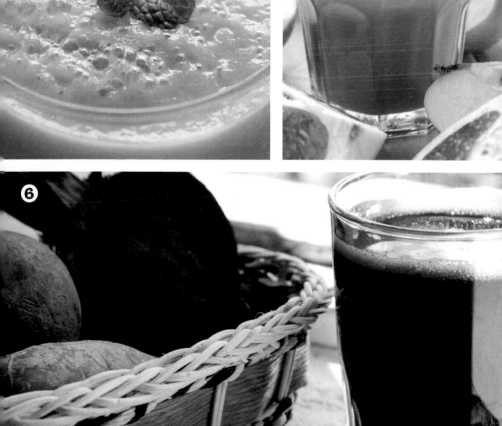

MORNING JUICES

No matter what you plan for the day ahead, starting out with a glass of juice will help you get the most out of it.

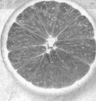

Orange

START YOUR DAY ON A HIGH

There is a morning juice to please every palate. Choose classic citrus blends, or try one of the many veggie options available.

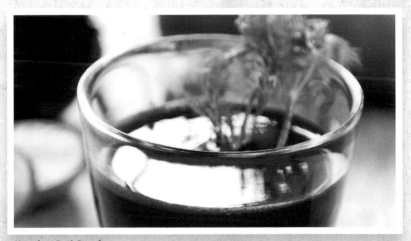

Morning Red Sunrise

Morning Red Sunrise

- 1 beet
- 1 purple carrot
- 1 cup strawberries
- 2 blood oranges
- 2 celery stalks

Wash all ingredients. Peel the blood oranges and the beet. Chop produce to fit through juicer, and then juice all ingredients.

Substitutions:
- Beet: *golden beet*
- Carrot: *sweet potato*
- Purple carrot: *carrot, sweet potato, golden beet*
- Strawberries: *berries*
- Blood orange: *orange, apple*
- Celery: *cucumber, lettuce, zucchini, watercress, spinach*

Sunburst Juice

- 1 orange
- 1 red bell pepper
- 4 carrots
- ½ lemon

Peel orange and lemon. Wash red pepper. Remove seeds and stem. Wash carrots. Juice all ingredients. Pour over ice.

Blueberry-Cabbage Power Juice

- ¼ medium red cabbage, sliced
- 1 large cucumber, peeled and cut into chunks
- 1 cup fresh blueberries
- 2 apples
- ice cubes (optional)

After thoroughly scrubbing all produce, put ingredients through a juicer.

Go Green

- 6 to 8 leaves kale
- 3 small apples
- 1 cucumber, peeled
- 2 to 3 stalks celery
- ½ lemon (no peel)
- 2 inches fresh ginger
- 1 cup water

After thoroughly scrubbing all produce, put ingredients through a juicer.

Green Magic

- 2 celery stalks
- 2 cucumbers
- 4 kale leaves

After thoroughly scrubbing all produce, put ingredients through a juicer.

Get Up & Go

- 4 small carrots
- 1 cucumber
- 1 apple
- 1 beet, thinly peeled
- ½-inch piece fresh ginger

After washing all produce, put ingredients through a juicer.

The Morning Drive

- 1 stalk broccoli
- 5 carrots

After thoroughly scrubbing all produce, put ingredients through a juicer.

Carrot, Cucumber, Apple, Beet & Ginger

- 1 cucumber, peeled
- 3 carrots, scrubbed well, tops removed, ends trimmed
- 1 beet, scrubbed well, with stem and 1 or 2 leaves
- 2 stalks celery
- 1 handful parsley
- 1- or 2-inch chunk ginger root, scrubbed, or peeled if old
- ½ lemon, peeled

After washing all produce, put ingredients through a juicer.

Morning Boost Juice

- 1 small-medium pink grapefruit, peeled
- 1 apple
- 3 carrots
- 1 teaspoon fresh ginger, peeled
- ½ lemon, peeled

After thoroughly scrubbing all produce, put ingredients through a juicer.

Vibrant Ginger Tonic

- 2 lemons, peeled
- 2-inch chunk ginger, peeled
- 4 large stalks celery (stems and leaves)
- pinch pink sea salt
- 1 small green apple or 2 teaspoons agave-maple syrup
- a dash of cayenne (optional)

Juice the lemon and ginger separately. Place juice aside. Juice the celery or celery-apple blend. Pour 1 to 2 parts ginger-lemon blend in each glass, and then add 5 parts green juice (customize the ratio however you'd like). Swirl in some maple-agave syrup for sweetness if you did not include an apple in your juice. Add a dash of optional cayenne on top.

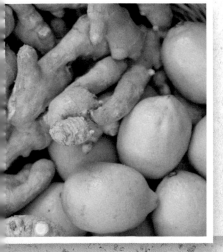

Lemons and ginger

NOON JUICES

Avoid the dreaded afternoon slump with a shot of high-nutrient juice.

Kale

KEEP IT GOING

Many of us get that tired feeling just about midday. You don't have to succumb to fatigue. These energizing juice recipes will help you keep functioning at top capacity.

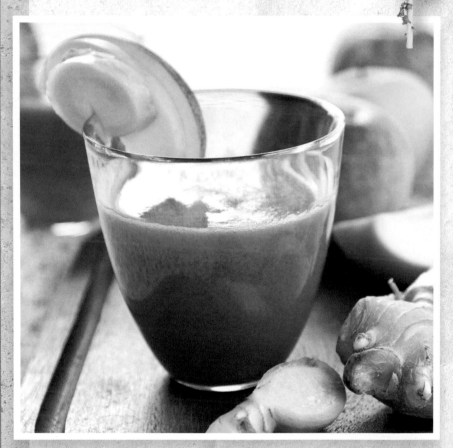

Bazingo

Bazingo

- 1 lemon
- 2 bunches parsley
- 2 apples
- 4-inch piece ginger
- 4 carrots

After washing all produce, put ingredients through a juicer.

THINK ABOUT IT!

Instead of reaching for that granola bar in your desk drawer or (even worse) heading for the vending machine for a snack, try adding ginger to a rich blend of fruits and veggies. It gives a healthy boost that won't mean an energy crash later.

Kale Energy Booster

- 1 cup kale
- 1 cucumber
- 1 apple
- ½ bunch parsley
- 3 carrots

After thoroughly scrubbing all produce, put ingredients through a juicer.

Number 9 Juice

- 2 celery stalks, leaves included
- 1 carrot, green top removed
- 1 leaf green cabbage
- 1 leaf chard (Swiss, rainbow, green, or red)
- 4 leaves kale
- 3 stems parsley
- ½ cucumber, peeled
- ½ lemon
- ½ apple

After washing all produce, put ingredients through a juicer.

High-Energy Boost Juice

- 6 carrots
- 4 celery stalks
- ½ bunch cilantro
- 2 tomatoes
- 1 lemon

After thoroughly scrubbing all produce, put ingredients through a juicer.

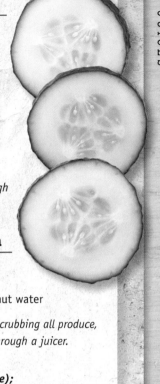

Coconut Splash

- ½ cantaloupe, peeled
- 8 ounces coconut water

After thoroughly scrubbing all produce, put ingredients through a juicer.

Cucumbers (above); cantaloupe (below)

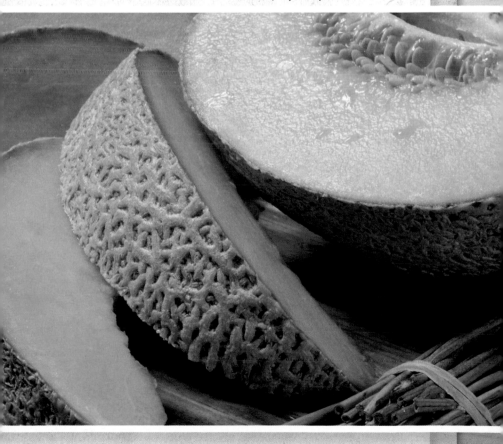

NIGHT JUICES

Juices certainly rev up your energy levels, but after a long day, you can enjoy a glass that can help you relax and recharge.

Celery

EVENING INDULGENCE

A glass of juice in the evening can help you end the day on a high note and help you get ready for tomorrow. Some fruits and veggies, like tart cherry juice that contains melatonin, can even help you fall asleep.

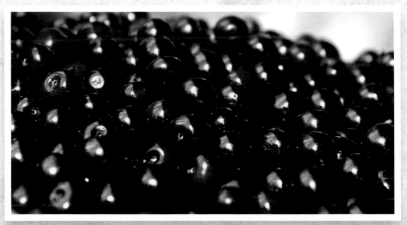

Tart morello cherries (above); Nighttime Energy Drink (opposite)

Cherry Chamomile Snoozer

- ½ cup tart cherries, pitted
- ½ cup boiling water
- 1 chamomile tea bag
- ½ teaspoon honey

Steep the chamomile tea bag in the boiling water for 20 minutes until cooled. Thoroughly wash the cherries, and put through a juicer. Add the cherry juice to the steeped tea, and sweeten with honey.

Sunset Blend

- 1 large sweet potato
- 2 small carrots
- 1 red bell pepper
- 2 large red beets
- 2 apples

After washing all produce, put ingredients through a juicer.

Rainbow Juice

- 5 celery stalks
- ½ medium cucumber
- 2 carrots
- 1 medium tomato
- ½ medium orange
- ½ medium peach

After thoroughly scrubbing all produce, put ingredients through a juicer.

THINK ABOUT IT!
Tart or sour cherries have the highest concentration of melatonin. Look for Early Richmond, Montmorency, and morello varieties.

Nighttime Energy Drink

- 5 carrots
- 2 celery stalks
- 1 cup parsley

After thoroughly scrubbing all produce, put ingredients through a juicer.

PREWORKOUT JUICES

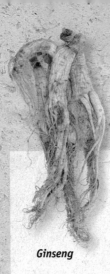

Ginseng

You need energy before a workout, and what better way to get the nutrients you need to power through than a glass of juice?

PREPARE YOURSELF

You'll want vegetables with complex carbohydrates that provide the best energy-producing fuel. Some veggies to put on your shopping list are carrots, a great source of antioxidant beta-carotene to protect against the depleting effects of exercise and increase oxygen in the blood, tissues, and brain; garlic to increase stamina; and ginseng, which is said to increase strength and boost energy.

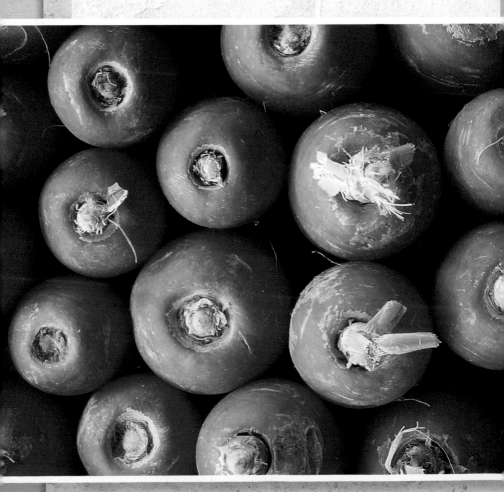

Natural Energy

- 1½ cups coconut water
- 2 cups spinach
- 1 cup kale
- 2 celery stalks
- 1 banana
- 1 to 2 tablespoons cinnamon

After thoroughly scrubbing all produce, blend all ingredients in a blender until smooth.

Battery Booster

- 4 carrots
- 1 clove garlic
- 1 teaspoon ginseng powder

After scrubbing the carrots, juice the carrots first and then the garlic; add the ginseng powder to the fresh carrot and garlic juice.

Carrots (below)

Golden Spicy Beet Juice

- 1 large or 2 small golden beets
- 3 small carrots
- 1 pear
- 1 large orange, peeled
- ½-inch piece ginger, peeled

After thoroughly scrubbing all produce, put ingredients through a juicer. Garnish with a dash of cayenne and a slice of raw beet.

Juicy Preworkout

- 3 apples
- 3 to 4 leaves kale
- 1 bunch romaine lettuce
- 1 bunch cilantro
- ¼ lemon
- a few leaves of mint
- 1 inch ginger (optional)

After thoroughly scrubbing all produce, put ingredients through a juicer.

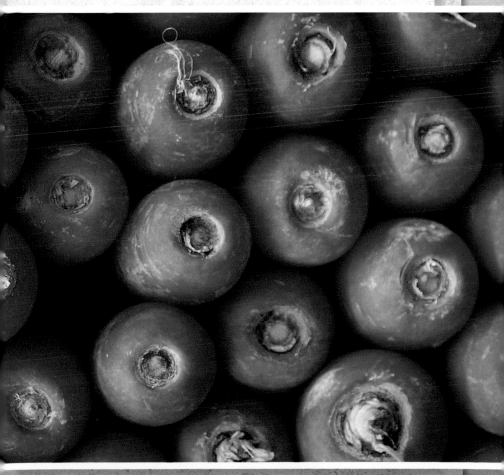

POSTWORKOUT JUICES

Limes

After a workout, it is essential to replace the nutrients and minerals, such as potassium, lost during high-energy activity.

RECOVER AND RECHARGE

Choose one of the following recipes that will help your body recover and recharge after a workout—without making you feel too full.

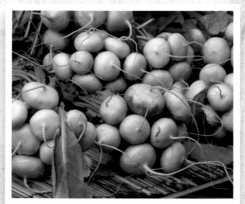

Turnips (left); Parsley Power (opposite)

Power Postworkout Juice

- ½ head romaine lettuce
- 4 leaves kale
- 4 carrots
- ½ bunch carrot tops
- 2 small apples
- 1 lime

After thoroughly scrubbing all produce, put ingredients through a juicer.

Parsley Power

- 1 large bunch parsley
- 2 carrots
- 1 apple
- 1 celery stalk

After thoroughly scrubbing all produce, put ingredients through a juicer.

Lemon, Pear, Celery & Cucumber Blend

- 1 pear
- 2 celery stalks
- 1 cup water
- juice of ½ lemon
- 1 cucumber
- ¼ teaspoon salt
- ¼ teaspoon pepper

After washing all produce, put ingredients through a juicer.

Turnips & Fennel Juice

- ½ turnip
- 3 carrots
- 1 apple
- ¼ fennel bulb

After thoroughly scrubbing all produce, put ingredients through a juicer.

Juicy Postworkout

- 2 green apples
- 1 celery stalk
- 1 small cucumber
- 2 tomatoes
- 1 orange

After thoroughly scrubbing all produce, put ingredients through a juicer.

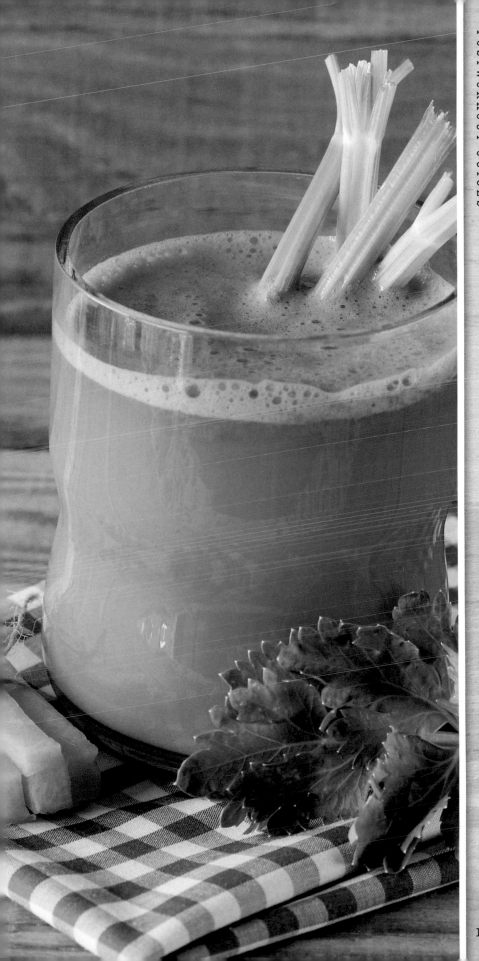

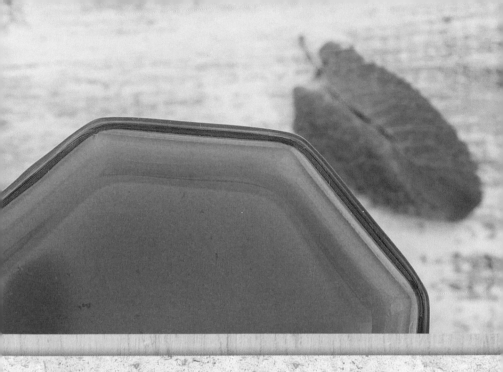

CHAPTER 4
CLEANSING JUICES

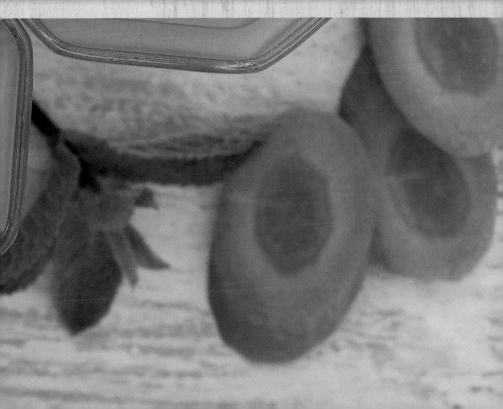

CLEANSING JUICES

Cleansing routines combine certain juices for different systems in the body with diet regimens over a specified length of time. Some target individual systems in the body, whether digestive or hepatic, while others—the master cleansers at the beginning of this chapter—wage an attack on all fronts. Many provide the first step for successful weight loss by cleansing your body before you embark on a new life of healthier foods.

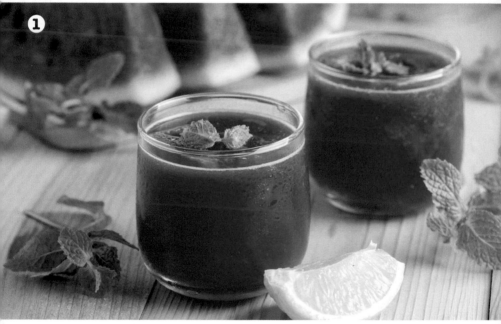

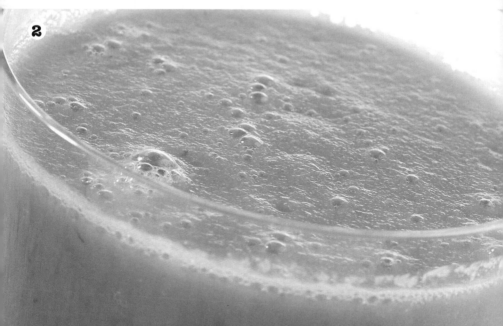

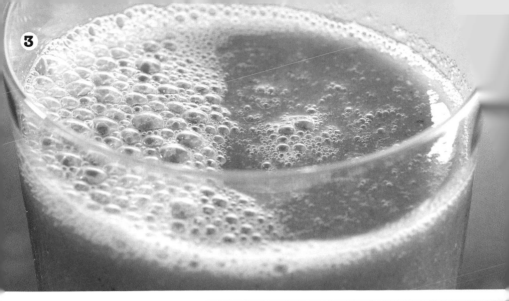

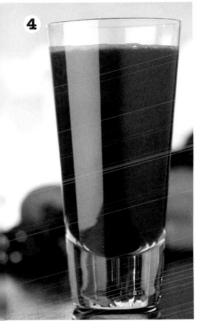

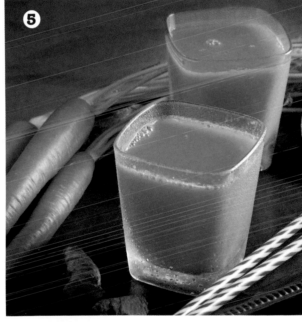

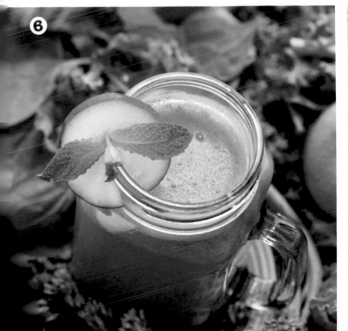

1 Watermelon-
   Lemon Detox
2 Carrot-Apple-
   Lemon Juice
3 Summer Melon
4 Fresh Nine
   Cleansing Juice
5 Orange Breather
6 Green Clean

MASTER CLEANSES

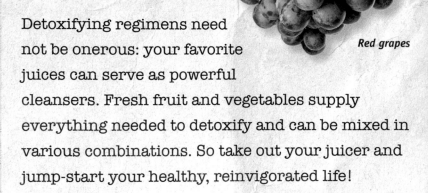

Red grapes

Detoxifying regimens need not be onerous: your favorite juices can serve as powerful cleansers. Fresh fruit and vegetables supply everything needed to detoxify and can be mixed in various combinations. So take out your juicer and jump-start your healthy, reinvigorated life!

CLEANSING AND FASTING

Certain cleansing routines involve consumption of only a single juice (over a week or more) and no solid food, and are known as juice fasts; these may work for people who want to clear their system and start losing weight quickly. Other fasting regimens use a variety of juices that target different systems over a shorter period of time, and these juices can either be part of a juice fast or used with other foods or juices in a juice-heavy diet.

A five-day alkaline cleanse incorporates a wide variety of juices, of which the following recipes are just a small sample:

ALKALINE CLEANSES

With this popular kind of cleanse, you consume only raw, fresh, alkaline juices, smoothies, and soups for 3 to 10 days. Its aim is for you to load up on foods that are rich in alkalizing nutrients and avoid eating acid-producing ones. Proponents claim that this helps your body to maintain its PH balance, which helps it to detoxify, cleanse, and rebuild itself.

Broccoli, Carrot & Parsley

- 2 handfuls broccoli
- 1 handful parsley
- 3 carrots
- 2 apples
- a little bit of flaxseed oil

After thoroughly scrubbing all produce, put ingredients through a juicer.

Green Clean

- 1 cucumber
- 2 apples
- 1 bunch kale
- a few large handfuls spinach
- 1 lemon, peeled

After thoroughly scrubbing all produce, put ingredients through a juicer.

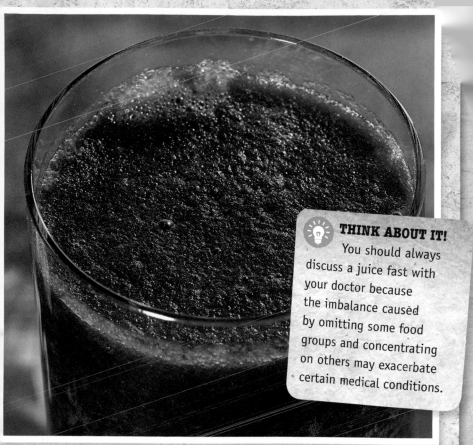

THINK ABOUT IT!
You should always discuss a juice fast with your doctor because the imbalance caused by omitting some food groups and concentrating on others may exacerbate certain medical conditions.

Scarlet Rhapsody

Scarlet Rhapsody

- 1 green apple
- ½ large cucumber
- ½ medium beet
- ½ inch ginger (optional)

Process all ingredients through a juicer. If you are using it as part of a juice fast, strain it and dilute with an equal quantity of filtered water. If not fasting, you can consume it without straining.

Red Dawn Cleanser

- 1 apple
- 3 leaves kale
- 1 beet
- 1 large bunch red grapes
- ¼ red cabbage
- ½ inch ginger

After thoroughly washing all produce, put ingredients through a juicer.

Lemonade Diet

- 2 tablespoons fresh-squeezed lemon or lime juice
- 2 tablespoons grade-B organic maple syrup
- a pinch of cayenne pepper
- 10 ounces filtered water

Mix the ingredients in a large glass. Drink six or more servings a day, a saltwater flush of 2 teaspoons of salt in a quart of water in the morning, and an herbal laxative tea at night for 10 days. This lemonade fast was created by Stanley Burroughs in 1941.

In Threes

- 3 cucumbers
- 3 cups spinach
- 3 cups parsley
- 3 celery stalks
- 1 lemon

After thoroughly washing all produce, put ingredients through a juicer.

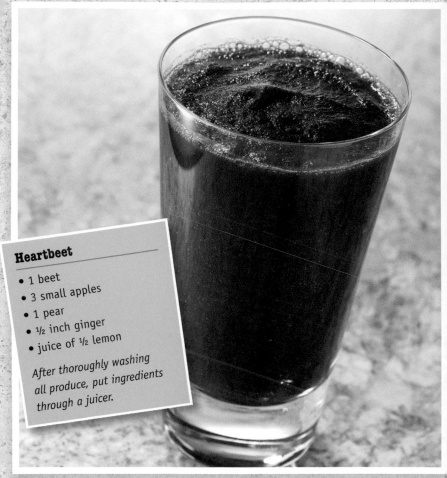

Heartbeet

- 1 beet
- 3 small apples
- 1 pear
- ½ inch ginger
- juice of ½ lemon

After thoroughly washing all produce, put ingredients through a juicer.

Heartbeet

Super-Green Cleanser

- 8 kale leaves
- 2 large handfuls parsley
- 1 large cucumber
- 3 celery stalks (plus leaves)
- 1 zucchini
- ½ lime

Wash all vegetables. Peel lime for a less bitter flavor. Put produce through your juicer and enjoy.

Cucumber Fennel

- 1 cucumber
- 1 piece fennel
- 1 lemon, peeled
- 1 stalk celery

After thoroughly washing all produce, put ingredients through a juicer.

Green Alfalfa

- 2 big handfuls spinach
- 3 stalks celery
- 1 head Little Gem lettuce
- 1 small green pepper
- ½ cucumber
- 1 handful alfalfa sprouts

After thoroughly washing all produce, put ingredients through a juicer.

Drink Your Veggies

- 2 pears
- 1 inch ginger
- 4 medium carrots
- 3 celery stalks
- 1 baby beet
- ½ cup parsley (stems and leaves)
- 2 teaspoons fresh lemon juice

After thoroughly washing all produce put ingredients through a juicer.

TARGET: BLOOD

Blood is life, and the right juices can help you cleanse it of health-depleting heavy metals, waste, and toxins.

Beetroot

THINK RED

Since the Middle Ages, beets have been used to treat illnesses related to blood. And they do act as nature's blood cleaners, increasing its oxygen-carrying capacity. Try the following beet-based recipes:

To the Beet of Your Heart

- 1 beet
- 2 leaves red cabbage
- 4 small carrots
- ½ lemon
- 1 orange
- ¼ pineapple
- 2 handfuls spinach

After thoroughly washing all produce, put ingredients through a juicer.

Just Beet It

- 2 medium apples
- 1 beet
- 6 small carrots
- 3 large stalks celery
- 1 small cucumber
- ½ inch ginger

After thoroughly washing all produce, put ingredients through a juicer.

Spicy Red Tang

- 1 beet
- 3 large carrots
- 2 large stalks celery
- 1 inch ginger, peeled
- ½ lime
- 1 jalapeño pepper
- 2 cups spinach

After thoroughly washing all produce, put ingredients through a juicer.

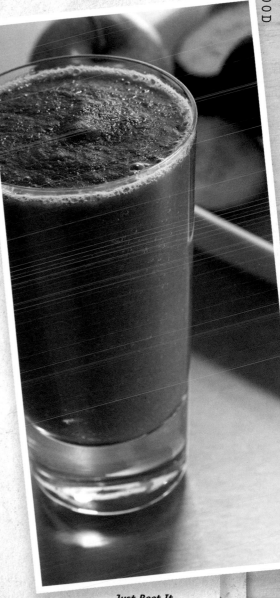

Just Beet It

TARGET: GI TRACT

Apples

The gastrointestinal tract, from mouth to colon, digests food and moves the unused wastes out of the body—but the highly processed foods so common in our diet today can take days to digest. The wastes that then build up in the colon need to be flushed out. Juicing is the natural way to speed digestion and flush wastes.

COLON

Keeping the colon cleansed is essential for good health. Juices offers several benefits, including supplying folic acid and, if you include the "bits" in your juice, can provide fiber, which is necessary for overall intestinal and colon health.

PRUNE-APPLE SPRING CLEAN

One of the simplest colon cleansers doesn't necessitate a juicer at all. Start the day with a large glass of unfiltered prune juice. Follow this with a large glass of water at room temperature. Then alternate between apple juice and water every half hour throughout the day.

Fresh Nine Cleansing Juice

- 3 beets
- 4 carrots
- 3 celery stalks
- 3 cucumbers
- 3 lemons, peeled
- 3 handfuls lettuce
- 3 handfuls parsley
- 3 handfuls kale
- 2 inches ginger

Wash all ingredients carefully and juice together. This recipe should produce enough juice to drink one 8-ounce glass every hour, for eight hours. Add extra cucumber if required.

Berry Cleanser

- 2 large apples
- ½ lime
- 4 cups strawberries

After thoroughly washing all produce, put ingredients through a juicer.

Carrot-Apple-Lemon Juice

- 3 medium carrots
- 2 apples
- ½ lemon

After thoroughly washing all produce, put ingredients through a juicer.

Berry Cleanser (opposite)

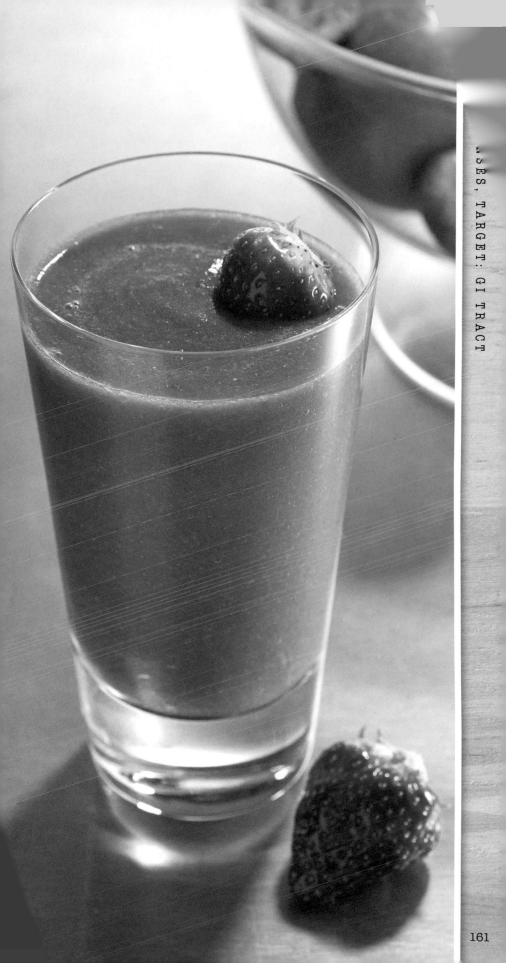

Colon Cleanser

- 3 handfuls spinach
- 4 green apples
- 2 handfuls parsley (optional)

Juice together apples and spinach and, if desired, parsley. Drink one cup not strained every four hours, for maximum benefit.

Celery Parsley Detox

- 1 medium apple
- ½ beet
- 3 medium carrots
- 2 stalks celery
- 1 handful parsley

After thoroughly washing all produce, put ingredients through a juicer.

STOMACH

This group of recipes will cleanse your stomach. Think carrots, apples, and ginger for this type of detox.

Tummy Detox

- 2 tablespoons fresh ginger, peeled and chopped
- 1 medium beet, scrubbed and coarsely chopped
- 4 medium carrots, scrubbed and sliced
- 1 medium apple, cored and cubed
- 1 cup water

In a blender, combine ginger, beet, carrots, apple, and water; blend, scraping down sides occasionally, until smooth. Strain juice and, if desired, thin with additional water.

Vegetable Detox Juice

- 4 carrots
- 4 kale leaves
- 3 celery stalks
- 2 beets
- 1 turnip
- ½ bunch spinach
- ½ cabbage
- ½ bunch parsley
- ½ onion
- 2 garlic cloves
- a dash of cayenne powder

Mix all ingredients with water and puree in a blender.

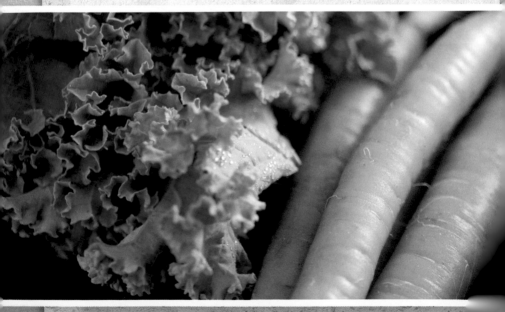

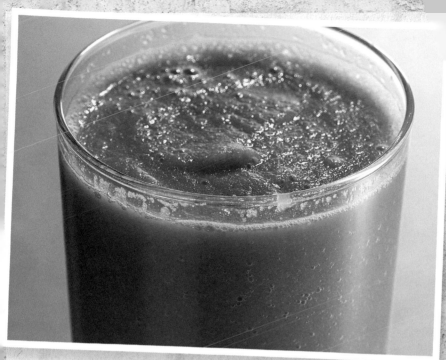

The Belly Cleanser

Twisty Fruit Punch

- 3 medium apples
- 4 kiwis
- ¼ lemon, with rind
- ¼ lime, with rind
- 2 oranges, peeled
- 1 pineapple, peeled and cored

Process all ingredients in a juicer, shake or stir, and serve.

Kale, carrots, and red and golden beets

The Belly Cleanser

- 5 carrots
- 2 apples
- 12 spinach leaves

After thoroughly washing all produce, put ingredients through a juicer.

THINK ABOUT IT!

Think of cleansers as an invigorating way of doing a spring-cleaning of your body—not unlike that much-needed spring-cleaning of your home, armed with vacuum, dust cloths, and trash bags! Spring-cleaning your home may be a matter of choice. Spring-cleaning and detoxifying your body is not.

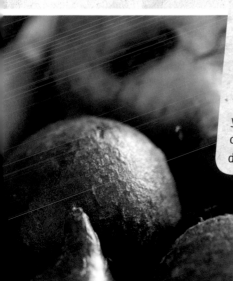

TARGET: LIVER

Over time and as the result of many bad habits, your system gets clogged, affecting the many processes that clean your body.

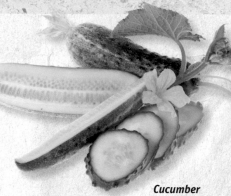

Cucumber

The ability of the liver—the metabolism powerhouse that processes, stores, and manufactures most of the chemicals passing through your body—to detoxify your system and produce bile to break up fats, is reduced.

THE USUAL SUSPECTS

When it comes to taking care of the liver, look for the usual veggie suspects: leafy greens, beets, and carrots. Also add to your shopping list some lemons, cucumbers, grapefruits, and ginger root, which are all excellent liver cleansers.

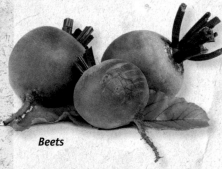

Beets

Apple, Beet & Carrot Blend

- 1 beet, rinsed, lightly peeled, and quartered
- 1 apple, lighted peeled, cored, and quartered
- 1 inch ginger, peeled
- 4 carrots, rinsed and peeled
- ¼ cup unfiltered apple juice (optional)

After thoroughly washing all produce, put ingredients through a juicer.

Liver Cleanser

- 1 large apple
- 1 beet
- 4 carrots
- 1 celery stalk
- ½ inch ginger

After thoroughly washing all produce, put ingredients through a juicer.

The Super Salad

- 1 cucumber
- 1 lemon
- 1 medium green onion/scallion
- 1 handful parsley
- ½ medium sweet red pepper
- 3 small tomatoes

After thoroughly washing all produce, put ingredients through a juicer.

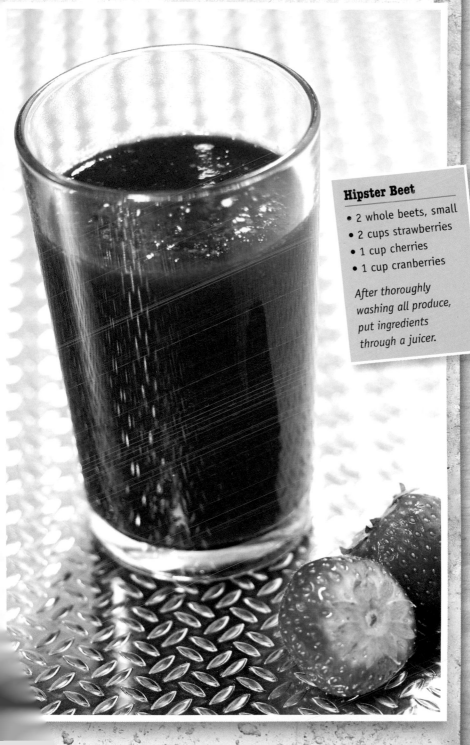

Celery Cooler

- 2 large celery stalks
- 1 handful cilantro
- 1 small cucumber
- 1 medium tomato

Juice tomato, celery, cucumber, and cilantro in that order.

Pizza Party

- ½ head medium cauliflower
- 1 small cucumber
- 2 cups cherry tomatoes
- a dash of dried basil

After thoroughly washing all produce, put ingredients through a juicer.

Hipster Beet

- 2 whole beets, small
- 2 cups strawberries
- 1 cup cherries
- 1 cup cranberries

After thoroughly washing all produce, put ingredients through a juicer.

TARGET: KIDNEYS

Why perform a kidney cleanse? There are many good reasons, one of which is that it flushes toxins and wastes from your body. *Strawberries* This results in reduced bloating and a lower chance of developing kidney infections.

SWEET DETOX

If you decide to try a kidney-detoxing program, you will find that there are plenty of sweet, flavorful fruits to blend together, such as watermelons, pineapples, and strawberries.

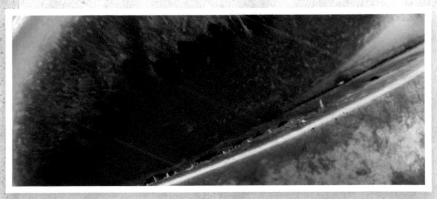

Watermelon

Yosemite Falls Cleanser

- 1 wedge watermelon
- ½ pound red grapes

After thoroughly washing all produce, put ingredients through a juicer.

Spring Clean

- ½ lemon
- 3 tomatoes
- 1 large wedge watermelon
- 1 handful parsley

After thoroughly washing all produce, put ingredients through a juicer.

Watermelon-Lemon Detox

- ½ watermelon, rind included
- 1 lemon, peeled

After thoroughly washing all produce, put ingredients through a juicer.

Summer Melon

- 1 medium tomato
- 1 large wedge watermelon

After thoroughly washing all produce, put ingredients through a juicer.

Pineberry Cleanser (opposite

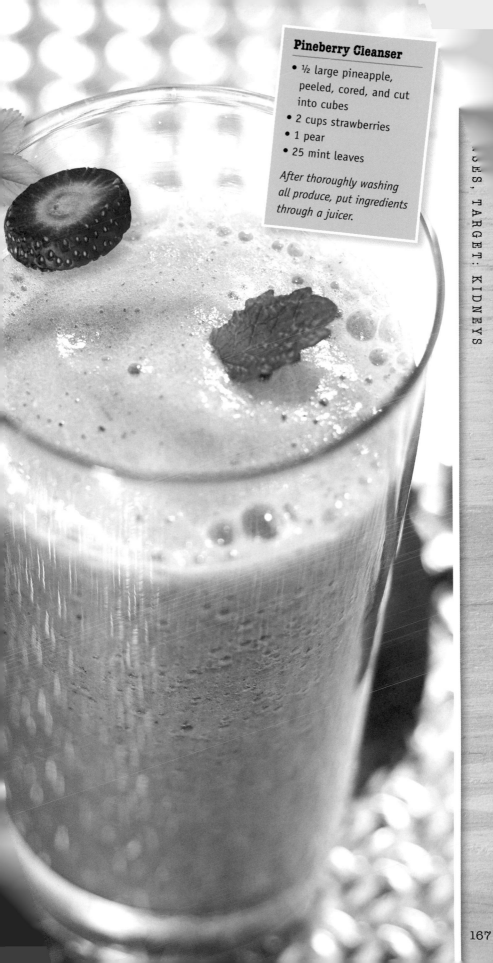

Pineberry Cleanser

- ½ large pineapple, peeled, cored, and cut into cubes
- 2 cups strawberries
- 1 pear
- 25 mint leaves

After thoroughly washing all produce, put ingredients through a juicer.

TARGET: LUNGS

In order to function at your peak levels, you need oxygen, so add a few juices that target your lungs and respiratory system.

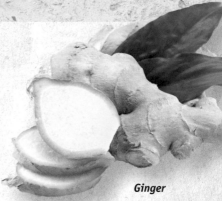

Ginger

TAKE A DEEP BREATH

One of the keys to better breathing is keeping your airways clear and unrestricted. Look for vegetables and fruits that are carotenoid-rich, such as carrots. Carotenoids act to heal and protect lung cells and help maintain the mucous membranes in lung tissue. And don't overlook the anti-inflammatory properties ginger or the vitamin C-packed citrus fruits that can also reduce mucus.

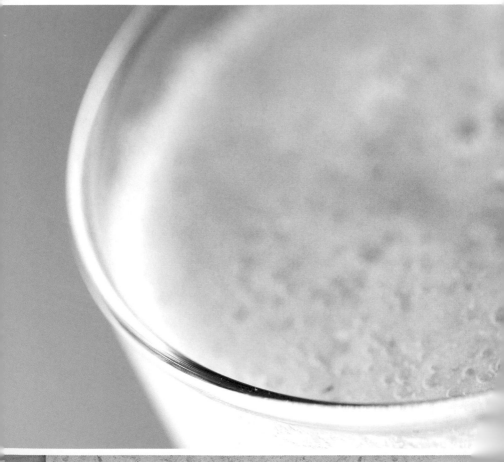

Lung Power Cleansing Juice

Summer Cooler

- 2 medium apples
- 5 Swiss chard leaves
- 6 celery stalks
- 1 bunch parsley
- 1 lemon, peeled
- ½ inch ginger
- 1 inch fresh turmeric
- at least 2 watermelon rinds

After thoroughly washing all produce, put ingredients through a juicer.

Orange Breather

- 3 carrots
- ½ inch fresh ginger
- ½ inch fresh turmeric
- ½ grapefruit, peeled

After thoroughly washing all produce, put ingredients through a juicer.

Lung Power Cleansing Juice

- 1 head celery
- 2 to 4 Fuji apples
- 1 lemon
- ½ inch ginger
- 1 bunch wild watercress

After thoroughly washing all produce, put ingredients through a juicer.

Radiant Radish Cleanser

- 1 large radish
- 2 apples
- 1 pear
- ½ jicama
- 1 lime, peeled
- 1 handful cilantro
- a pinch sea salt (optional)

After thoroughly washing all produce, put ingredients through a juicer.

THE DETOX DEBATE

Debate rages over whether detox fasts or diets actually provide any genuine health benefits. On one hand, healthy bodies should be capable of flushing toxins from the system very efficiently, without fasting, which itself can result in malnourishment and potentially dangerous health risks; further, fasting may lead to increased weight over time as the body switches into famine mode and slows the metabolic rate accordingly. On the other hand, hard fasting has long been practiced in certain cultures for a variety of reasons, including medical and religious, and it seems many people do actually feel better and less sluggish after a short fast. Whether that is the power of suggestion at work, or whether they have indeed successfully detoxed, or whether they are simply carrying less semidigested food around and hence feel lighter—or maybe a combination of all three—remains unknown. Fasting for weight loss or detoxification purposes is not suitable for children, adolescents, pregnant or breastfeeding women, or the elderly, and should not be undertaken by anyone—especially those with preexisting medical conditions—without first consulting with their doctor or nutritional adviser.

TARGET: SKIN

A malfunctioning system reveals itself in the health and vitality of your skin. A range of juices can help rejuvenate and revitalize it, giving you a refreshed, healthy glow.

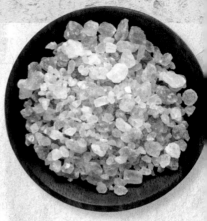

Himalayan sea salt

SALT AND PEPPER

To target the health of your skin, look for fresh red peppers or healthy, bright-green veggies, like spinach and romaine, and add a pinch of salt. Fruits like apples and pineapples round off your grocery list.

Red Pepper Skin Cleanser

- 2 red peppers
- 2 carrots
- 1 apple
- 1 broccoli spear

After thoroughly washing all produce, put ingredients through a juicer.

Perfect Skin Juice

- ½ bunch spinach
- ½ bunch celery
- ½ large cucumber
- 1 head romaine lettuce
- ⅓ bunch fresh parsley
- a pinch of Himalayan sea salt

After thoroughly washing all produce, put ingredients through a juicer.

Cucumber, Celery, Mint, Apple & Pineapple Refresher

- 1 cucumber
- 2 celery stalks
- 2 green apples
- 2 pineapple slices
- 1 cup mint leaves

After thoroughly washing all produce, put ingredients through a juicer.

Red Pepper Skin Cleanser (left); Cucumber, Celery, Mint, Apple & Pineapple Refresher (opposite)

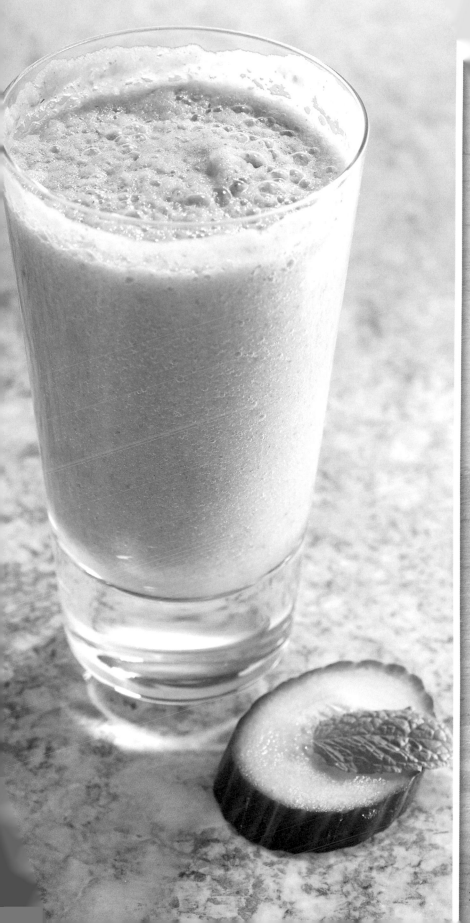

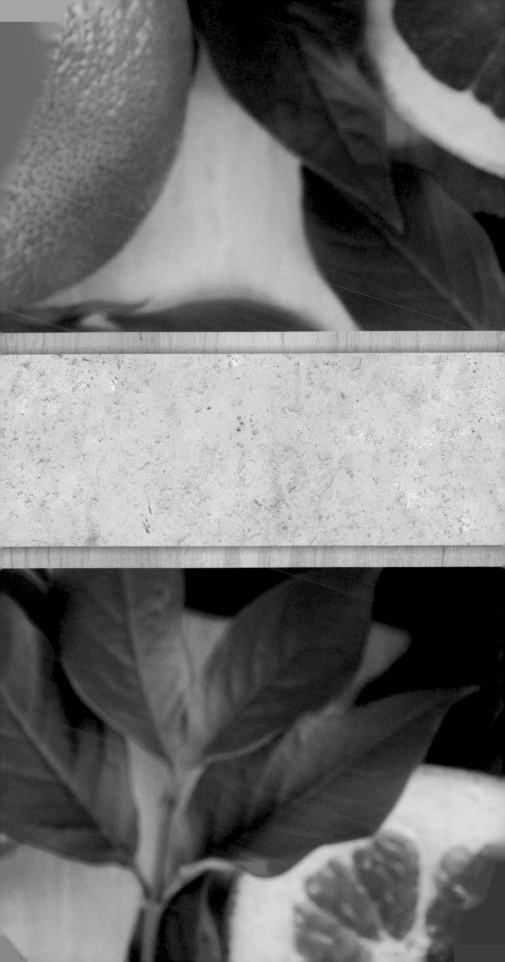

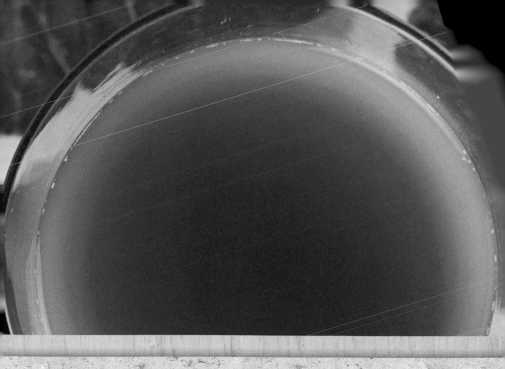

CHAPTER 5

JUICE REMEDIES

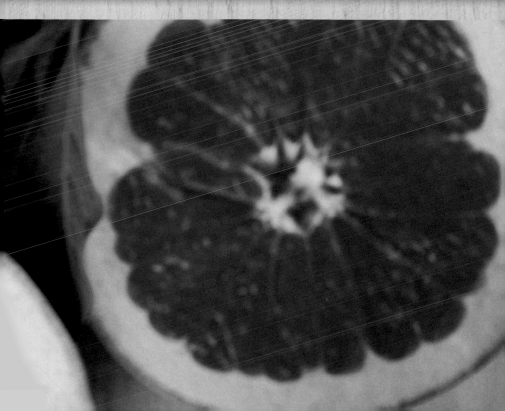

JUICE REMEDIES

Juices are used as cleansers to purge and purify the system or as healthful alternatives to a junk-laden diet, but they also provide commonsense health benefits and relief from the symptoms of common ailments through their active ingredients—from carrots, beets, and parsley to apples and citrus fruits. Whether your problem is allergies or arthritis, insomnia or migraines, consider these recipes for a delicious and healthful solution.

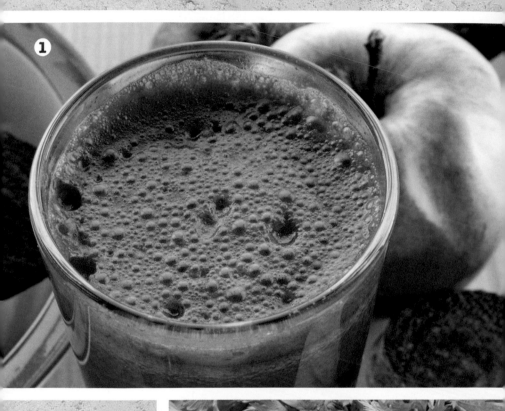

1

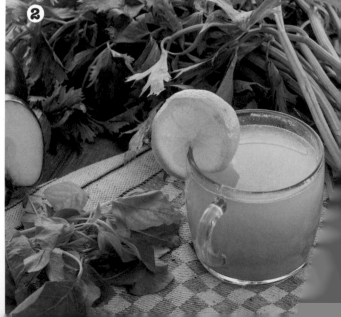

2

1 **Beet It**
2 **The Iron Lady**
3 **Carrot, Celery, Garlic & Parsley Juice**
4 **Blueberry, Watermelon & Cranberry Cleanser**
5 **Minty Berry Juice**
6 **Minus-Sinus Reliever**

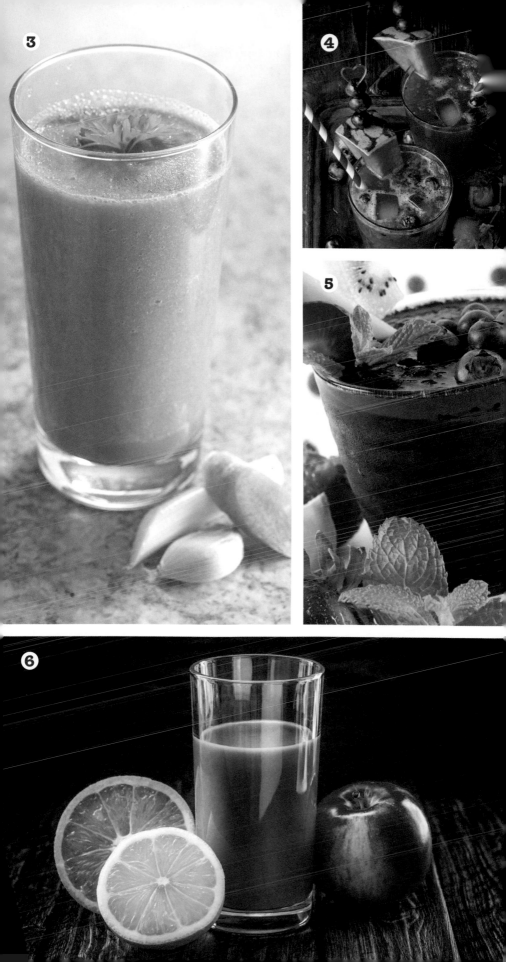

A JUICE FOR WHAT AILS YOU

The curative powers of a wide range of vegetable and fruit products have been recognized for centuries.

A HISTORY OF SUCCESS

From the use of pomegranate juice in ancient Greece as an aphrodisiac, to the combination of pomegranates and figs as an elixir to promote physical strength and prowess (recorded in the Dead Sea Scrolls), the juices of many fruits and vegetables have a history of medicinal use. Spaniards planted the first Florida orange trees in the 1500s, but it wasn't until the early twentieth century that pasteurization, coupled with the transcontinental railroad, provided orange juice across the country as a popular breakfast beverage that supplies a healthy dose of vitamin C.

Juicing as a nutritional and alternative treatment took off after home juicers were invented in the 1950s, making it possible to create instant juice combinations with a wide range of healthful effects in your own kitchen. In more recent years, a wide range of juice bars will create anything on request, and even the corner café has a juicer and can offer a freshly made glass of carrot juice. In addition, there are many commercially prepared juices on the market, so even if you don't have your own kitchen equipment, you can obtain one of these juices to help ease your symptoms.

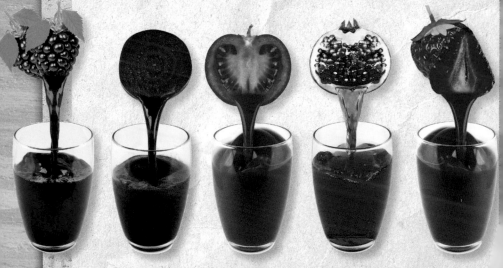

From left to right: blackberry, beet, tomato, pomegranate, and strawberry juices

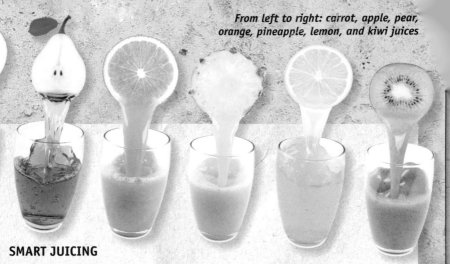

SMART JUICING

If you are under medical supervision for an existing condition, juices should be used only as complementary therapies to your regular treatment until you have established whether they work for you. You should never attempt to replace medical treatment with juicing until you have discussed it with your physician. Certain ingredients—for example, grapefruit juice—have a well-established capacity for interfering with the metabolism of prescribed treatments, bringing them to a toxic level. Fruit juices, higher in natural sugar than whole fruits and without the fiber, can cause a spike in blood sugar level, so vegetable juices can be safer for people with diabetes.

Other ingredients are natural panaceas for a host of different symptoms and conditions. For example, it has been found that the daily consumption of apples and apple juice protects against asthma and increases bone density, while lemon juice helps control high blood pressure and respiratory disorders. Explore the following pages to find recipes to target a wide range of conditions, including ones that will stop a migraine in its tracks and ones that help relieve acid reflux.

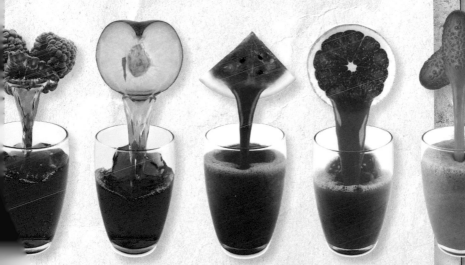

From left to right: raspberry, plum, watermelon, grapefruit, and spinach juices

TARGET: AGING

Aging is a natural process of life, but how you age isn't a given. Along with healthy practices like exercise, the right foods—such as nutrient-rich juices—can help you keep your mind sharp and your body in shape.

Blackcurrants

FOREVER YOUNG

To counter the effects of premature aging, you need to eat a balanced diet with high-quality nourishment, including the antioxidant vitamins A, C, and E. Choose juices that combine plenty of green, orange, and yellow vegetables. For instance, carrots contain luteolin, a flavonoid that can reduce the inflammation that leads to cognitive decline. Dark berries, such as blackcurrants, can also help stave off the signs of premature aging, as can citrus fruits, which are rich in vitamin C.

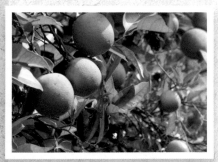

Oranges ripening on tree

Carrot-Parsley Juice

- 3 carrots
- 4 broccoli florets
- 1 handful parsley

After washing all produce, roughly chop the carrots and break the broccoli into chunks. Reserve a sprig of parsley for decoration. Juice the carrots and broccoli separately, and combine the juices in a glass. Garnish with a sprig of parsley.

Avocado-Tomato Juice

- ½ avocado
- 4 medium tomatoes
- 2 sprigs cilantro

Remove the stone from the avocado, and scoop out the flesh. Combine the ingredients in a blender (avocados do not juice well). Garnish with cilantro.

Strawberry-Blackcurrant Tonic

- 5 ounces blackcurrants
- 5 ounces strawberries

Rinse the blackcurrants and remove the stems. Rinse and hull the strawberries. Juice each ingredient and combine the juices in a glass.

Apple-Grape Juice

- 5 ounces grapes
- 5 ounces blackcurrants
- 1 apple

After washing all produce, put ingredients through a juicer.

Blackcurrant Orange Juice (opposite

Blackcurrant Orange Juice

- 2 oranges
- 5 ounces blackcurrants

Peel the oranges and divide them into segments to fit in the feed tube. Rinse the blackcurrants and remove the stems. Juice each ingredient separately, and combine the juices in a tall glass.

TARGET: ALLERGIES

Sneezing, sniffling, runny eyes, and runny nose . . . for too many of us, spring and fall herald not the joys of the outdoors, but the discomfort of seasonal allergies.

BLOCKING HISTAMINE

To suppress allergy symptoms, you want to block histamines. Go for fruits and veggies rich in vitamin C, one of the best histamine blockers. Raw honey, which contains propolis, will also bolster your immune system. Also add ginger to your shopping list for its anti-inflammatory properties; parsley, a natural diuretic that blocks histamine; and green apples, which contain quercetin, a flavonoid that reduces allergic inflammation.

THINK ABOUT IT!

Sneezing and other allergy symptoms are the body's natural response to what it perceives as a threat to your immune system. It is histamines that start the process to rid your body of irritating allergens.

Parsley Lemonade

- 2 cups flat-leaf parsley
- 1 small cucumber
- 2 lemons, peeled
- 1 green apple
- 1 teaspoon honey
- 1 inch ginger (optional)

After thoroughly washing all produce, put ingredients through a juicer.

Dandelion Leaf Relief

- 2 cups fresh dandelion greens or 6 leaves (not the flowers)
- 5 celery stalks
- 1 cup spinach
- 2 cucumbers
- 2 apples
- 1 lime or lemon
- ½ inch ginger (optional)

After thoroughly scrubbing all produce, put ingredients through a juicer.

Minus-Sinus Reliever

- 1 large orange, peeled
- ½ lemon, de-seeded and peeled
- 1 apple
- 1 inch ginger, peeled
- a dash of ground cayenne

After thoroughly scrubbing all produce, put ingredients through a juicer.

Vitajuice

- 3 large red beets
- 4 small carrots
- 2 celery stalks
- 4 plum tomatoes
- 4 cups parsley, roughly chopped
- 1 jalapeño, ribs and seeds removed
- 8 red radishes

After thoroughly washing all produce, put ingredients through a juicer.

Vitajuice (opposite)

Ginger Shooter

- 1 large pear
- 1 inch ginger, peeled
- 1 tangerine
- 1 tablespoon lemon juice

After thoroughly scrubbing all produce, put ingredients through a juicer.

Japple Ginger Juice

- 5 Jazz apples
- ½ to 1 lemon, peeled
- 1 inch ginger, peeled
- a dash of cayenne (optional)

After thoroughly scrubbing all produce, put ingredients through a juicer.

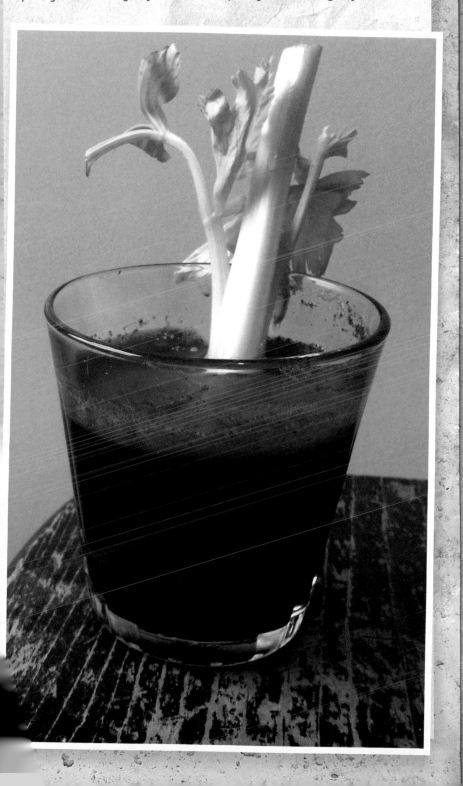

TARGET: ASTHMA

The symptoms of asthma—attacks of wheezing, coughing, and shortness of breath—range from mildly debilitating to outright life-threatening.

JUICING FOR BREATH

During an asthma attack, mucus and other secretions begin to clog the lungs' small airways. This kind of blockage, if not cleared, can lead to suffocation. One way to avoid these frightening attacks is to maintain a healthy diet that will keep them from even happening. Fruits and vegetables high in vitamin C and antioxidants can help you stave off attacks, and fortunately the list of anti-asthma juices is quite long and varied. Stock up on veggies like beets, carrots, celery, cucumbers, fennel, kale, pumpkin, radish, spinach, tomato, watercress, and wheatgrass. Mix up blends with fruits like blueberry, pineapple, pomegranate, strawberry, and watermelon, and flavor them with herbs and spices like cayenne, cilantro, ginger root, or lemongrass.

Blueberry Breeze

Blueberry Breeze

- 3 leaves basil (fresh)
- 1½ cups blueberries
- 2 pinches of ground cayenne
- ½ lime
- 5 cups watermelon, diced

After thoroughly scrubbing all produce, put ingredients through a juicer.

Melon Tea

- 1 large wedge watermelon
- ½ cup green tea, chilled
- ½ lemon

After thoroughly scrubbing all produce, put ingredients through a juicer.

Hang On Juice

- 1 beet
- 3 large celery stalks
- 3 cups spinach
- 1 teaspoon spirulina (dried)

After washing all produce, put ingredients through a juicer.

Jazzy Ginger Zinger

- 2 green apples
- 3 small carrots
- ½ inch ginger
- ½ lemon (with rind)

After washing all produce, put ingredients through a juicer.

TARGET: ANEMIA

Anemia leaves the sufferer mentally and physically tired, but this condition can be avoided with a diet rich in iron and vitamins B and C.

BOOST YOUR BLOOD

Anemia occurs when blood lacks sufficient hemoglobin, the red blood cells that transport oxygen from the lungs to the rest of the body. This causes the heart to pump extra hard to deliver the oxygen to where it is needed, leaving you exhausted and possibly dizzy and short of breath. Juicing with iron-rich and vitamin-packed veggies can help prevent anemia, keeping your blood healthy and flowing.

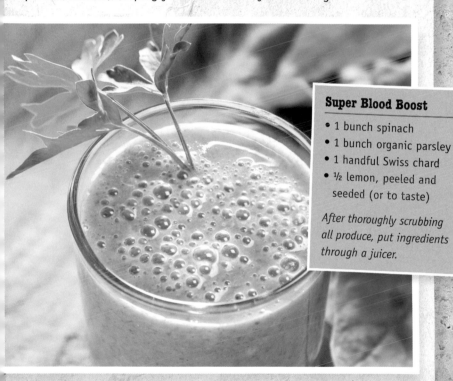

Super Blood Boost

- 1 bunch spinach
- 1 bunch organic parsley
- 1 handful Swiss chard
- ½ lemon, peeled and seeded (or to taste)

After thoroughly scrubbing all produce, put ingredients through a juicer.

Super Blood Boost

Minty Berry Juice

- 2 cups blueberries
- 2 kiwis, peeled
- 20 strawberries
- 2 cups mint leaves

After thoroughly washing all produce, put ingredients through a juicer.

The Iron Lady

- 1 bunch spinach
- 1 bunch parsley
- 1 handful Swiss chard
- 1 apple, cored
- ½ inch ginger

After thoroughly scrubbing all produce, put ingredients through a juicer.

TARGET: ARTHRITIS

Pineapple

For many people, especially as they age, the daily aches and pains of arthritis keep them from living life to the fullest. Fortunately, there are plenty of juice recipes to help alleviate these symptoms.

ANTIOXIDANT BOOSTERS

Antioxidants can help neutralize free radicals that lead to painful inflammation. Look for fruits and veggies packed with vitamin C, like citrus, pineapple, and carrots.

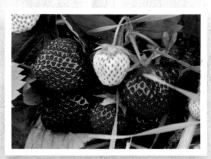

Ripening strawberries (above); Tango in the Tropics (opposite)

> **THINK ABOUT IT!**
> The free radical theory of aging posits that free radicals, which are unstable atoms, damage or break down cells over time. This damage might be related to many age-related diseases, such as arthritis and Alzheimer's, as well as vision decline.

Goldfinger

- 1 golden beet
- 1 pear
- 3 large carrots
- 4 large celery stalks
- 1 small cucumber
- ½ inch ginger

After thoroughly scrubbing all produce, put ingredients through a juicer.

Dragon Fire

- 4 leaves red cabbage
- ½ lemon with rind
- 3 small pears

After thoroughly scrubbing all produce, put ingredients through a juicer.

Good & Green Juice

- 2 large green apples
- 8 large stalks celery
- 1 lemon with peel
- 1 small tangerine, peeled

After thoroughly scrubbing all produce, put ingredients through a juicer.

Pear, Strawberry, Pineapple & Mint Juice

- 1 pear
- 15 leaves peppermint
- ½ pineapple
- 15 strawberries

After thoroughly scrubbing all produce, put ingredients through a juicer.

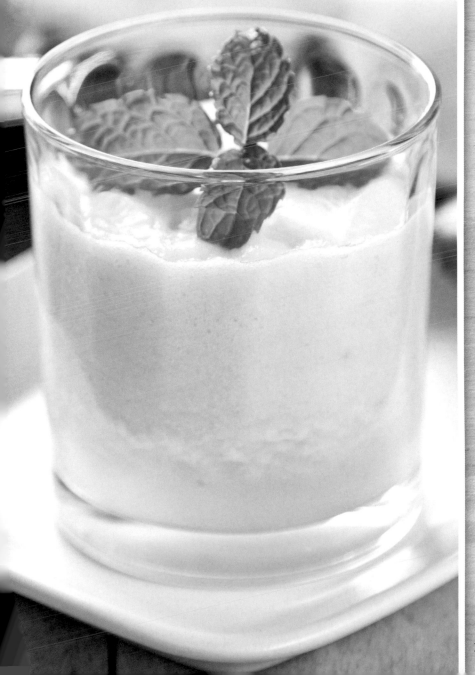

Tango in the Tropics

- 2 peaches, pits removed
- 2 pears
- ½ pineapple

After thoroughly scrubbing all produce, put ingredients through a juicer. Garnish with mint leaves.

TARGET: DIGESTIVE SYSTEM

A poor diet can put a lot of stress on your digestive system, leading to diarrhea, constipation, gas, heartburn, and nausea.

Sweet potato

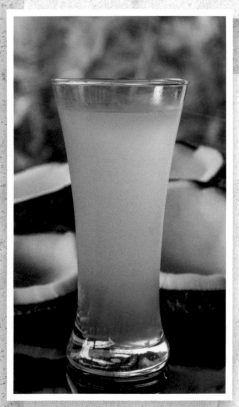

Coconut water

DIARRHEA

We all know diarrhea is unpleasant, keeping you from getting through a day or night. The inflammation of the bowel that triggers it can be caused by infection and food allergies, among other things. Diarrhea is a signal that your digestive system is malfunctioning or trying to remove something from your body. It can leave you depleted, so try creating juices that resupply lost nutrients.

Carrot, Cranberry & Blueberry Juice

- 2 carrots
- 1 cup cranberries
- 1 cup blueberries

After washing all produce, put ingredients through a juicer.

Stop the Runs

- 4 stalks celery
- 2 large carrots
- 1 large apple

After thoroughly scrubbing all produce, put ingredients through a juicer.

Spinach Carrot Juice

- 1½ cup filtered water or coconut water
- ½ cup pineapple
- 1 cup spinach
- 4 carrots
- 1 cup ice

Place all ingredients into the blender in the order listed, secure lid, and blend until smooth.

CONSTIPATION

Constipation, a medical condition that causes slow bowel movement and the inability to pass stool, leaves you feeling bloated and gassy, too uncomfortable to eat anything that will make you feel even more blocked. Juices are an efficient way to get the relief you need. Try blends with carrots, prunes, plums, apples, and pears.

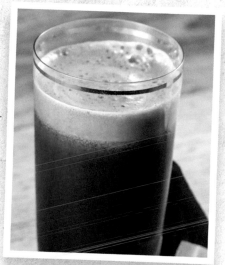

Carrot Cleanser

Peach, Plum & Apricot Juice

- 4 plums
- 3 peaches
- 2 apricots

Remove pits, and juice. Softer, ripe plums, peaches, and apricots produce more of a puree than juice.

Carrot Cleanser

- 1 medium apple
- 4 medium carrots
- 2 celery stalks
- 1 small cucumber
- ½ inch ginger

After thoroughly scrubbing all produce, put ingredients through a juicer.

Fruit Punch

- 4 apples
- 4 kiwis
- ½ lime
- 2 oranges, peeled
- 1 pineapple

After thoroughly scrubbing all produce, put ingredients through a juicer.

The Lemon Mover

- 2 apples
- 8 medium carrots
- 1 inch ginger
- 1 lemon

After thoroughly scrubbing all produce, put ingredients through a juicer.

Sweet Soother

- 2 apples
- 2 beets
- 2 carrots
- 1 red pepper
- 1 sweet potato
- 1 small celery stalk
- ½ cucumber
- ½ inch ginger

After washing all produce, put ingredients through a juicer.

Spiced Prune Juice

- 5 to 6 prunes
- ½ teaspoon honey
- ½ teaspoon cumin
- 1 cup warm water

Soak the prunes in a cup of warm water for 5 minutes, then remove the pith and toss the prunes into a blender along with the water. Add honey and cumin powder, and blend until thoroughly combined.

BLOATING AND GAS

Excess gas in your intestines can cause that uncomfortable bloating feeling coupled with unsightly belly bulging that makes you look like you've gained a bit of weight. Your juicing goal is to alleviate this issue by removing the toxic waste and promoting the growth of healthy intestinal flora. A few proven bloat and gas banishers are lemon, cucumber, and celery.

Pear

Wheatgrass & Ginger Juice

- 1 bunch wheatgrass (about a handful)
- 1 lemon
- 4 apples
- 2 carrots
- 2 inches ginger

After thoroughly scrubbing all produce, put ingredients through a juicer.

Gut Ease

- 2 pears
- 2 carrots
- ½ pineapple
- ½ inch ginger

After thoroughly scrubbing all produce, put ingredients through a juicer.

The Green Doctor

- 2 cups spinach
- ¼ cucumber
- ¼ head celery
- 1 bunch parsley
- 1 bunch mint
- 4 carrots
- 2 apples
- ¼ orange
- ¼ lime
- ¼ lemon
- ¼ pineapple

After thoroughly scrubbing all produce, put ingredients through a juicer.

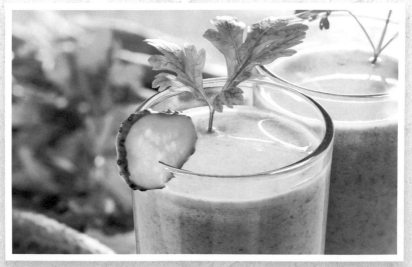

The Green Doctor

HEATBURN

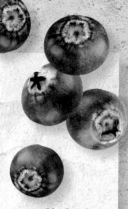

Despite its name, heartburn isn't about your heart. Instead, it's that burning feeling you get in your chest that is the result of acidic fumes or gases from half-digested food flowing upward and back into the esophagus. Prevention is the best cure for heartburn, but there are many juice combos that can help relieve it and, better yet, prevent it.

Blueberries

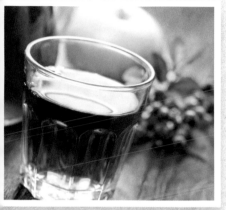

Blue Apple Burn Relief

> **THINK ABOUT IT!**
> Citrus juices tend to be acidic, so avoid them if you suffer from acid reflux.

Tropical Delight

- 1 papaya
- 1 guava
- 2 mangoes

After thoroughly scrubbing all produce, put ingredients through a juicer.

Blue Apple Burn Relief

- 2 cups blueberries
- 1 apple

After thoroughly scrubbing all produce, put ingredients through a juicer.

Green Extinguisher

- 2 green apples
- ½ inch ginger
- 1½ large English cucumbers
- 2 to 3 broccoli stems
- 1 handful leftover kale stems

After thoroughly scrubbing all produce, put ingredients through a juicer.

Alkaline Firefighter

- ½ cucumber
- 1 cup spinach
- 1 cup kale
- 1 cup parsley
- ½ apple

After thoroughly scrubbing all produce, put ingredients through a juicer.

Magic Alkaline Greens

- 1 cup of broccoli heads
- 2 stalks celery (including leaves)
- 4 large carrots
- 1 inch ginger (optional)

After thoroughly scrubbing all produce, put ingredients through a juicer.

Alkaline Paradise

- 1 cup spinach
- ½ cucumber
- 2 celery stalks (including leaves)
- 4 carrots
- ½ apple

After thoroughly scrubbing all produce, put ingredients through a juicer.

NAUSEA

Whatever the cause—morning sickness, a stomach bug, adverse food interaction, or something else—nausea can be a nightmare. But you can fight that queasy feeling with an array of juices, including ones that contain cucumbers, lemons, limes, beets, or green apples. Don't forget to add some ginger, too; it will help settle your stomach.

Cucumbers

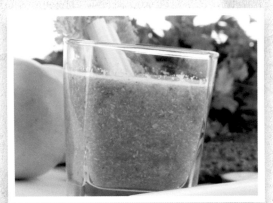

Ginger Ninja (left); Better Digestion (opposite)

Ginger Ninja

- 3 green apples
- 2 celery sticks
- 1 large cucumber or 2 smaller cucumbers
- 1 lime
- 2 inches ginger

After thoroughly scrubbing all produce, put ingredients through a juicer.

Substitutions:
- Green apple: *other varieties of apple, pear*
- Celery: *zucchini, lettuce, fennel*
- Cucumber: *celery, zucchini, lettuce*
- Lime: *grapefruit, lemon*
- Ginger: *mint*

Better Digestion

- 1 cucumber
- ½ lemon
- 1 spring onion
- 1 handful parsley
- 1 small red pepper
- 3 small whole tomatoes

After thoroughly scrubbing all produce, put ingredients through a juicer.

Spicy Beet Juice

- ½ to 1 small beet
- 1 small carrot
- ¼ yellow bell pepper
- 2 lemon wedges, with rind
- 2 large romaine lettuce leaves
- jalapeño pepper and cilantro, according to taste

After thoroughly scrubbing all produce, put ingredients through a juicer.

Digestion Aid

- 1 cucumber
- 1 medium fennel bulb
- 1 handful fresh mint leaves
- 1 inch ginger
- 2 celery stalks
- 1 apple (optional)

After thoroughly scrubbing all produce, put ingredients through a juicer.

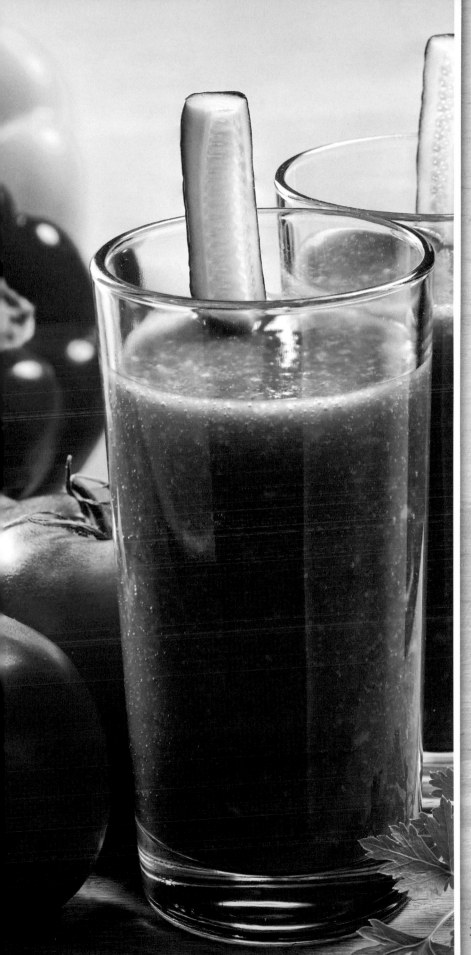

TARGET: DIABETES

Swiss chard

For those with type 2 diabetes, juicing can be a good way to take in beneficial nutrients, such as magnesium, chromium, and chlorophyll, as well as fiber.

NECESSARY NUTRIENTS

Magnesium, which ensures the proper function of insulin receptors, can be found in spinach or Swiss chard. Spinach also supplies chlorophyll, which promotes healthy immune system functioning; wheatgrass, broccoli, and kale are also good sources. Chromium helps balance blood sugar, and spinach is a good source. Get fiber from cabbage, citrus, and celery, among others.

Superb Defender

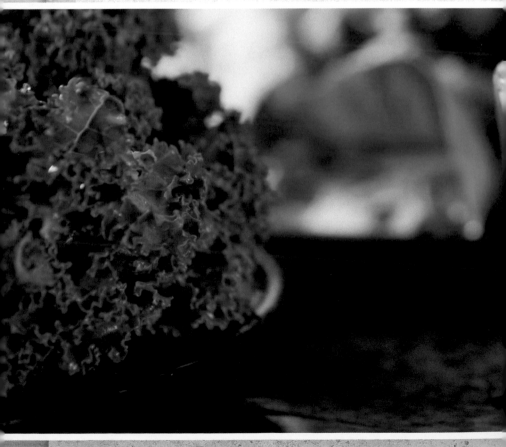

Carrot Digestif

- 5 carrots
- ½ pineapple
- 2 large white cabbage leaves

After thoroughly scrubbing all produce, put ingredients through a juicer.

Greek Goddess Juice

- 1 pear
- 2 celery stalks
- 3 kale leaves
- ½ avocado
- 1½ green apples
- 1½ cup water
- juice of 1 lime
- 1 cucumber, peeled and deseeded
- ¼ teaspoon salt
- ¼ teaspoon pepper
- ⅛ teaspoon cumin powder

After thoroughly scrubbing all produce, put ingredients through a juicer.

Green Grapefruit

- 4 large kale leaves
- 2 handfuls spinach or Swiss chard
- 2 sticks celery
- 1 grapefruit, peeled

After thoroughly scrubbing all produce, put ingredients through a juicer.

Superb Defender

- 5 large kale leaves
- 1 handful spinach or Swiss chard
- 4 carrots
- 1 cup broccoli heads
- 1 orange

After thoroughly scrubbing all produce, put ingredients through a juicer.

THINK ABOUT IT!
Juicing for diabetes can be a tricky proposition. Most fruit juices contain too much fructose—the natural sugars in fruits.

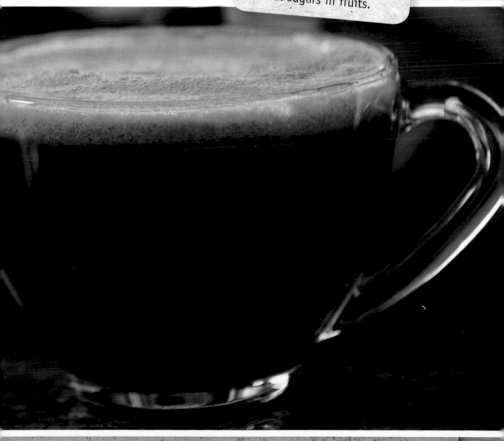

TARGET: HAIR LOSS

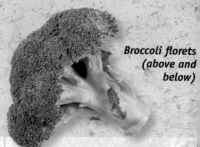

Broccoli florets (above and below)

A healthy diet is essential for preventing hair loss. Your follicles need vitamins A and C, iron, zinc, and B-vitamins to keep from shedding, and these nutrients can also promote hair growth.

HAIR-RAISING NUTRIENTS

Look for fruits and vegetables, such as carrots, that are rich in vitamin A, which might work to increase the rate of hair growth and can make hair shinier and healthier.

Hair-Growth Tonic

- 5 carrots
- 2 apples
- ½ cup alfalfa sprouts
- 1 handful dark green kale

After thoroughly washing all produce, put ingredients through a juicer.

Great Green Hair Regimen

- 3 large broccoli florets
- 2 to 3 green apples, seeded
- 1 handful spinach
- 1 lime, peeled

After thoroughly washing all produce, put ingredients through a juicer.

Hair Repair Juice

- 2 ounces wheatgrass
- 1 small handful parsley
- 1 handful cilantro
- 4 carrots, cleaned of greens and skin
- 1 stalk celery
- ½ cup fennel, chopped
- ½ apple, seeded

After washing all produce, put ingredients through a juicer.

Hair-Enhancing Juice

- 1 cup sprouts
- 1 cabbage leaf or 2 brussels sprouts
- 1 cup broccoli florets
- 2 medium carrots
- 2 slices red onion
- 1 medium beet with greens
- 2 slices watermelon
- 2 apples
- ½ to 1 clove garlic (optional)

After thoroughly scrubbing all produce, put ingredients through a juicer.

Healthy Hair Tonic

- 1 handful parsley
- 1 handful spinach
- 4 to 5 carrots, greens removed
- 2 stalks celery

After thoroughly washing all produce, put ingredients through a juicer.

Healthy Hair Tonic (opposite)

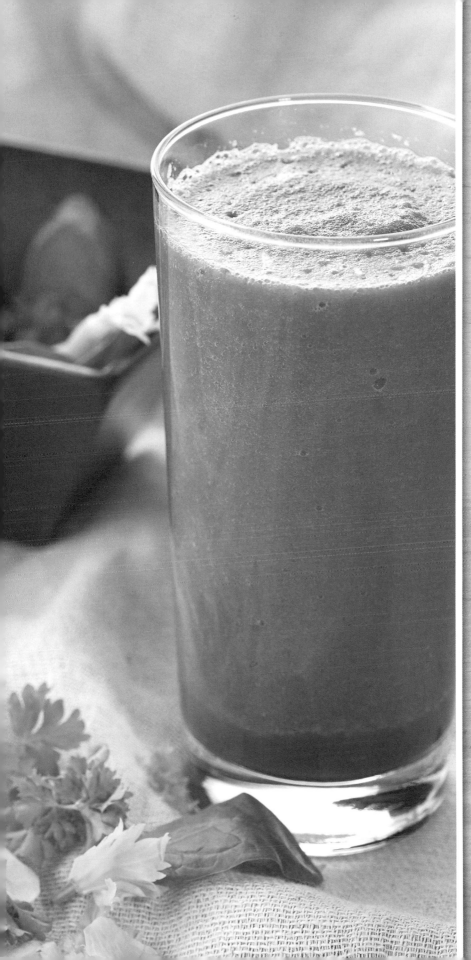

TARGET: HYPOGLYCEMIA

Hypoglycemia, or low blood sugar, results from the overproduction of insulin, which causes your level of blood glucose to drop. Its list of effects is long. Hypoglycemia may leave you feeling achy, hungry, or dizzy. Headaches are common, and you might feel like your brain is fuzzy and also suffer from fatigue, insomnia, palpitations, sweating, digestive disorders, or nervous tension.

Tomato (above and below left)

BALANCE BLOOD GLUCOSE

Juicing can help you keep your blood glucose level from dropping too low. Just about all greens are good choices, as are fruits like apples, grapefruit, and tomatoes.

GraLemPa Juice

- 1 grapefruit
- 1 lemon
- 1 large piece papaya

After thoroughly scrubbing all produce, put ingredients through a juicer.

Broccoli, Artichoke, Fennel & Parsley Blend

- 1 stalk broccoli
- 2 Jerusalem artichokes, cut into pieces
- ¼ head fennel
- 3 sprigs parsley

After thoroughly scrubbing all produce, put ingredients through a juicer.

Watercress, Tomatoes & Parsley Juice

- 3 stalks celery
- 3 tomatoes
- 1 small bunch fresh parsley
- 1 handful watercress
- ½ lemon

Thoroughly clean all produce, then juice them together.

Carrot, Celery, Garlic & Parsley Juice

- 2 carrots
- 2 celery stalks
- 1 garlic clove
- 3 sprigs parsley

After thoroughly scrubbing all produce, put ingredients through a juicer.

Speared Apple Juice

- 2 green apples
- 6 asparagus spears

Wash produce thoroughly, then juice apples and asparagus spears together.

Spinach & Celery Juice

- 3 green apples
- 2 stalks celery
- 1 large bunch baby spinach

After scrubbing clean all produce, juice some of the spinach first. Then alternate among celery, apples, and spinach to help flush spinach out of the juicer. Makes two glasses, one to enjoy now and one for later.

French Green Beans & Brussels Sprouts

- 1 cup French green beans
- 8 brussels sprouts
- 1 lemon, peeled

After thoroughly scrubbing all produce, put ingredients through a juicer.

Green Carrot Juice

- 6 spinach leaves
- 1 handful parsley
- 2 stalks celery
- 5 carrots

Thoroughly scrub all produce, peel the carrots, then juice all ingredients together.

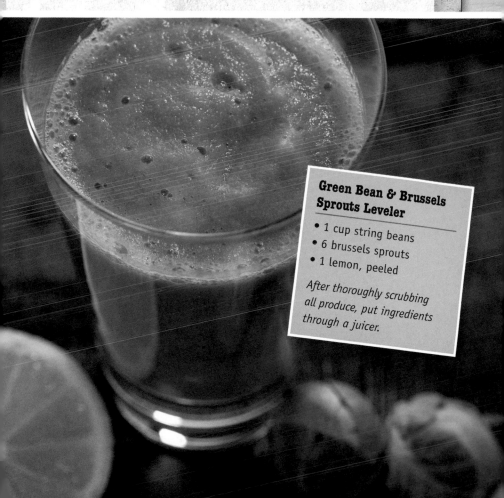

Green Bean & Brussels Sprouts Leveler

- 1 cup string beans
- 6 brussels sprouts
- 1 lemon, peeled

After thoroughly scrubbing all produce, put ingredients through a juicer.

Green Bean & Brussels Sprouts Leveler

TARGET: IMMUNE SYSTEM

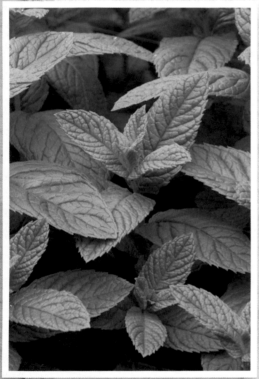

Ginger

Keeping your immune system functioning in top form improves your overall health. Eating a well-balanced diet that provides essential vitamins and minerals is the best way to bolster immunity.

IMMUNE BOOSTERS

To boost your immune system, get out your juicer and create recipes that include fruits, such as apples, limes, and oranges, and vegetables like carrots and beets. You can then spice it up with cleansing ginger root.

The Orange Genie

- 3 small apples
- 12 small carrots
- 1 large orange

After thoroughly scrubbing all produce, put ingredients through a juicer.

Red Devil

- 2 small beets
- 2 inches ginger
- 3 cucumbers
- ½ lemon

After thoroughly scrubbing all produce, put ingredients through a juicer.

Mint leaves (above); Moheeto (opposite)

Hard-2-Beet

- 1 beet
- 2 apples
- 1 pear
- 1 inch ginger
- ½ lemon

After thoroughly scrubbing all produce, put ingredients through a juicer.

Beet It

- 1 beet
- 1 clove garlic
- 2 apples

After thoroughly scrubbing all produce, put ingredients through a juicer.

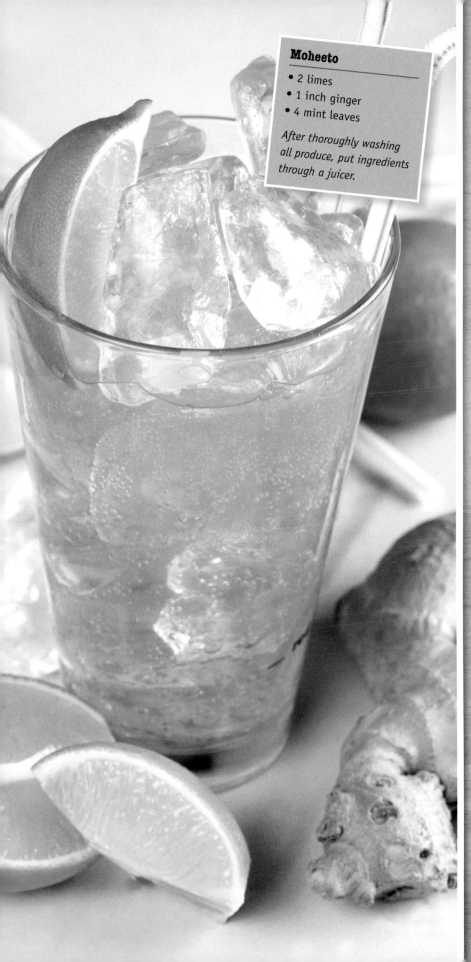

Moheeto

- 2 limes
- 1 inch ginger
- 4 mint leaves

After thoroughly washing all produce, put ingredients through a juicer.

TARGET: INSOMNIA

Cherries

If you have trouble falling asleep or staying asleep, you know how depleting insomnia can be. Rather than reaching for pills, try a juicing to help you get a good night's rest.

BEDTIME JUICES

Lack of sleep is not just a nuisance; over time, insomnia can affect your daytime dexterity, cognitive function, and mental focus. Try juices made with melatonin-rich tart cherries, celery (which will calm your nerves), or avocado, which may help you sleep better.

Sweet Dreams Juice

- 2 large oranges, peeled
- ½ lemon, peeled
- ½ bunch organic watercress
- 8 stalks celery
- ½ head romaine lettuce

After thoroughly scrubbing all produce, put ingredients through a juicer.

Ultimate Sleeper

- 1 cup tart cherries, pitted
- 1½ cucumbers
- 1 banana
- 1 cup spinach
- ½ avocado

Juice the cherries and cucumber, then blend with the other ingredients.

Insomnia Soother

- ½ cabbage
- 1 large zucchini
- ½ inch ginger
- 3 cups broccoli florets
- 1 large head green lettuce
- 6 medium carrots
- 1 apple
- 1 pear

After thoroughly washing all produce, put ingredients through a juicer. Makes three glasses of a strong mixture; drink one before dinner, one after—and the third only if you're still tossing and turning.

Ultimate Sleeper (opposite); tart cherries, avocados, and spinach (below)

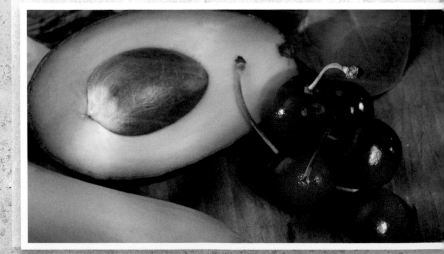

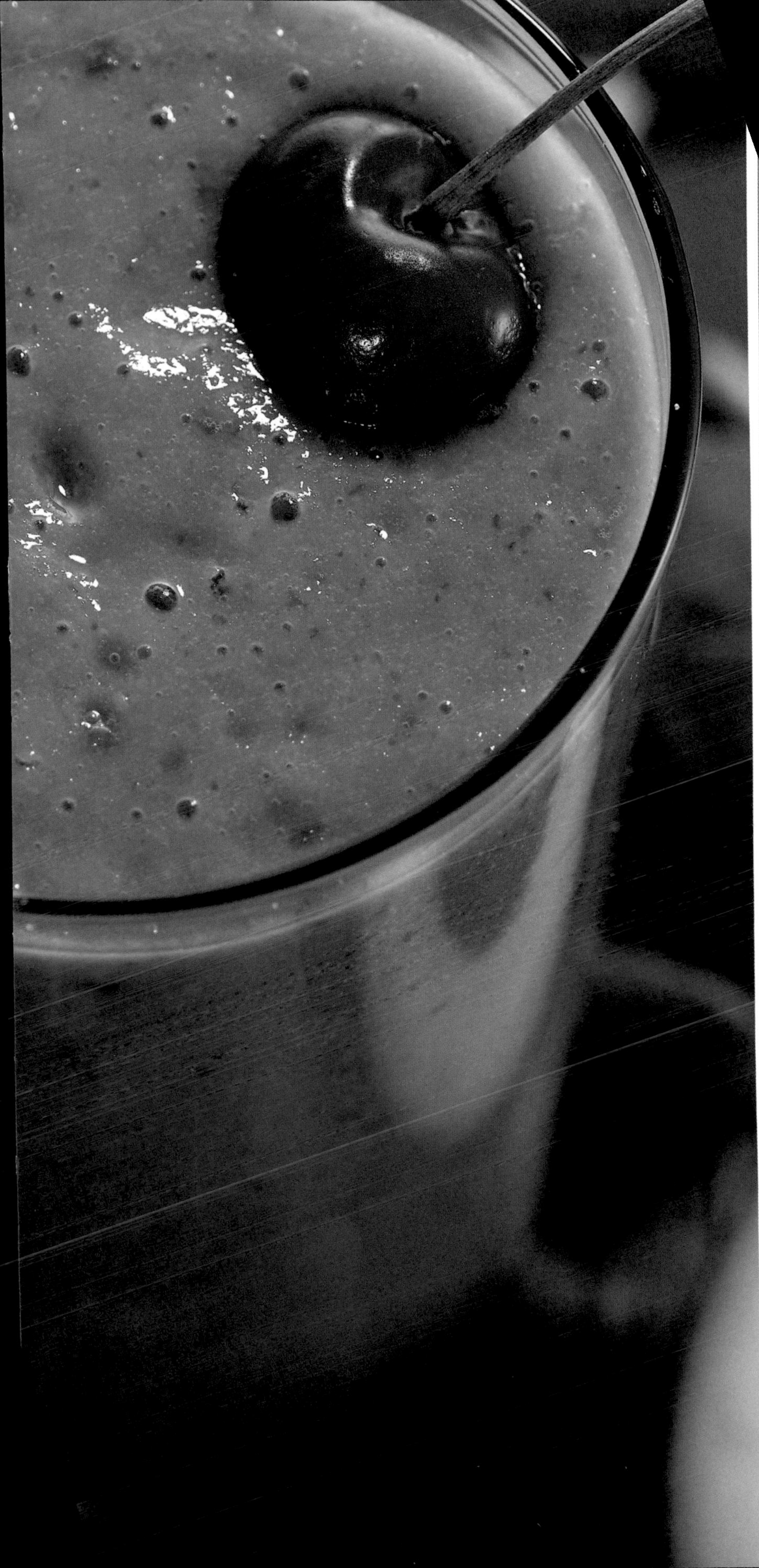

TARGET: MIGRAINES

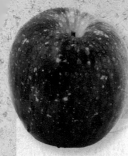

Fuji apple

The cause of the debilitating, throbbing pain of migraine headaches, as well as the visual auras, is up for debate. What is not up for debate is the fact that they can leave sufferers immobile for hours, if not days. Juicing nutrient-rich raw fruits and vegetables might relieve some of the pain.

USEFUL JUICES

Research suggests that juices made from apples, celery, spinach, lemon, cucumber, and ginger may help migraine sufferers if consumed on a daily basis.

Migraine Soother

- 16 ounces filtered water or coconut water
- 1 cup pineapple
- 1 cup kale (3 to 4 leaves)
- 1 stalk celery
- ½ lemon, juiced
- 1 cup cucumber
- ½ inch ginger
- 1½ cups ice

After thoroughly scrubbing all produce, put ingredients in a blender and process until smooth.

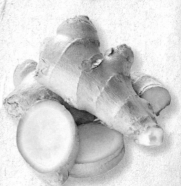

Slices of ginger root (above); Carrot-Top (opposite)

Carrot-Spinach Juice

- 5 bunches spinach
- 4 carrots

After thoroughly washing all produce, put ingredients through a juicer.

Tropikale Ease

- ½ pineapple
- 3 to 4 kale leaves
- 1 stalk celery
- ¼ lemon
- ½ cucumber
- ½ inch ginger

After thoroughly scrubbing all produce, put ingredients through a juicer.

Clear Skies

- 4 kale leaves
- 2 handfuls spinach
- 3 celery stalks with leaves
- ¼ inch ginger
- 1 cucumber (peeled if not organic)
- 2 Fuji apples

After thoroughly scrubbing all produce, put ingredients through a juicer.

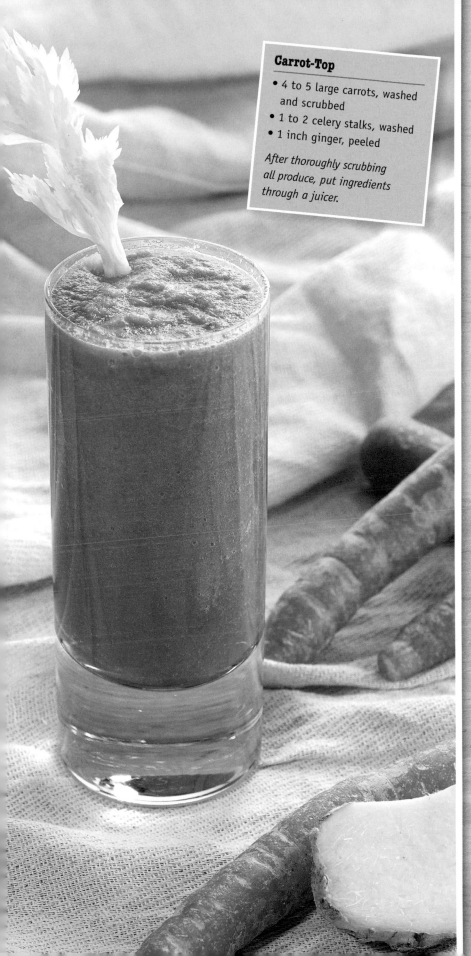

Carrot-Top

- 4 to 5 large carrots, washed and scrubbed
- 1 to 2 celery stalks, washed
- 1 inch ginger, peeled

After thoroughly scrubbing all produce, put ingredients through a juicer.

TARGET: SKIN HEALTH

Skin, the largest human organ, is a channel for the body to rid itself of toxins. Any blockages can result in several skin problems that can keep people from enjoying life to the fullest. Whether it's acne, eczema, or psoriasis, there are juice recipes that can help relieve these uncomfortable, even painful, conditions.

Pineapple

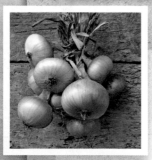

Onions (above); Kale Clear (opposite)

ACNE

For acne, you want to create juices loaded with anti-inflammatory and antioxidant vitamin C, such as those made with cantaloupe or pineapple. The vitamin A in the cantaloupe perks up your overall health, as well as your skin. Healthy greens can supply phytonutrients that help build and repair skin collagen and connective tissue, which can help reduce scarring.

Coconut Cleanser

- ½ cantaloupe
- 1 glass of coconut water
- ½ cucumber

Peel and juice the cantaloupe, then juice the cucumber and mix with the coconut water.

Onion & Carrot Clear

- 4 medium carrots
- ½ medium onion
- 1 handful parsley

After thoroughly scrubbing all produce, put ingredients through a juicer.

Ginger Sweet Potato Blend

- 1 sweet potato, peeled
- 1 large carrot, end removed
- 1 large slice pineapple, peeled, cored, about ½ cup fruit
- ¼-inch slice ginger root, peeled

After thoroughly scrubbing all produce, put ingredients through a juicer.

Carrot Clear-Up

- 6 medium carrots
- 2 cloves garlic
- 1 handful parsley

After thoroughly washing all produce, put ingredients through a juicer.

Kale Clear

- 1 cup kale
- 1 cucumber
- 2 apples
- ½ bunch parsley
- 3 carrots

After thoroughly washing all produce, put ingredients through a juicer.

ECZEMA

Eczema, an inflammatory skin condition, expresses as red, dry, and itchy skin on the face, hands, elbows, wrists, and knees. Not only can it be painful and unsightly, it also leaves the sufferer at risk of bacterial and viral infections. When choosing your fruits and veggies for eczema relief, be sure they are pesticide free.

Pear

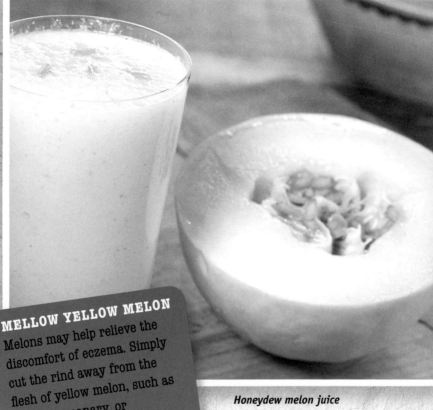

MELLOW YELLOW MELON

Melons may help relieve the discomfort of eczema. Simply cut the rind away from the flesh of yellow melon, such as a Korean, canary, or honeydew. Add flesh (and seeds) to juicer, and enjoy.

Honeydew melon juice

Honeydew-Pear Blend

- 1 pear, skin removed
- ½ honeydew melon
- ½ cucumber
- 1 handful mint leaves
- ice, as needed

After thoroughly washing all produce, put ingredients through a juicer.

Green Relief

- ¾ cucumber
- ½ avocado
- 1 handful watercress
- 1 sprig parsley

Remove the stone from the avocado and scoop the flesh into the blender. Either juice the cucumber and watercress and add the juices to a blender with the avocado, or put all the ingredients in the blender and whiz to a smooth consistency.

PSORIASIS

For psoriasis sufferers, the plagues of thickened, scaly skin can be both painful and embarrassing. Juicing can help prevent and relieve the unsightly patches. Try beta-carotene-rich carrots, anti-inflammatory ginger, and antioxidant-rich citrus fruits or pumpkin.

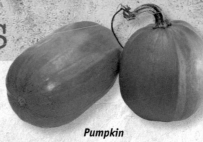

Pumpkin

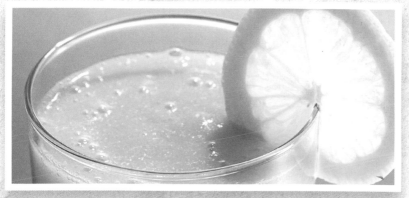

Citrus Relief

Jack & Jill

- 3 carrots
- ½ small pumpkin
- 2 oranges

After thoroughly scrubbing all produce, put ingredients through a juicer.

Citrus Relief

- 1 grapefruit
- 3 oranges
- ¼ lemon slice

Use a citrus juicer for this one, then mix the juices in a glass.

Carrot-Apple Skin Relief

- 1 carrot
- 2 green apples
- 1 bunch spinach
- 3 to 4 leaves kale
- ¼ lemon slice

After thoroughly scrubbing all produce, put ingredients through a juicer.

Ginger & Veggies

- 2 carrots
- 1 medium beet
- 1 bell pepper
- ¼ lemon slice

After thoroughly scrubbing all produce, put ingredients through a juicer.

Green Therapy

- 2 carrots
- 1 bunch spinach
- 1 cup broccoli
- 1 orange bell pepper
- ¼ lemon slice
- 1 inch ginger

After thoroughly scrubbing all produce, put ingredients through a juicer.

Wheatgrass & Lemon Juice

- 1 ounce wheatgrass juice
- 1 squeeze lemon juice

Buy or make wheatgrass juice, and squeeze the lemon into the glass.

TARGET: UTIs

Many of us are all-too familiar with the uncomfortable symptoms of urinary tract infections (also known as UTIs): back pain, painful urination, tenderness in the pelvic area, and cloudy urine. To prevent and treat this infection, it is essential to stay hydrated. On top of drinking plenty of water, try juicing to get relief.

Pineapple

LIQUID RELIEF

Although they are not the miracle cure that they are often touted to be, cranberries are antioxidant and contain beneficial phytonutrients. Citrus fruits should also go on your shopping list—vitamin C can fight a UTI. Pineapples and blueberries also pack a vitamin-C punch, as does hydrating watermelon.

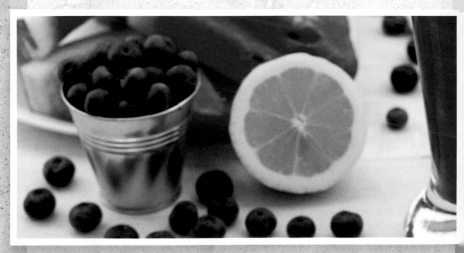

Watermelon, lemon, and blueberries

Blueberry, Watermelon & Cranberry Cleanser

- 1½ cups blueberries
- 2 cups watermelon, deseeded
- ½ cup cranberries
- ½ lemon, peeled

After thoroughly scrubbing all produce, put ingredients through a juicer.

Apple, Orange & Guava Juice

- 1 apple
- 1 orange
- 2 cups guava nectar

After thoroughly scrubbing all produce, put ingredients through a juicer.

Guava Delight (opposite)

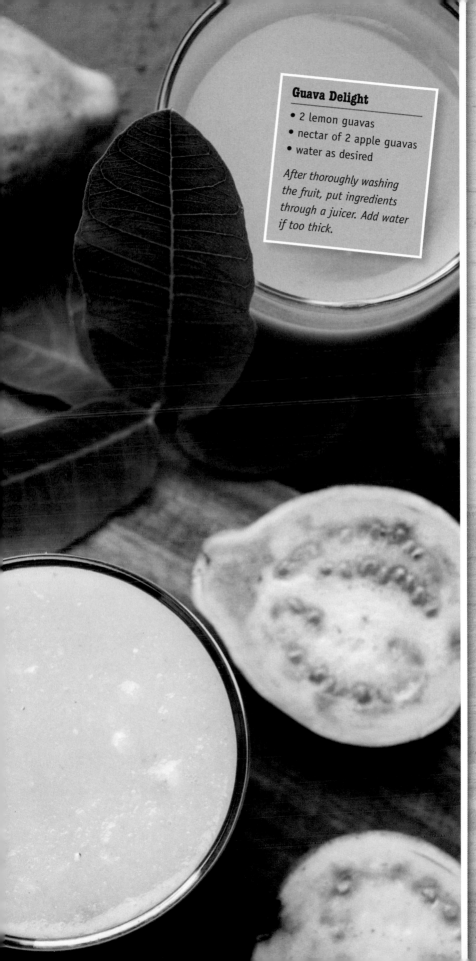

Guava Delight

- 2 lemon guavas
- nectar of 2 apple guavas
- water as desired

After thoroughly washing the fruit, put ingredients through a juicer. Add water if too thick.

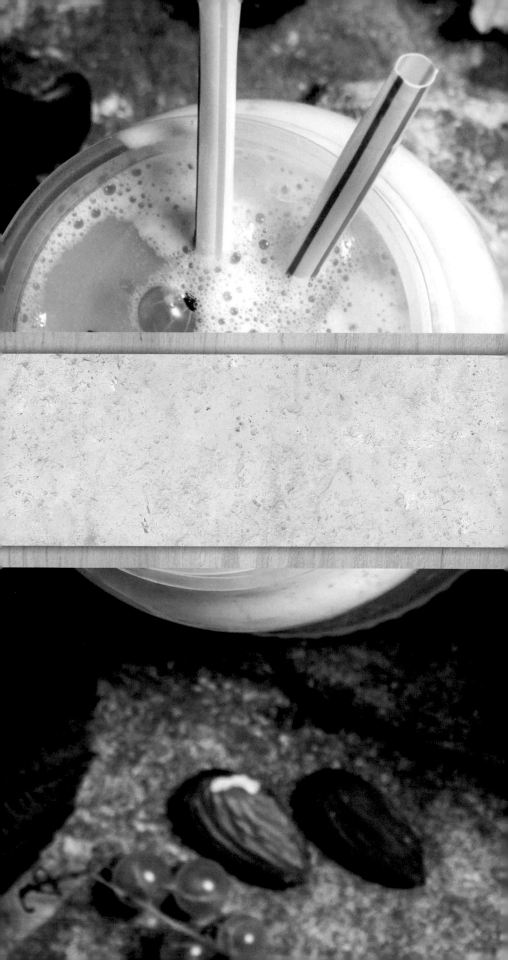

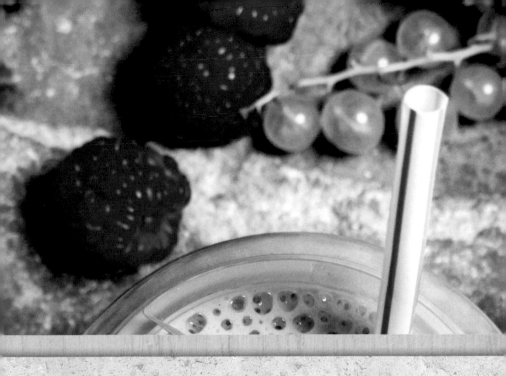

CHAPTER 6

SMOOTHIES
FOR EVERYONE

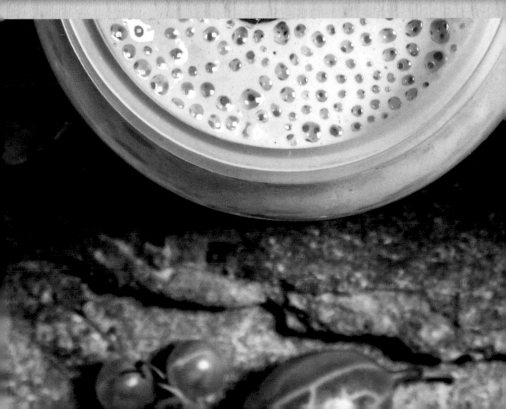

SMOOTHIES FOR EVERYONE

Smoothies offer a totally different experience from juices, with their slushy or creamy consistency. Smoothies also have the potential to be far more caloric than juices—although they don't have to be. Fruit- and veggie-based smoothies can be the foundation of a life-changing weight-loss regimen. Smoothies for dessert or after-dinner coffee are nothing less than decadent.

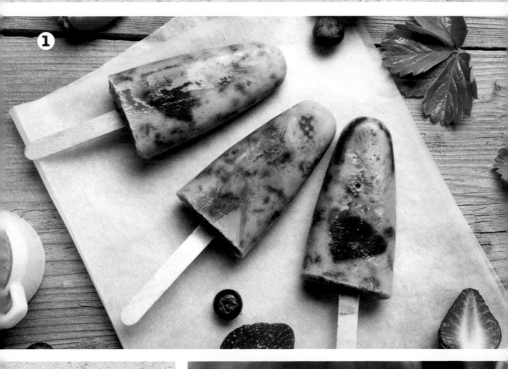

1. Strawberry & Blueberry Smoothie Pops
2. Ripe peaches
3. Big Apple Smoothie
4. Fresh plums
5. Watermelon Mint Smoothie
6. Spicy Green Smoothie

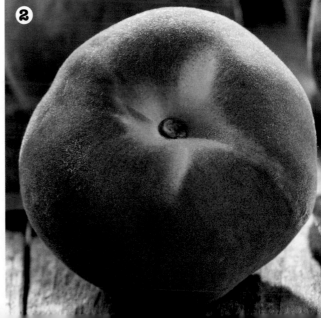

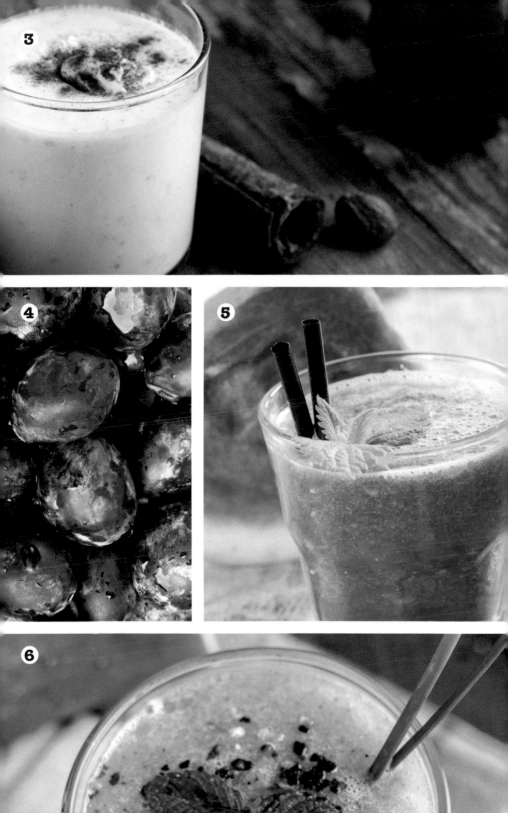
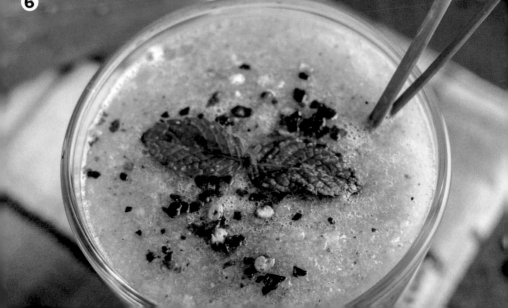

FRUITY AND CREAMY

The pairing of fruit and dairy is classic—just think of strawberries and cream. These concoctions can be as decadent as a dessert or as healthy as a power drink.

Almonds

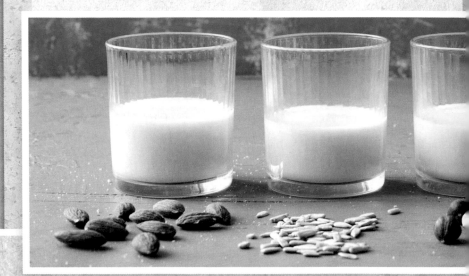

CHOOSE YOUR MILK

Dairy products are highly nutritious. Cow's milk, for example, is a complete food because it contains all the nutrients necessary to sustain life. To provide a creamy base for smoothies, use whole, low-fat, or even lactose-free milk. There are also many nondairy milks that are delicious in their own right. Most of the "creamy" recipes in this book suggest alternatives, such as almond milk, because they blend well in smoothies without making them too heavy. Here are a few of the favorites:

- *Soy milk:* Soy milk is the least processed of the dairy alternatives, and it's high in protein and low in saturated fats.

- *Coconut milk:* With a "mouth feel" similar to dairy milk, this milk has a distinct coconut flavor. It is high in saturated fat and very low in protein

and calcium compared to dairy milk. It is, however, suitable for vegans if they are able to obtain their calcium from other sources.

- *Oat milk:* Made from ground oats and water, oat milk contains some dietary fiber and various

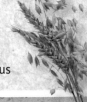

CHOOSE YOUR FRUIT

Just stop by the local farmers' market or browse your grocery produce aisle to find the freshest fruits, and then get out your blender. Combine your choice with your favorite milk for a nutritious meal or snack. You are really only limited by your imagination.

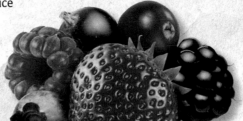

Assorted berries

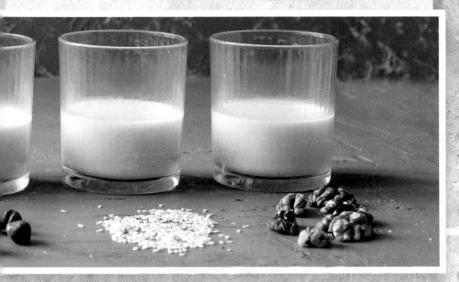

A few of the many nondairy alternative milks available, from left to right: almond, oat, hazelnut, rice, and walnut. They are all suitable for people who are lactose-intolerant, and they are generally lower in calories than whole cow's milk.

vitamins and minerals. It is low in calcium, although commercial varieties are often fortified with it. It has a taste similar to cow's milk.

- *Rice milk:* Made from boiled rice, brown rice syrup, and brown rice starch, it contains more carbohydrates than cow's milk. It has a light, sweet flavor, but a slightly watery consistency.

- *Almond milk:* Made from the ground nuts and, perhaps, a sweetener, almond milk is rich in vitamin E but has less protein and calcium than cow's milk—however,

it does offer the highest level of calcium of all the nut milks.

- *Other nut milks:* Cashew milk has a subtle flavor and is a good source of fiber, copper, magnesium, and antioxidants. With a nuttier flavor than cashew or almond milks, hazelnut milk is a good source of B vitamins and an excellent source of antioxidant vitamin E. You can also use walnut milk, which has the silky texture of most nut milks.

SO-GOOD SOY

Soy is one of the classic smoothie bases, with a silky texture and mild taste that lets fruit flavors take center stage.

Soy beans

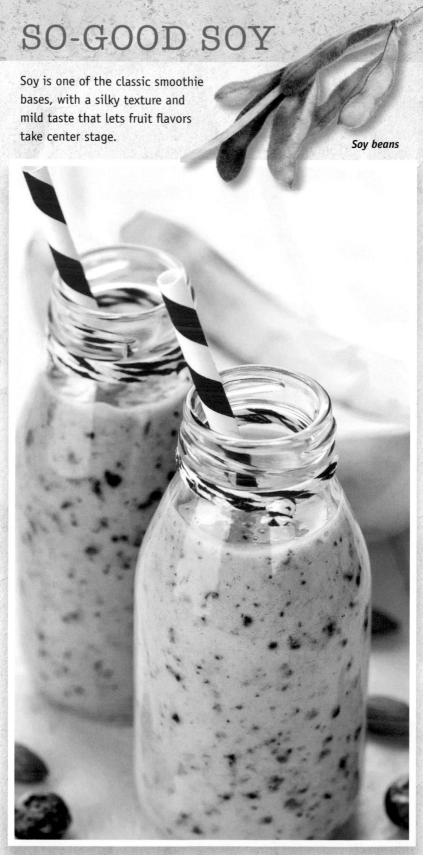

Wild Berry Soy Smoothie

THE HEALTHY WAY TO INDULGE

Juices may win the prize for offering nutrition-packed combos of fruits and veggies, but the process of juicing extracts the pulp, leaving a product that is high in natural sugars but low in fiber. Smoothies, on the other hand, keep their fiber because you toss the entire fruit or vegetable into the blender, and it all gets pulverized together rather than being pulped.

A smoothie's creamy or slushy consistency is provided by soft fruits or veggies that would merely clog up a juicer, such as bananas or avocados, or by juices, yogurt, tofu, or milk. But each of these foods provides important nutrients that are necessary for proper functioning, such as omega-3 oils from avocados or probiotics from yogurt. Any time you want to reach for a cool, thick drink, satisfy your craving with a healthy—and totally delicious—fruit smoothie.

Wild Berry Soy Smoothie

- 1 cup frozen blueberries
- 1 cup vanilla soy milk
- 1 banana, frozen
- 3 to 4 dashes of cayenne
- 1 teaspoon almond butter
- ½ cup coconut water
- 4 ice cubes

Put all of the ingredients into a blender, and blend until smooth.

Fruity Vanilla Soy Smoothie

- ½ cup pineapple cubes
- 1 small banana
- ½ cup frozen raspberries
- ½ cup fresh-squeezed orange juice
- ¼ cup carrot juice
- ½ cup vanilla soy milk
- 1 tablespoon honey

Put all of the ingredients into a blender, and blend until smooth.

Pear Soy Smoothie

- 1 banana
- ½ cup soy milk
- ½ cup unsweetened apple juice
- ¼ cup pear, peeled and chopped
- ¼ cup blueberries

Put all of the ingredients into a blender, and blend until smooth.

Strawberry-Banana Vanilla Soy Smoothie

- 1 cup strawberries
- ¾ cup vanilla soy milk
- ¾ tablespoon honey
- ¼ teaspoon vanilla extract
- 1 banana

Put all of the ingredients into a blender, and blend until smooth.

Melon & Mango Soy Smoothie

- 1 mango, cut into small pieces
- 2 cups seedless watermelon
- ½ cup vanilla soy milk
- 1 tablespoon honey
- 4 ice cubes

Put all of the ingredients into a blender, and blend until smooth.

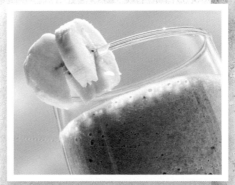

Strawberry-Banana Vanilla Soy Smoothie

STARRING BANANA

With their soft, mild-flavored flesh, bananas are naturals in smoothies. You can rely on their own creamy consistency or combine them with yogurt or the milk of your choice.

Banana slice

Banana Apple Smoothie

- 1 frozen banana, peeled and chopped
- ½ cup orange juice
- 1 Gala apple, peeled, cored, and chopped
- ¼ cup milk

Wash all produce, then put all of the ingredients into a blender, and blend until smooth.

Buttermilk & Banana Smoothie

- 1 cup low-fat buttermilk
- 2 ripe bananas, cut into 2-inch-thick rounds
- 11 dried pitted dates
- 1 teaspoon honey
- a pinch of salt
- 1 cup ice

Put all of the ingredients into a blender, and blend until smooth.

Berry, Banana, Agave Smoothie

- 1 cup plain fat-free yogurt
- ⅓ cup fresh or frozen blueberries, thawed
- 2 teaspoons light agave nectar
- 1 chilled, sliced ripe banana

Put all of the ingredients into a blender, and blend until smooth.

Banana Honey Smoothie

- 1 cup freshly squeezed orange juice (about 6 oranges)
- 2 tablespoons raw honey
- 1 tablespoon freshly squeezed lemon juice
- 2 teaspoons finely grated fresh ginger
- 2 ripe bananas

Put all of the ingredients into a blender, and blend until smooth.

Banana Strawberry Smoothie

- 1 banana, broken into chunks
- 1 teaspoon banana extract
- ¾ cup milk
- 8 ounces strawberry yogurt
- 2 teaspoons white sugar

Put all of the ingredients into a blender, and blend until smooth.

Banana Berry Smoothie

- 1 banana
- 1 cup frozen raspberries
- ¾ cup orange juice
- ¼ cup vanilla yogurt

Put all of the ingredients into a blender, and blend until smooth.

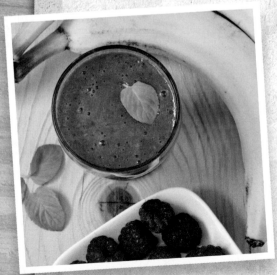

Banana Berry Smoothie (above); Banana Smoothie (opposite)

Banana Smoothie

- 1½ bananas, sliced
- ½ cup pineapple juice
- 1½ teaspoons honey

Put all of the ingredients into a blender, and blend until smooth.

CITRUS COMBOS

Tart, tangy, and deliciously flavorful, citrus fruits like oranges and grapefruits, whip up into vitamin-C rich smoothies. They blend best with yogurt and vegan milks.

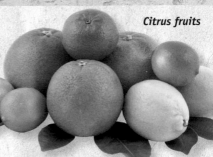

Citrus fruits

Almond-Orange Smoothie

- 1 cup vanilla almond milk
- ½ cup orange juice
- juice of 1 lemon
- juice of 1 lime
- 1 handful ice
- 1 tablespoon honey

Put all of the ingredients into a blender, and blend until smooth.

Cran-Orange Power Smoothie

- 1 cup cranberry juice
- 1 large banana
- 1 medium orange, peeled and segmented
- ½ cup strawberries, hulled
- ¼ cup raspberry sherbet
- 1 cup ice cubes
- ¼ cup whey protein powder

Wash all produce, then put all of the ingredients into a blender, and blend until smooth.

Grapefruit Surprise

- 2 red grapefruits
- 8 large strawberries
- 2 ripe bananas
- 8 ounces strawberry-banana yogurt
- 2 tablespoons honey
- 1 cup crushed ice

Juice grapefruit, and measure 1⅓ cups juice. Add strawberries. Cut bananas into chunks. Combine all the ingredients in a blender and whirl until smooth.

Strawberry, Orange & Coconut Smoothie

- 2½ cups hulled strawberries
- 1 orange, peeled
- ½ cup coconut milk
- 4 ice cubes (optional)

Wash all produce, then put all of the ingredients into a blender, and blend until smooth.

C-Vit Smoothie

- 1 large pink grapefruit, peeled, seeded, and cut into chunks
- ½ cup crushed pineapple, canned or fresh
- ½ cup fresh strawberries
- ½ cup nonfat Greek yogurt
- ½ cup ice

Wash all produce, then put all of the ingredients into a blender, and blend until smooth.

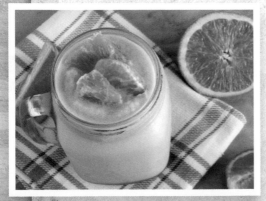

Almond-Orange Smoothie

APPLE TREATS

There is an apple for everyone, from the tart McIntoshes and Granny Smiths to the sweet Fuji, Honeycrisp, and Red Delicious varieties. Try combining them with veggies to sweeten more savory smoothies.

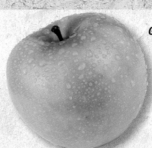

Granny Smith apple

Big Apple Smoothie

- 2 sweet apples, cored and sliced
- 2 large scoops vanilla yogurt
- ¼ cup vanilla soy milk
- ½ teaspoon pure vanilla extract
- ½ tablespoon pure maple syrup
- ¼ teaspoon ground cinnamon
- pinch of ground nutmeg

Put all of the ingredients into a blender, and blend until smooth.

Apple Avocado Smoothie

- 2 Granny Smith apples, cored and sliced
- ½ ripe Hass avocado
- ½ cup apple juice
- ½ cup ice
- 3 sprigs mint leaves
- 1 teaspoon fresh-squeezed lime juice

Wash all produce, then put all of the ingredients into a blender, and blend until smooth.

Cardamom Apple Smoothie

- ½ cup apple, chopped and cored but not peeled
- ½ cup low-fat plain yogurt
- 1 tablespoon honey
- a pinch of ground cardamom
- ½ cup unsweetened apple juice
- ½ banana
- 2 to 3 ice cubes

Wash apple, then put all of the ingredients into a blender, and blend until smooth.

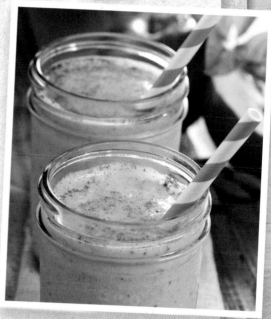

Cardamom Apple Smoothie

YOGURT FOR HEALTH

Yogurt and other fermented foods are an important part of the diet, and can make an excellent base for a creamy smoothie or smoothie bowl. Yogurts with probiotics (healthy bacteria) help to keep our gut flora in balance and our digestive and immune systems functioning well. Yogurt is also an excellent source of high-quality protein, calcium, B-group vitamins, and all the other nutrients found in dairy milk. People with lactose intolerance may find it easier to tolerate yogurt than milk because the bacteria partly digest the lactose.

BERRY GOOD

With their tartly sweet tastes and vibrant colors, summer fruits like strawberry, raspberry, blackcurrant, and blackberry make great additions to a creamy smoothie.

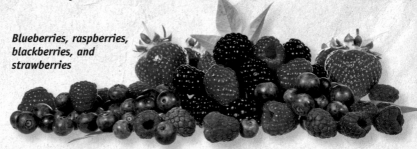

Blueberries, raspberries, blackberries, and strawberries

Strawberry-Apple Smoothie

- 1 cup frozen strawberries
- 1 apple, cored and peeled
- ½ cup low-fat milk
- ½ cup strawberry, vanilla, or other fruit yogurt
- 2 teaspoons honey
- 2 teaspoons ground flaxseeds

Put all of the ingredients into a blender, and blend until smooth.

Blackberry Yogurt Smoothie

- 1 cup fresh blackberries
- ½ frozen banana
- 6 ounces low-fat Greek yogurt
- 4 ice cubes
- ½ to ¾ cup unsweetened almond milk or other type of milk

Wash all produce, then put all of the ingredients into a blender, and blend until smooth.

Cinnamon Blackberry Smoothie

- 1½ cups frozen blackberries
- ½ cup low-fat plain yogurt
- ½ cup low-fat buttermilk
- 1 tablespoon honey
- ⅛ teaspoon ground cinnamon

Wash all produce, then put all of the ingredients into a blender, and blend until smooth.

Blueberry Breakfast Smoothie

- 1 cup blueberries
- ½ cup low-fat vanilla yogurt
- ½ cup skim milk
- 2 tablespoons honey
- 5 ice cubes

Wash all produce, then put all of the ingredients into a blender, and blend until smooth.

Berry Yogurt Smoothie

- 1 handful blueberries
- 1 handful blackcurrants
- 5 tablespoons natural yogurt
- 6 tablespoons apple juice

Wash all produce, then put all of the ingredients into a blender, and blend until smooth.

Tropical Berry Smoothie

- 1 cup blueberries
- ½ cup chopped mango
- ½ cup beets, cooked and chopped
- ¼ avocado
- 1 cup coconut milk
- 1 tablespoon fresh lemon juice
- ½ cup ice

Put all of the ingredients into a blender, and blend until smooth.

Raspberry-Blackberry Smoothie (opposite)

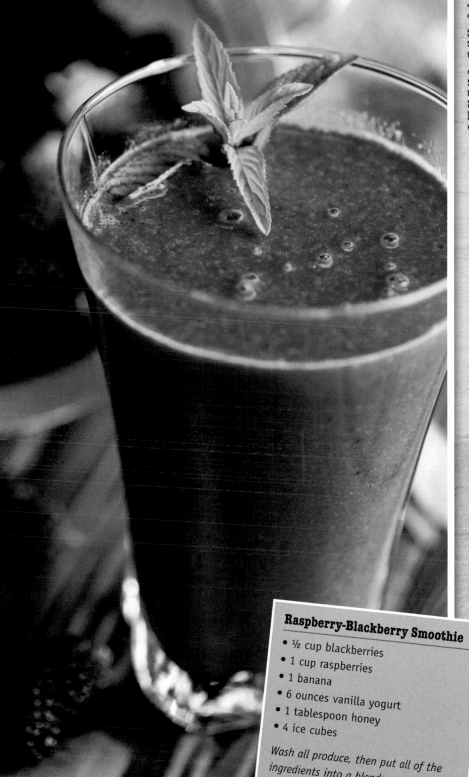

Raspberry-Blackberry Smoothie

- ½ cup blackberries
- 1 cup raspberries
- 1 banana
- 6 ounces vanilla yogurt
- 1 tablespoon honey
- 4 ice cubes

Wash all produce, then put all of the ingredients into a blender, and blend until smooth.

PLUMMY BLENDS

Juicy, ripe plums are delicious in creamy smoothies. To retain nutrients and fiber, just roughly chop them with their skins still on before dropping them into the blender.

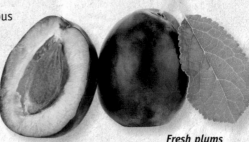

Fresh plums

Plum Yogurt Smoothie

- 1 cup vanilla yogurt
- 1 plum, pitted
- ½ banana
- ¼ cup almond milk
- ice, as needed

Put all of the ingredients into a blender, and blend until smooth.

Plum, Red Grape & Almond Milk Smoothie

- 2½ small or 2 large plums, pitted and sliced (about ¾ cup sliced)
- ½ cup red grapes, rinsed
- 1 to 2 teaspoons rose geranium syrup
- 1 tablespoon almond meal
- ⅛ teaspoon vanilla extract
- ¼ cup almond milk
- 3 to 4 ice cubes

Place all of the ingredients in a blender, and blend until frothy, about one minute.

Vanilla & Plum Buttermilk Smoothie

- 2 cups sugar
- 1 vanilla bean, halved with scraped seeds reserved
- 5 plums, quartered, pitted
- ½ cup buttermilk
- 1½ cups small ice cubes

Put 4 cups water, sugar, and halved vanilla bean with scraped seeds into a large saucepan. Bring to a boil over medium-high heat, stirring until sugar has dissolved. Add plums. Reduce heat to medium-low, and simmer until plums are tender, about 15 minutes. Using a slotted spoon, transfer plums to a plate to cool completely; remove bean, and discard poaching liquid. Puree cooled plums in a blender. Add buttermilk and small ice cubes, and then blend until smooth.

Vanilla & Plum Buttermilk Smoothie

POMEGRANATE POTIONS

Pomegranate seeds

With hard-to-harvest seeds, pomegranates may be finicky fruits to work with, but the antioxidant benefits the juicy seeds provide make any extra effort worth it. And they taste great!

Prickly Pear-Pomegranate

- 1½ cups prickly pear, peeled and chopped
- seeds from 1 pomegranate
- ¾ cup freshly squeezed orange juice
- ¼ cup cashew milk
- ¼ cup banana, chopped
- 1½ teaspoons fresh ginger, peeled and minced
- 2 cups crushed ice

Put all of the ingredients into a blender, and blend until smooth.

Pink Pomegranate Smoothie

- 2 cups pure pomegranate juice (fresh squeezed or bottled fresh)
- 2 cups plain nonfat yogurt
- 2 large bananas, sliced crosswise

In a blender, combine the chilled nonfat yogurt with the pomegranate juice. Add the sliced bananas and puree until the mixture is creamy.

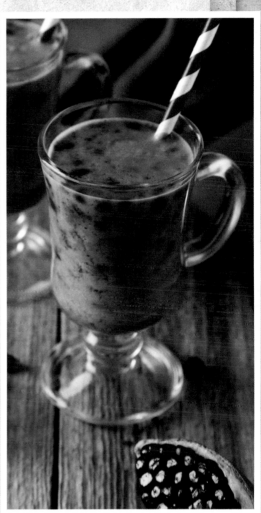

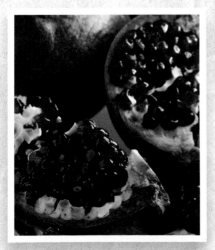

Pink Pomegranate Smoothie (above); quartered pomegranate (left)

Pomegranate-Berry Smoothie

- ½ cup chilled pomegranate juice
- ½ cup vanilla low-fat yogurt
- 1 cup frozen mixed berries

Put all of the ingredients into a blender, and blend until smooth.

TROPICAL DREAMS

If you like piña coladas . . . well, if you like any "umbrella" drink, just whip up a tropical fruit smoothie that ditches the alcohol but keeps the nutrients. And these once exotic fruits, like pineapples, papayas, mangoes, and guavas, are all readily available in most supermarkets.

Pineapple chunks

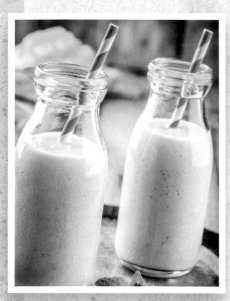

Mango-Lime Smoothie

Mango-Lime Smoothie

- 2 cups ripe mango chunks
- 2 to 3 tablespoons fresh lime juice
- 2 cups coconut water
- a pinch of cayenne powder

Wash all produce, then put all of the ingredients into a blender, and blend until smooth.

Mango-Pineapple Smoothie

- 1 cup frozen pineapple
- 1 cup frozen mango pieces
- 1 cup vanilla yogurt
- ⅓ cup milk (or more if needed)
- 2 teaspoons sugar
- 2 ice cubes, if needed

Put all of the ingredients into a blender, and blend until smooth.

Mango, Strawberry & Peach Smoothie

- 2 small peaches
- 1 mango
- 6 frozen strawberries
- 1 frozen banana
- ½ cup almond milk
- ¾ cup vanilla yogurt
- 6 ice cubes

Wash all produce, then put all of the ingredients into a blender, and blend until smooth.

Mango, Papaya & Pineapple Smoothie

- 1 cup frozen mango
- 1 cup frozen pineapple
- 1 cup papaya, peeled, seeded, and diced
- ½ cup low-fat Greek yogurt
- ½ to ¾ cup whole or skim milk, or orange juice

Wash all produce, then put all of the ingredients into a blender, and blend until smooth.

Mango-Papaya Smoothie

- 1¼ cups almond milk
- ½ cup coconut water (not coconut milk)
- 1 cup papaya, peeled and cubed
- 1 cup mango, peeled and cubed
- ½ cup ice

Wash all produce, then put all of the ingredients into a blender, and blend until smooth.

Pineapple Ginger

- 1 cup fresh or frozen pineapple, cut into 1-inch pieces
- 1-inch piece fresh ginger, peeled and minced
- ½ cup low-fat plain yogurt
- 1 cup pineapple juice
- ⅛ teaspoon ground cinnamon
- ½ cup ice (or as needed)

Put all of the ingredients into a blender, and blend until smooth.

Guava, Pineapple & Strawberry Smoothie

- ½ pineapple
- 1 handful strawberries
- 5 tablespoons natural yogurt
- 8 tablespoons guava juice

Put all of the ingredients into a blender, and blend until smooth.

Pineapple Berry Smoothie

- ½ cup mixed berries
- ½ cup water
- ½ cup ice
- ½ cup pineapple, diced
- 1 banana
- ½ cup Greek yogurt
- 1 tablespoon grated ginger

Put all of the ingredients into a blender, and blend until smooth.

Clementine, Banana & Pineapple Smoothie

- 8 clementines, segmented
- ½ cup fresh pineapple, cubed
- 1 banana, sliced
- 1 cup milk or plain yogurt
- 1 handful ice cubes

Put all of the ingredients into a blender, and blend until smooth.

Piña Banana Smoothie

- ½ cup coconut milk
- ½ cup plain or vanilla yogurt
- 1 medium banana
- 1 cup pineapple, chopped
- ¼ cup shredded coconut
- 1 teaspoon vanilla extract
- ¾ cup ice
- 1 tablespoon honey
- 2 tablespoons lime juice

Put all of the ingredients into a blender, and blend until smooth.

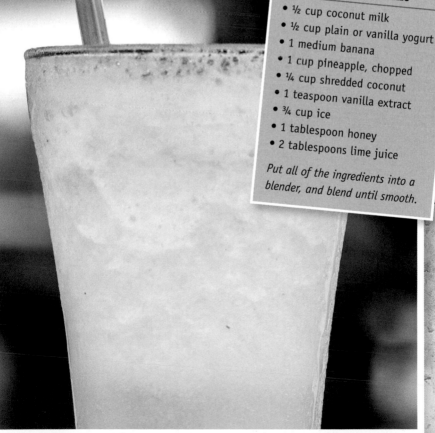

Piña Banana Smoothie

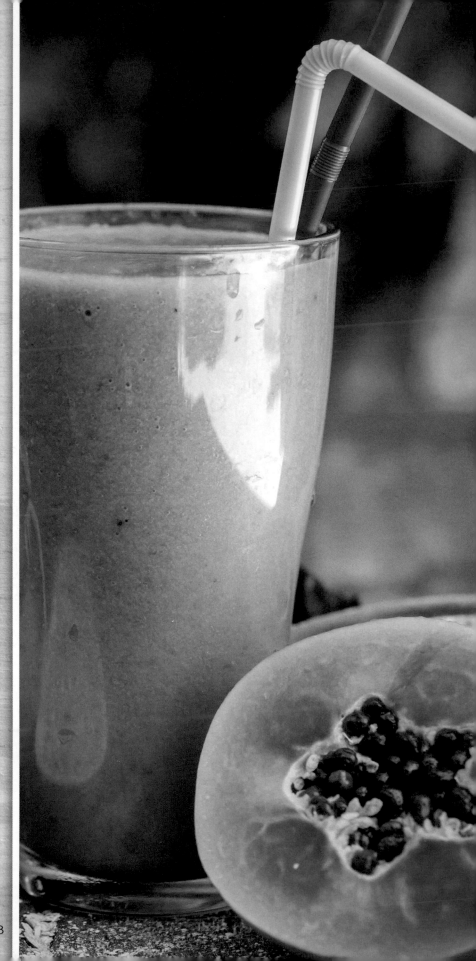

Strawberry-Papaya Smoothie

- ¾ cup chopped papaya, chilled
- ½ cup strawberry, chilled
- ½ cup plain fat-free yogurt
- ½ cup nonfat milk
- 1 tablespoon honey
- ½ cup ice cubes or crushed ice

In blender, combine yogurt and milk; add papaya, strawberries, and honey. Add ice cubes. Cover and blend until nearly smooth.

Caribbean Dream

- ½ cup papaya
- ½ cup mango
- 1 orange
- 1 inch ginger
- 2 tablespoons fine-cut, dried unsweetened coconut
- ¼ teaspoon nutmeg
- 2 tablespoons sugar or sugar substitute
- 1¼ cups cream or milk

Put all of the ingredients into a blender or food processor and whiz on pulse and then high until smooth. Add 6 ounces of light rum for a cocktail version of this smoothie.

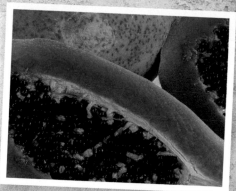

Papaya

Papaya Ginger Smoothie

- 2½ cups papaya chunks
- 1 cup ice cubes
- ⅔ cup nonfat plain yogurt
- 1 tablespoon finely-chopped, peeled fresh ginger
- 1 tablespoon honey
- juice of 2 lemons
- 16 fresh mint leaves, plus 4 sprigs, for garnish

Refrigerate papaya until very cold, at least 1 hour or overnight. Blend papaya, ice, yogurt, ginger, honey, and lemon juice in a blender. Add up to ¼ cup water, 1 tablespoon at a time, until mixture is smooth and thinned to desired consistency. Blend in mint leaves. Garnish with mint

Papaya Berry Smoothie

- 1 cup papaya, peeled and seeded
- 1 cup frozen mixed berries
- ½ cup skim milk or soy milk
- 1 tablespoon honey (optional)

Put all of the ingredients into a blender, and blend until smooth.

Orange Sunset Smoothie

- ½ cup guava, seeds removed
- 2 medium carrots, chopped
- 1 medium banana, peeled
- 2 medium peaches
- 1 teaspoon fresh ginger, grated
- 1 cup coconut water

Put all of the ingredients into a blender, and blend until smooth.

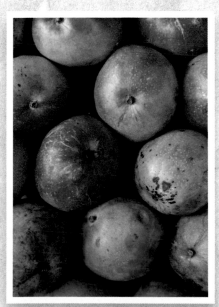

Ripe Florida mangoes (above); Papaya Ginger Smoothie (opposite)

FROSTY FRUIT

Let fruit flavors and textures come to the forefront with frosty smoothies that combine your favorite fruits and veggies.

ICE, ICE SMOOTHIE

Throw ice and fruit into a blender for a frosty treat.

Frosty smoothies are a refreshing, healthy treat. Certain fruits, such as bananas, avocados, and papayas, add a creamy thickness to a smoothie all on their own, or add crushed or cubed ice to fruits and veggies to get a slushy consistency.

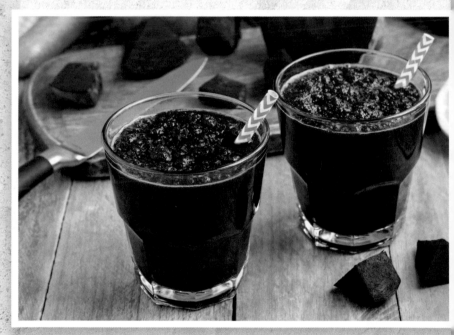

Purple Apple Slushy

Purple Apple Slushy

- 1 Granny Smith apple, cored and sliced
- 2 beets, about 8 ounces total, peeled and cut into chunks
- 2 carrots, about 4 ounces total, peeled and cut into chunks
- 1 cup ice cubes
- ¾ cup sweetened cranberry juice

Put all of the ingredients into a blender, and blend until smooth.

Apple Sunshine Smoothie

- ½ apple, seeded, halved
- 1 orange, quartered, including white part of peel
- ½-inch slice pineapple, with core
- 1 medium carrot
- ½ cup cold water
- 1 cup ice cubes

Wash apple, then put all of the ingredients into a blender, and blend until smooth.

Pineapple-Pomegranate Frosty

- ½ pineapple, chopped
  (including the core)
- 1½ cups pomegranate seeds
- a few handfuls ice

*Put all of the ingredients into a
blender, and blend until smooth.*

Papaya Peach Nectar Smoothie

- 1 medium, ripe papaya, peeled
  and seeded
- ¾ cup peach nectar
- juice of 1 lime
- 1 cup ice

*Add all the ingredients to the
blender. Pulse intermittently until it
begins to swirl. Blend on high until
smooth, about 20 seconds.*

Papaya Smoothie Shots

- 1 small papaya, peeled, seeded,
  and diced
- 1 banana, sliced
- 15 ice cubes
- ½ cup sliced strawberries
- pineapple wedges and/or
  maraschino cherries, for garnish

*Combine the papaya, banana,
strawberries and ice in a blender
and puree until smooth. Pour into
2-ounce shot glasses and garnish
with pineapple and/or cherries.*

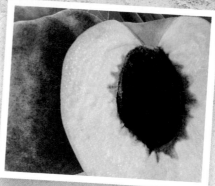

Peaches

Pineapple Passion Smoothie

- ½ pineapple
- 2 bananas
- 2 passion fruits
- 8 tablespoons pineapple juice

*Put all of the ingredients into a
blender, and blend until smooth.*

Carrot-Mango Smoothie

- 1 mango, chopped
- 2 medium carrots, peeled and
  finely grated
- a dash of freshly grated nutmeg
- 1 cup water
- 2 tablespoons lime juice
- ½ cup ice cubes

*Wash all produce, then put all of the
ingredients into a blender, and blend
until smooth.*

Spiced Apple-Carrot Smoothie

- 2 Granny Smith apples,
  cored and sliced
- 2 medium carrots, ends trimmed,
  cut into one-inch lengths
- ½ to 1 inch ginger
- ½ navel orange, peel
  and pith removed
- ½ small banana, peeled
- ½ to 1 cup water
- ¾ cup ice cubes
- 1 tablespoon golden flaxseed meal
  (optional)

*Wash all produce, then put all of the
ingredients into a blender, and blend
until smooth.*

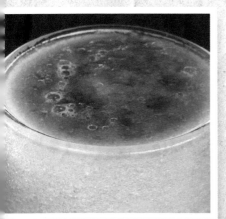

Apple Sunshine Smoothie

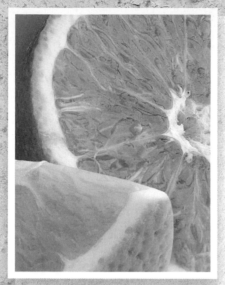

Orange slices

Grapefruit-Carrot-Ginger Smoothie

- 2 grapefruits, chopped (peel and pith removed)
- 5 carrots, chopped
- 1 inch fresh ginger, peeled and chopped

Press grapefruits, carrots, and ginger through a juice extractor. Stir and serve immediately.

Triple B with Acai Smoothie

- 2 medium bananas
- 1 blood orange
- ½ cup frozen blueberries
- ½ cup frozen blackberries
- 1 cup acai berry juice

Put all of the ingredients into a blender, and blend until smooth.

Golden Honey Smoothie

- 2 cups freshly squeezed orange juice (about 6 oranges)
- ¼ cup plus 1 tablespoon honey
- 1 tablespoon freshly squeezed lemon juice
- 2 teaspoons finely grated ginger
- 2 ripe bananas

Put all of the ingredients into a blender, and blend until smooth.

Sweet Grapefruit, Orange & Banana Smoothie

- 1 grapefruit
- 1 large orange
- 1 banana

Squeeze both the grapefruit and orange when you add them to your blender so that you have some free liquid to help blend. If you have difficulty blending this smoothie in your blender, add a little bit of water or extra squeezed orange juice.

Grapefruit Mango Smoothie

- fresh-squeezed juice from 3 grapefruits
- 1 mango, cubed
- 2 frozen bananas

Wash all produce, then put all of the ingredients into a blender, and blend until smooth.

Orange-Berry Smoothie

- 2 navel oranges, peel and pith removed, cut into chunks
- 1 cup frozen blueberries
- 1 cup frozen raspberries

Wash all produce, then put all of the ingredients into a blender, and blend until smooth.

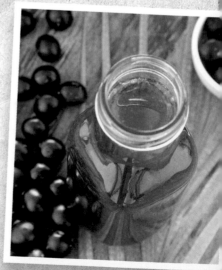

Acai juice

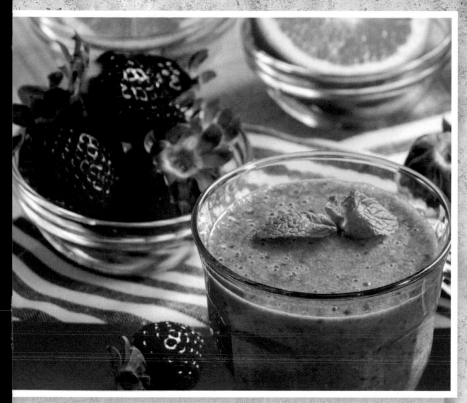

Magnificent Strawberry & Orange Smoothie

Magnificent Strawberry & Orange Smoothie

- ½ cup fresh strawberries, chopped
- ½ cup orange juice
- 5 cubes ice
- 1½ teaspoons sugar

Wash strawberries, then put all of the ingredients into a blender, and blend until smooth.

Strawberry-Grapefruit Slushy

- 1 grapefruit, peeled, seeded, and chopped
- 2 cups hulled strawberries, fresh or frozen
- 1 sweet apple (such as Honeycrisp or Pink Lady), cored and chopped
- 1 cup water
- 1-inch piece fresh ginger, peeled and chopped

Wash all produce, then put all of the ingredients into a blender, and blend until smooth.

Beet, Strawberry & Cranberry Smoothie

- ¾ cup cranberry juice, chilled
- ¼ cup cranberries, fresh or frozen
- 1 small beet, steamed
- ⅓ cup frozen strawberries
- 2 teaspoons honey or other sweetener, to taste
- ⅔ cup ice cubes

Put all of the ingredients into a blender, and blend until smooth.

Lemon-Melon Smoothie

- 1½ cups honeydew melon, diced
- ½ cup nonfat lemon yogurt
- 1 cup frozen green grapes
- 1 tablespoon fresh mint, chopped
- fresh lemon juice to taste (optional)

Combine the honeydew melon and lemon yogurt in a blender. Add the grapes and mint. Blend until smooth. Taste and add lemon juice if you like.

GREEN SMOOTHIES

"Green smoothies" aren't just vegetables—they can be any mixture of fruits, vegetables, or both, generally blended with fruit juice or water to achieve the desired consistency. And they don't even need to be the color green. The aim of the green smoothie is to get more vegetables into your body, as easily as possible. So if you really dig blueberries, make one of the berry smoothies and just throw in a handful of spinach to get used to the taste.

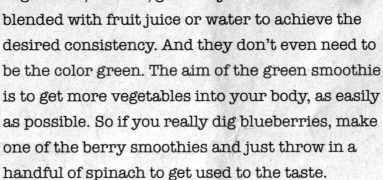

Parsley

THE HEALTHIEST ONES

Tired of a juice diet or, perhaps, of cleaning the juicer several times a day? If you want to make a switch, or at least take a break from your routine, you can get all of the benefits, including nutrients and healthy

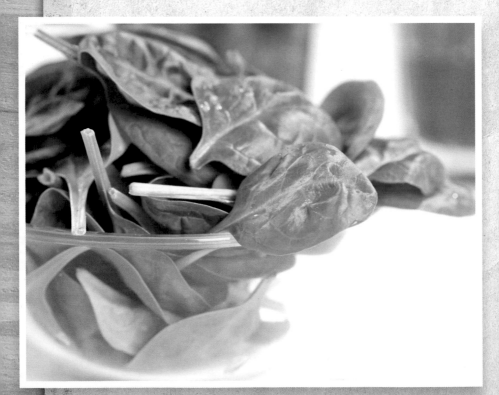

Fresh baby spinach leaves

weight loss, by throwing the same ingredients into a blender rather than a juicer. Even hard vegetables such as carrots can be cut into small pieces that can be tackled by a blender. Your kids will find smoothies every bit as delicious and scintillating as juices, and easier for them to make. If the smoothie tastes a little too "green" for you, add more fruit until you get used to the taste.

Green Tomatoes Smoothie

- 1 cup fresh parsley
- 3 stalks celery
- 3 Roma tomatoes
- ½ lemon, peeled and seeds removed
- ½ cup water
- 2 tablespoons dulse flakes

Wash all produce, then put all of the ingredients into a blender, and blend until smooth.

Spinach Smoothie with Avocado & Apple

- 1½ cups apple juice
- 2 cups spinach or kale, stemmed and chopped
- 1 apple, unpeeled, cored, and chopped
- ½ avocado, chopped

Combine the apple juice, spinach, apple, and avocado in a blender and puree until smooth, adding water to reach the desired consistency.

Healthy Start Smoothie

- 1 cup baby spinach
- 8 leaves romaine lettuce
- 2 dates, pitted
- 1 tablespoon sunflower seeds, soaked overnight
- 1 tablespoon sesame seeds, soaked overnight
- 1 banana
- 1 cup water
- 1 to 2 ounces lemon juice

Wash all produce, then put all of the ingredients into a blender, and blend until smooth.

Avocado Vanilla Smoothie

- 1 ripe avocado, chopped
- 1 cup no-sugar-added pear nectar, plus more as needed
- ½ teaspoon pure vanilla extract
- 1 cup ice cubes

Wash all produce, then puree all of the ingredients in a blender until smooth. If too thick, add more nectar to adjust consistency.

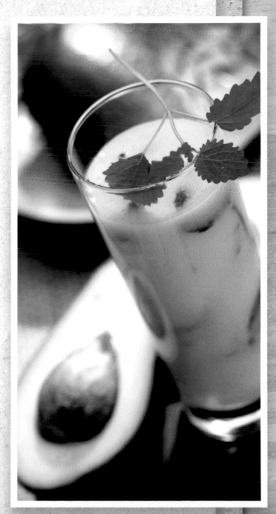

Spinach Smoothie with Avocado & Apple

GREEN AND FRUITY

A green smoothie doesn't have to be literally green. You just have to make it with nutrient-rich fresh veggies and fruits.

Spinach

UP YOUR VEGGIE INTAKE

Even if you dislike most green veggies, there is probably a combo that you can create that let's you get all their goodness while still tasting delicious. From apples to oranges and every other fruit, there is a green smoothie for everyone. You can also ditch the veggies entirely, and concoct healthy fruit smoothies that are no less "green." Green smoothies can be creamy or slushy, so add your favorite milk, yogurt, or a handful of ice to get the consistency just right.

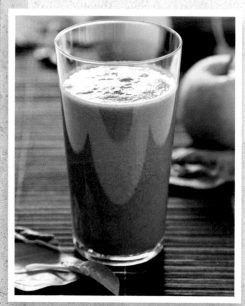

Apple-Grape Smoothie

- 2 medium apples, unpeeled and sliced
- 6 to 10 seedless grapes
- 1 tablespoon Greek yogurt
- ½ cup fresh milk (high calcium, low fat)
- 4 to 6 ice cubes

Wash the apples and grapes and drop them into a blender, pour in the milk and the yogurt, add the ice cubes, and then blend until smooth.

Apple & Almond Smoothie

Apple & Almond Smoothie

- 1 apple, sliced
- 1 cup almond milk
- 1 handful spinach
- ½ teaspoon cinnamon
- pinch of nutmeg
- 1 cup ice

Wash all produce, then put all of the ingredients into a blender, and blend until smooth. Garnish with a pinch of cinnamon and enjoy.

Apple-Lemonade Smoothie

- 1 cup water (or ½ cup water and ½ cup ice)
- 1 lemon, peeled and seeded
- 1 apple, cored, peeled, and sliced
- 1 banana
- 1 to 2 cups baby spinach
- a little honey, stevia, or maple syrup to sweeten (optional)
- ½ inch ginger (optional)

Wash all produce, then put all of the ingredients into a blender, and blend until smooth.

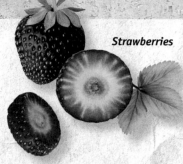

Strawberries

Strawberry-Mango Smoothie

- 2½ cups strawberries
- 1 cup pineapple
- 1 large ripe mango, peeled
- ½ to 1 head romaine lettuce
- 8 ounces filtered water

Wash all the produce, then start by adding the liquid to your blender, followed by the soft fruit. Add the greens to your blender last. Blend on high for 30 seconds or until the smoothie is creamy.

Green Pineapple & Coconut

- 1 cup fresh pineapple, chopped
- ¼ cup coconut milk
- ¼ cup vanilla- or coconut-flavored yogurt
- 1 tablespoon sweetened flaked coconut
- 3 to 4 ice cubes (optional)

Blend all ingredients until smooth. Sprinkle top with flaked coconut.

Kale & Pineapple Almond Milk Smoothie

- 1 banana, sliced into chunks, frozen is ideal
- 1 heaping cup fresh pineapple chunks
- 1 giant handful coarsely chopped kale leaves, center rib removed
- 1 cup cold almond milk
- 1 tablespoon honey (optional, for added sweetness)

Wash all the produce, then put all of the ingredients into a blender, and blend until smooth.

Pineapple-Spinach Smoothie

- ¼ cup plain, nonfat Greek yogurt or a nondairy alternative
- 1 tablespoon honey
- 2 cups lightly packed baby spinach
- ½ large apple, chunked
- 1 handful raw almonds (about 20)
- 1 cup frozen pineapple
- 3 to 4 ice cubes
- 1 cup unsweetened almond milk

Wash all produce, then put all of the ingredients into a blender, and blend until smooth.

Ban-Pin-Spin Smoothie

- 2 cups pineapple, cut into chunks
- 1 cup (8 ounces) vanilla almond milk or coconut milk
- 2 ripe bananas, peeled and sliced
- 1 to 2 cups baby spinach
- 1 cup crushed ice
- 2 tablespoons shredded toasted coconut (optional)

Blend all ingredients. Garnish with additional pineapple and toasted coconut, if desired.

Pineapple-Mango Smoothie

- 1 cup frozen pineapple
- 1 cup frozen mango pieces
- 1 cup vanilla yogurt
- ⅓ cup milk (or more, if needed)
- 2 teaspoons sugar
- 2 ice cubes (optional)

Place all of the ingredients in a blender, and blend until smooth. Add more milk if too thick or ice if too thin.

Fresh lemon

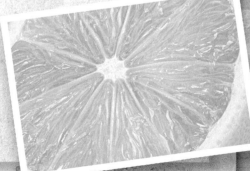

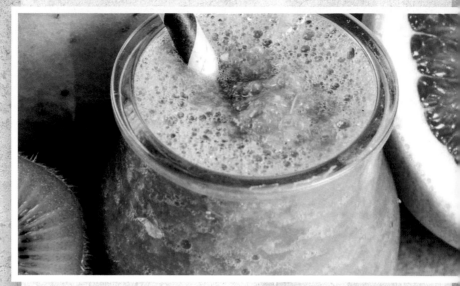

Grapefruit-Apple-Kiwi Smoothie

Orange-Banana Smoothie

- 1 large orange,
  peeled and segmented
- ½ banana, cut into chunks
- 6 large strawberries
- 2 cups spinach
- ⅓ cup plain Greek yogurt

Wash all the produce, then put all of the ingredients into a blender, and blend until smooth.

Orange-Blackcurrant Smoothie

- 1 pint blackcurrants
- 1 ripe mango
- 1 head butter lettuce
- 2 cups orange juice

Wash all the produce, then put all of the ingredients into a blender, and blend until smooth.

Orange & Green Smoothie

- 2 cups spinach, packed
- 1 mango
- 2 oranges, peeled and seeded
- 1 sprig fresh rosemary, leaves only

Wash all the produce, then put all of the ingredients into a blender, and blend until smooth.

Orange Smoothie

- 2 cups arugula
- ½ orange bell pepper
- 2 oranges, peeled and seeded
- 1 banana to make it sweeter,
  if desired

Wash all the produce, then put all of the ingredients into a blender, and blend until smooth.

Kale, Orange & Banana

- 1 orange, peeled
- ½ cup water
- 1 leaf kale, torn
  into several pieces
- 2 ripe bananas, peeled

Put all of the ingredients into a blender, and blend until smooth.

Kale-Orange Smoothie

- 1 cup kale
- 1 cup orange juice
- 2 tablespoons mint leaves
- 2 tablespoons cilantro
- 2 tablespoons parsley
- 1 cup ice

Wash all the produce, then put all of the ingredients into a blender, and blend until smooth.

Tangerine-Papaya Smoothie

- 2 tangerines, peeled and deseeded
- 2 cups papaya, cubed
- 2 cups fresh baby spinach
  (or other leafy green)
- 8 ounces tangerine juice

Wash all the produce, then put all of the ingredients into a blender, and blend until smooth.

Grapefruit-Apple-Kiwi Smoothie

- 1 grapefruit
- 1 kiwi
- 1 apple
- 1 medium banana
- 2 cups low-fat milk
- 2 tablespoons low-fat
  vanilla yogurt
- 1 teaspoon peanut butter
- 1 teaspoon flax seed
- 3 ice cubes

Wash all the produce, then put all of the ingredients into a blender, and blend until smooth.

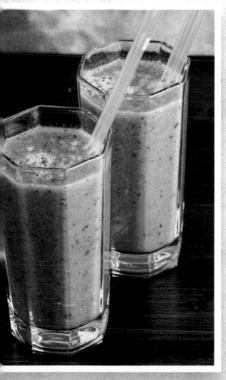

Citrus Energy Blast Smoothie

Tangerine-Coconut Smoothie

- 2 tangerines, peeled and deseeded
- 1 young green or Thai coconut
- 1 banana
- 2 cups fresh baby spinach
- 4 to 6 ounces of coconut water
- 2 celery stalks (optional)

Wash all the produce, then put all of the ingredients into a blender, and blend until smooth.

Citrus Energy Blast Smoothie

- 1 orange, peeled and chopped,
  seeds removed
- 1 lemon, peeled and chopped,
  seeds removed
- 6 spinach leaves
- 2 carrots, peeled and chopped
- 1½ cup almond milk
- 1 peach, peeled and chopped

Wash all the produce, then put all of the ingredients into a blender, and blend until smooth.

Citrus-Mango Smoothie

- 1½ mangoes
- ½ cup pineapple chunks
- ⅓ cup strawberries
- 2 large handfuls baby spinach
- 1 banana
- 1 orange
- 1 tablespoon agave nectar
- ⅓ cup water
- 1 cup ice

Wash all the produce, then put all of the ingredients into a blender, and blend until smooth.

Green Grapefruit Smoothie

- 4 to 5 kale leaves, chopped
- 2 large ripe bananas, frozen
- 1 grapefruit, peeled and cut
- 1 cup water

Wash all the produce, then put all of the ingredients into a blender, and blend until smooth.

Carrot-Apricot Smoothie

- 2 apricots
- 1 apple
- 2 cups fresh baby spinach (or other leafy green)
- 2 whole carrots
- ½ cup water

Wash all the produce, then put all of the ingredients into a blender, and blend until smooth.

Peaches & Cream Green Smoothie

- 1 cup almond milk
- 1 banana
- 2 cups spinach
- 1¼ cup frozen peach slices

Wash all the produce, then put all of the ingredients into a blender, and blend until smooth.

White Peach, Orange & Romaine Smoothie

- 2 oranges, peeled and chopped
- 1 white peach, pitted and chopped
- 4 to 6 large romaine lettuce leaves
- 1 cup ice

Wash all produce, then add oranges to blender, followed by peach, romaine, and ice. Blend on high until smooth.

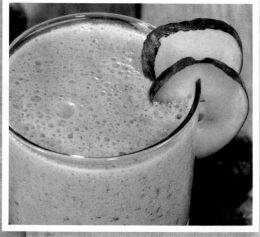

Plum-Banana Smoothie

Blueberry-Kale Smoothie

- 2 cups frozen blueberries
- 1 tablespoon Greek yogurt
- 2 to 3 cups nonfat milk
- 1 banana
- 1 cup kale
- honey (drizzled to taste)
- flaxseed (optional)

Wash all the produce, then put all of the ingredients into a blender, and blend until smooth.

Plum-Mango-Spinach Smoothie

- ½ mango
- 1 carrot
- 2 cups fresh baby spinach
- 2 plums
- 1 cup water
- ice, as needed

Wash all the produce, then put all of the ingredients into a blender, and blend until smooth.

Plum-Banana Smoothie

- 2 plums, deseeded
- 1 banana, peeled
- 2 cups fresh baby spinach (or other leafy green)
- ½ vine tomato
- ½ to 1 cup water, depending on desired consistency

Wash all the produce, then put all of the ingredients into a blender, and blend until smooth.

Plum-Watermelon Smoothie

- 2 plums, deseeded
- 2 cups watermelon
- 1 banana
- 2 cups fresh baby spinach (or other leafy green)
- 2 celery stalks, chopped
- ½ cup water, if needed

Wash all the produce, then put all of the ingredients into a blender, and blend until smooth.

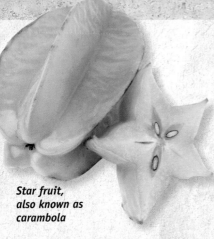

Star fruit, also known as carambola

Spinach & Strawberry Smoothie

- 1 cup water
- 1 cup spinach
- 3 cups strawberries
- 1 cup oats
- ¼ cup cashew nuts
- 7 leaves mint

Wash all the produce, then put all of the ingredients into a blender, and blend until smooth.

Star Fruit-Banana Smoothie

- 1 large star fruit, deseeded
- 1 banana, peeled
- ½ teaspoon pure vanilla extract
- 2 cups fresh baby spinach or other leafy green
- 8 ounces filtered water or coconut water

Wash all the produce, then put all of the ingredients into a blender, and blend until smooth.

Piña Carambola Smoothie

- 1 cup pineapple chunks
- 1 cup star fruit chunks
- 1 cup pineapple guava chunks
- 1 banana
- ½ bunch chard
- 2 cups water

Wash all the produce, then put all of the ingredients into a blender, and blend until smooth.

Piña Carambola Smoothie

Sweet & Sour Smoothie

- 1 cup collard greens, stems removed
- ½ cup alfalfa sprouts
- ½ pineapple
- 1 banana
- 3 medjool dates, pitted
- 3 tablespoons lemon juice
- 1 cup water

Wash all the produce, then put all of the ingredients into a blender, and blend until smooth.

Spinach-Kale-Pear Smoothie

- 1 heaping cup spinach leaves
- 1 heaping cup kale leaves, chopped
- ½ pear
- 1 frozen banana
- 1½ cups cold almond milk (or soy milk or orange juice)
- 1 tablespoon honey

Wash all produce, then remove kale leaves from the rough center stalk and coarsely chop. In a blender, combine kale, spinach, and almond milk. Blend until no big kale bits remain. Stop blender and add banana, honey, and pear. Blend until smooth.

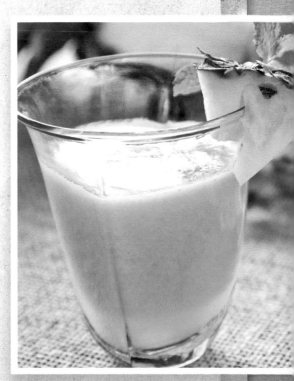

Green Magic

- 6 romaine leaves, chopped
- 4 kale leaves, chopped
- ½ cup fresh parsley sprigs
- ½ cup chopped pineapple
- ½ cup chopped mango
- 1 inch fresh ginger, peeled and chopped

Wash all the produce, then put all of the ingredients into a blender, and blend until smooth.

Spicy Green Smoothie

- 2 cups spinach
- 12 cloves garlic
- juice of 1 lemon
- ½ cucumber (add more if the smoothie is too hot)
- ¼ teaspoon cayenne pepper
- ½ teaspoon minced jalapeño pepper
- 1 cup water

Wash all the produce, then put all of the ingredients into a blender, and blend until smooth.

Blue-Green Smoothie

- 1 bunch dandelion greens
- 1 bunch fresh parsley
- 1 cup fresh blueberries
- 1 pear
- 3 cups water

Wash all the produce, then put all of the ingredients into a blender, and blend until smooth.

Dandelapple Smoothie

- 3 cups fresh dandelion greens
- 2 cups apple juice
- 1 cup water
- 1 fresh mango
- 1 ripe peach

Wash all the produce, then put all of the ingredients into a blender, and blend until smooth.

Romaine-Watermelon Smoothie

- 4 cups fresh watermelon chunks, rind removed
- 1 banana
- 5 leaves romaine lettuce
- juice of ½ lemon

Wash all the produce, then put all of the ingredients into a blender, and blend until smooth.

Sweet Romaine Smoothie

- 1 cup ice
- 1 cup nondairy milk
- 1 cup strawberries
- 1 banana or 1 cup mango chunks or 1 small mango
- 1 cup pineapple
- 1 apple
- 1 cup chopped romaine lettuce
- 2 tablespoons pumpkin seeds
- ½ cup dried apricots
- 1 cup oats

Wash all produce, then blend the ingredients in the order listed. Ground the oats into flour to make smoother. Add more water if required.

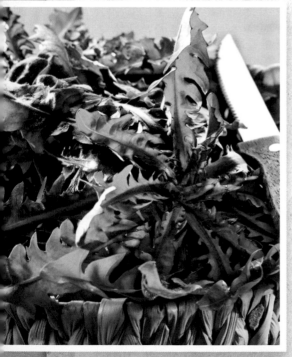

Freshly cut dandelion greens (above); Dandelapple Smoothie (opposite)

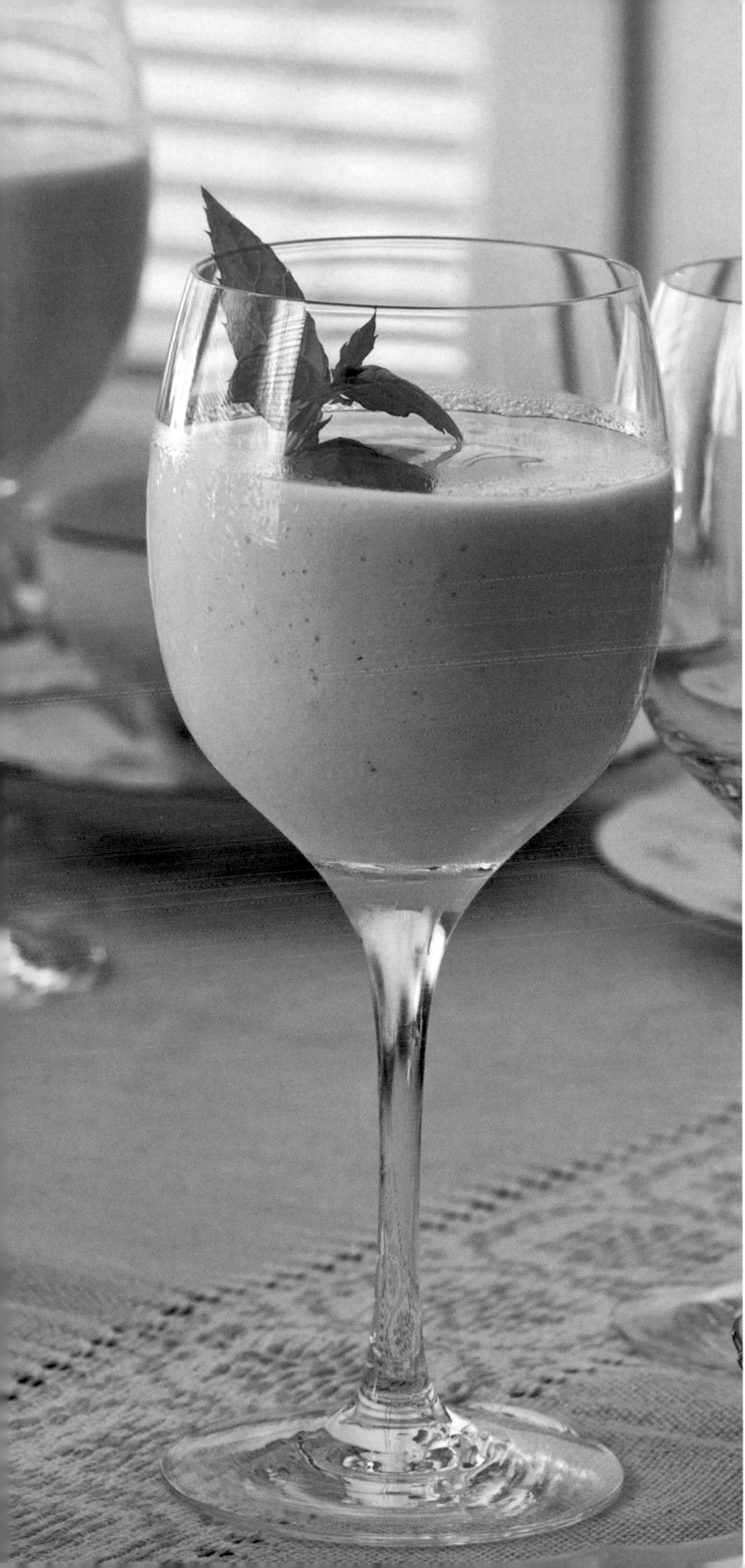

APPETIZER SMOOTHIES

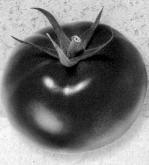

Tomato

A smoothie can be a sophisticated starter at your next dinner party.

FROSTY ELEGANCE

Vichyssoise and a variety of other fruit- or vegetable-based concoctions can be served in a bowl with a spoon, while pineapple and lemon juice combined with sparkling wine makes a delicious cocktail. To achieve their subtlety, these recipes have more ingredients than most of the other smoothies in this book.

TOMATO GAZPACHO

- 2 pounds tomatoes, chopped
- 1 cucumber, peeled and diced
- ¼ cup olive oil
- 2 slices day-old bread
- 1 tablespoon garlic, minced

Combine tomatoes with cucumber, olive oil, day-old bread, and garlic in a food processor or blender; process until chunky-smooth.

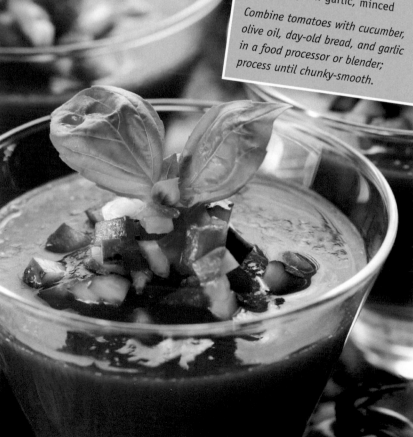

Watermelon Gazpacho

- ½ pound tomatoes, chopped
- 1½ pounds watermelon, seeded and cubed
- 1 cucumber, peeled and diced
- 1 handful mint leaves
- ¼ cup olive oil
- 2 tablespoons lemon juice

Combine tomatoes with watermelon, cucumber, mint leaves, and olive oil in a food processor or blender; process until chunky-smooth. Add lemon juice. Garnish with chopped mint.

Radish Gazpacho

- 1 pound tomatoes, chopped
- 1 pound radishes with leaves, chopped
- 1 cucumber, peeled and diced
- ¼ cup olive oil
- 1 slice day-old bread
- a few scallions, chopped
- 2 tablespoons lime juice
- ¼ teaspoon Worcestershire sauce

Combine tomatoes and radishes with cucumber, olive oil, day-old bread, scallions, lime juice, Worcestershire sauce, and water as needed in a food processor or blender; process until chunky-smooth. Garnish with a drizzle of fresh lime juice.

Vichyssoise Smoothie

- 2 tablespoons butter
- 3 potatoes, peeled and cubed
- 3 leeks, trimmed and chopped
- 4 cups stock
- ½ cup cream
- ½ chive, chopped, for garnish

Wash all produce, then melt butter in a large pot. Add potatoes and leeks. Cook for about 3 minutes, stirring until softened. Add stock. Boil, cover, lower the heat, and simmer until vegetables are tender, about 20 minutes. Puree, then let cool. Stir in cream before serving. Garnish with chopped chives.

Sparkling Wine & Pineapple

- 2 cups sparkling wine
- 3 cups pineapple, freshly grated
- 2 tablespoons lemon juice
- toasted coconut, for garnish

Combine sparkling wine, pineapple flesh, and lemon juice in a bowl; stir gently, and serve immediately. Garnish with toasted coconut.

Melon & Mint Delight

- 2 cups yogurt
- ¼ cup milk
- 1 cup mint leaves, chopped
- 1 medium ripe cantaloupe or honeydew melon
- 2 tablespoons lime juice
- 1 teaspoon chili powder

In a bowl, whisk together yogurt, milk, and mint leaves until mint is fragrant; strain and discard solids. In another bowl, combine the grated flesh of the melon, lime juice, and chili powder; refrigerate bowls for 2 hours, stirring once. To serve, spoon yogurt onto melon and stir. Garnish with mint leaves.

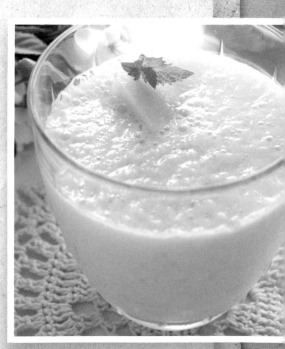

Melon & Mint Delight (above); Tomato Gazpacho (opposite)

PROTEIN SMOOTHIES

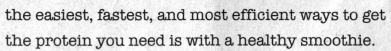

Whey protein powder

Protein is essential to build, maintain, and repair our bodies. One of the easiest, fastest, and most efficient ways to get the protein you need is with a healthy smoothie.

HEALTHY ADDITIONS

Use any of these recipes to start your day, fuel up before a workout, or replenish your muscles after you've finished training. In any of the following shakes, feel free to add a tablespoon of ground flaxseed, and go with extra or no ice.

PROTEIN SUPPLEMENTS

Protein supplements can be broadly classified into two groups: those that provide protein only, and those that provide both protein and carbohydrates. Both types often include additional ergogenic (performance-boosting) ingredients, such as vitamins, minerals, creatine, specific amino acids, and proposed fat metabolizers.

Protein-only supplements are typically 90% protein by weight, while those with added carbohydrates vary (with the protein content as little as 10% up to 50%). Protein that contains essential amino acids in a proportion similar to that required by humans is said to have a high biological value (HBV). There is a wide range of protein supplements available. Use only the amount specified by the manufacturer, and keep in mind that it is generally necessary to increase water intake when ingesting these.

• **Whey protein:** This is a HBV protein that is rapidly digested, and is comprised of approximately 20% dairy protein. Whey is rich in branched-chain amino acids, especially leucine, the amino acid primarily responsible for stimulating protein synthesis. Recent evidence suggests that whey protein may offer greater satiety than other whole proteins, alluding to a potential role in weight loss as well as weight gain. There are three main forms of whey protein:

Vanilla-flavored whey protein powder

Scoops of whey protein isolate and egg white powder sound like odd ingredients in a book of raw foods, specifically juices and smoothies designed to make up for an inability to consume the recommended number of servings a day. Yet these are standard—and essential—ingredients in many protein smoothies. Both are dried forms of protein-rich material, milk and egg whites respectively, and jump-start your morning. Protein smoothies are particularly intended to give you a burst of energy to get going (or, indeed, before a bodybuilding workout or any other physical exercise), and have been credited in increases in lean muscle.

Protein shaker set. A wire ball mixing whisk helps make sure the powder blends completely.

Whey protein concentrate (WPC): Derived from the first filtering step in the production of whey protein isolate, it is typically 70 to 80% protein by weight with small amounts of lactose (milk sugar) and fat. It is cheaper than whey protein isolate.

Whey protein isolate (WPI): Further filtration of WPC produces this powder that is approximately 90% protein by weight, with negligible amounts of carbohydrates (lactose) and fat.

Whey protein hydrolysate (WPH): This is derived from either WPC or WPI and claims to assist in even more rapid digestion and absorption, with greater insulin response. Evidence to date is conflicting. The process of hydrolysis used to produce the powder is more expensive and produces a bitter taste.

• **Casein or calcium caseinate:** This HBV protein makes up about 80% of the protein in milk. Casein forms clots in the stomach, slowing digestion and the delivery of amino acids to the body. Casein hydrolysates are also available, resulting in a more rapidly digested and absorbed protein.

• **Soy protein:** This HBV protein is rapidly digested. As with whey, soy protein is available as both a soy concentrate and a soy isolate, and is often used in supplements made up of protein from mixed sources because it is cheaper than whey. There is evidence to suggest that women with existing or pre-existing breast cancer should be cautious in consuming large quantities of soy foods. Talk to your doctor before incorporating soy into your diet.

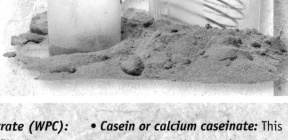

Soy protein powder

Burn Smoothie

- 1½ cups water or unsweetened almond milk
- 2 scoops egg white powder or whey protein isolate
- 8 strawberries
- 1 tablespoon raw almond butter or ground flaxseed
- 6 ice cubes

Wash all the produce, then put all of the ingredients into a blender, and blend until smooth.

Daddy Shake

- 1½ cups fresh orange juice
- 2 scoops egg white powder or whey protein isolate
- 1 banana
- 2 tablespoons almond butter or natural peanut butter
- 6 ice cubes

Put all of the ingredients into a blender or shaker, and blend until smooth.

Preworkout Shake

- 1 to 1½ cups water
- 1 banana
- 4 ice cubes

Put all of the ingredients into a blender, and blend until smooth.

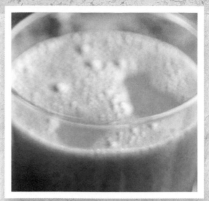

Orange juice

Rise & Shine Smoothie

- 1½ to 2 cups fresh-squeezed orange juice
- 2 scoops egg white powder or vanilla whey protein powder
- 1 banana
- ¼ cup Greek yogurt
- 2 teaspoons organic vanilla extract
- 1 tablespoon ground flaxseed
- 1 tablespoon lecithin (optional)

Put all of the ingredients into a blender, and blend until smooth.

Tropical Surprise Shake

- 1½ cups water or orange juice
- 1 scoop whey protein isolate
- ¼ cup each of as many fruits as you can find in the fridge
- 1 banana
- 6 ice cubes

Wash all the produce, then put all of the ingredients into a blender, and blend until smooth.

Blueberry Boost

- 1 cup unsweetened vanilla almond milk
- 1 frozen banana
- ½ cup blueberries
- 1 scoop unflavored or vanilla protein powder

Wash all the produce, then put all of the ingredients into a blender, and blend until smooth.

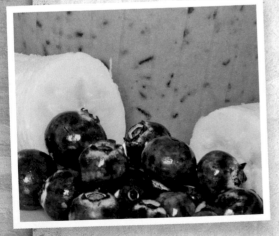

**Blueberry Boost (above);
Preworkout Shake (opposite)**

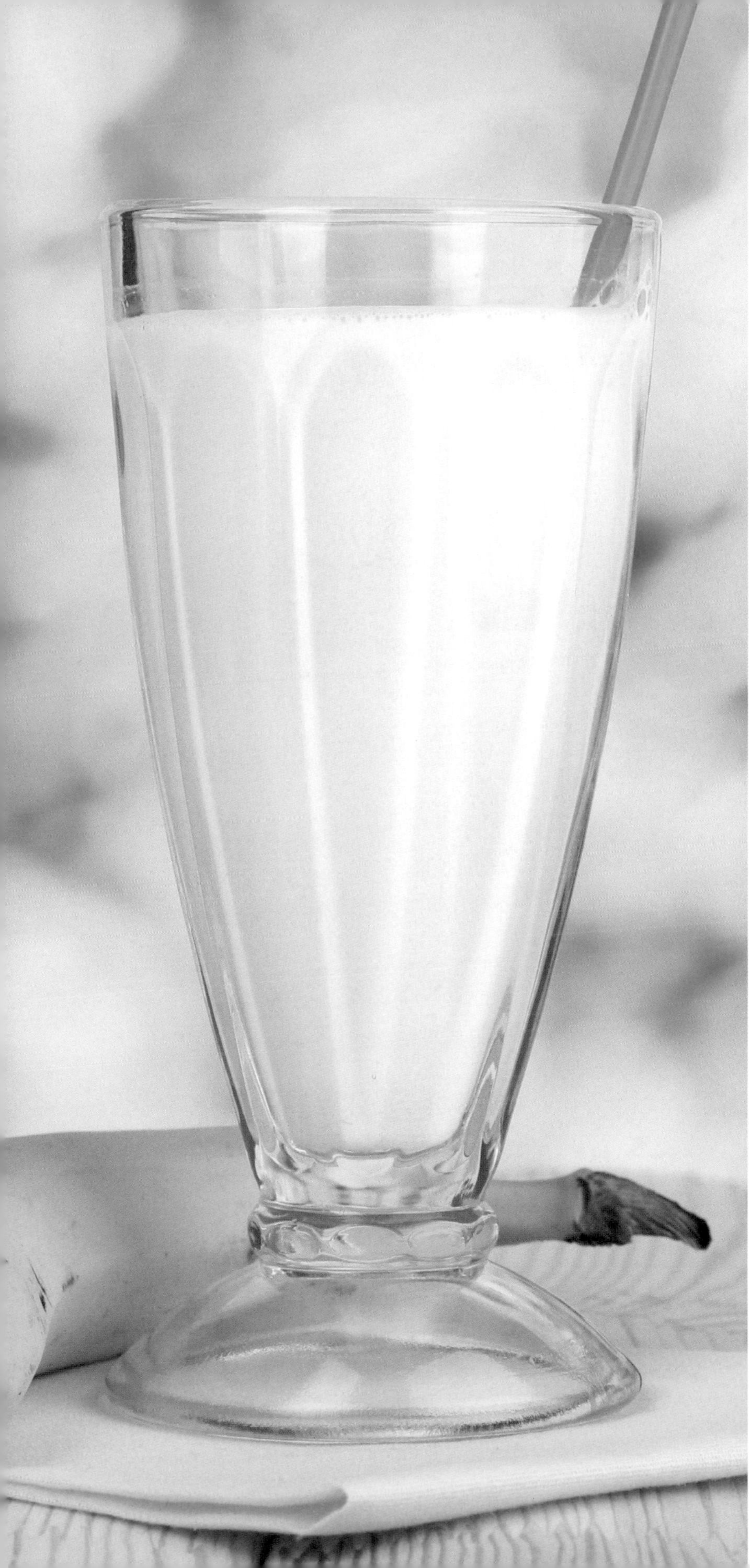

Kiwi-Spirulina Smoothie

- 2 kiwis (peel on or off)
- ½ cup pineapple or ½ banana
- ½ cup cucumber
- 1 handful spinach
- ½ lemon or lime, peeled
- 1 to 2 tablespoons chia seeds
- 1 teaspoon spirulina powder
- 1 cup coconut water or nut milk

Put all of the ingredients into a blender, and blend until smooth.

Blueberry-Spirulina Smoothie

- 1 frozen banana
- ½ cup frozen blueberries
- ½ cup frozen raspberries
- 1 cup spinach
- 1 cup coconut water
- 1 teaspoon spirulina powder

Put all of the ingredients into a blender, and blend until smooth.

SPIRULINA

Spirulina is blue-green algae found in salt water and is promoted as a source of dietary protein, vitamin A, B vitamins (especially B12), and iron. Similar products have been around for a long time and are said to be beneficial for many conditions, ranging from hay fever to the prevention of precancerous growths in the mouth. So far, however, there isn't enough evidence to determine whether or not they are effective. Other claims say spirulina is a good appetite suppressant and boosts energy levels.

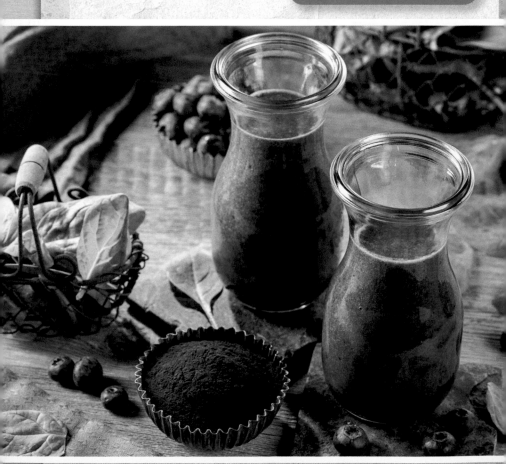

Blueberry-Spirulina Smoothie

Tropical Boost

- 1 cup unsweetened vanilla almond milk
- 1 cup frozen pineapple
- 1 teaspoon shredded coconut or coconut milk
- ½ cup frozen blueberries
- 1 scoop unflavored or vanilla protein powder

Put all of the ingredients into a blender, and blend until smooth.

Piña Colada Protein Smoothie

- ½ cup pineapple, chopped
- ½ frozen banana
- 1 scoop vanilla protein
- ½ cup unsweetened coconut milk
- ½ cup water
- crushed ice

Put all of the ingredients into a blender, and blend until smooth.

Strawberry Papaya Smoothie

- ½ cup strawberries
- 1 cup papaya, sliced
- 1 cup nonfat plain Greek yogurt
- ½ cup water
- crushed ice

Wash all the produce, then put all of the ingredients into a blender, and blend until smooth.

Chocolate Chip Smoothie

- 1 cup unsweetened chocolate almond milk
- 1 tablespoon natural almond
- 1 frozen banana (peel before freezing)
- 1 tablespoon cacao nibs
- 1 cup raw spinach
- 1 scoop chocolate protein powder
- a dash of red pepper flakes
- whipped cream, for garnish

Wash all the produce, then put all of the ingredients into a blender, and blend until smooth.

Peanut Butter Banana Smoothie

- 1 cup frozen banana, sliced
- 1 ounce natural peanut butter
- ½ cup 1% milk
- 1 tablespoon honey

Put all of the ingredients into a blender, and blend until smooth.

Watermelon Mint

- 1 cup watermelon, cubed
- ½ cup liquid egg whites
- mint sprigs
- crushed ice

Wash all the produce, then put all of the ingredients into a blender, and blend until smooth.

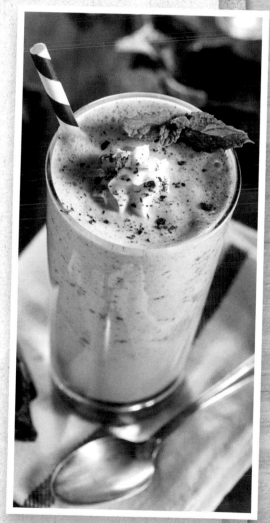

Chocolate Chip Smoothie

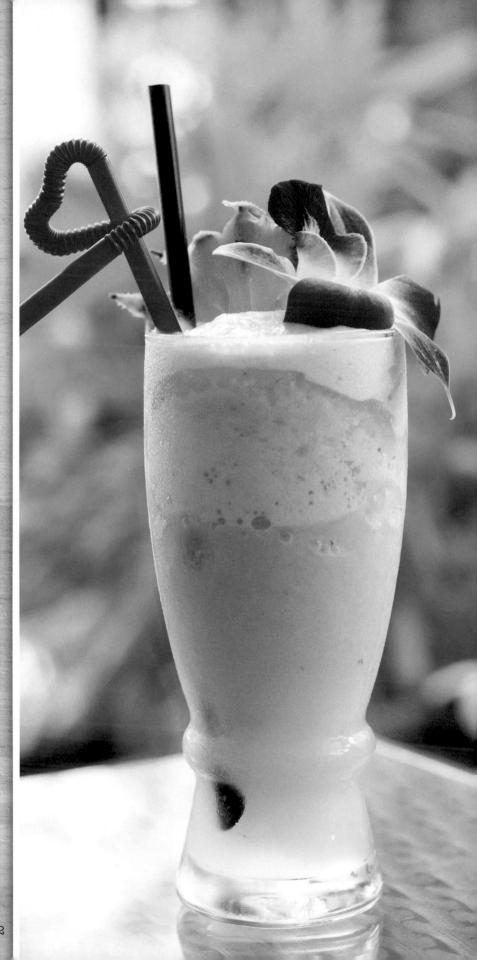

Strawberry-Banana Protein Smoothie

- 1 banana
- 1¼ cups fresh strawberries, sliced
- 10 whole almonds
- 2 tablespoons water
- 1 cup ice cubes
- 3 tablespoons chocolate-flavored protein powder

Place the banana, strawberries, water, and almonds into a blender. Blend to mix, then add the ice cubes and puree until smooth. Add the protein powder, and continue mixing until evenly incorporated, about 30 seconds.

Cranberry-Coco Blast

- 1 tablespoon dried, unsweetened cranberries
- ½ cup frozen cherries
- ½ tablespoon chia seeds
- ½ tablespoon flaxseeds
- ⅓ cup nonfat plain Greek yogurt
- ½ cup unsweetened coconut milk
- crushed ice

Put all of the ingredients into a blender, and blend until smooth.

Coco-Mango Cooldown

- 1 cup mango, chopped
- ½ cup unsweetened coconut milk
- 1 scoop vanilla protein powder

Wash all the produce, then put all of the ingredients into a blender, and blend until smooth.

Coolatta Shake

- 1 scoop chocolate or vanilla whey protein powder
- 6 ounces unsweetened almond milk (or milk of choice)
- 4 ice cubes
- 1 tablespoon Nutella
- 1 to 2 teaspoons instant coffee

Put all of the ingredients into a blender, and blend until smooth.

Cranberry-Orange Power Protein Smoothie

- 1 cup cranberry juice
- 1 large banana
- 1 medium orange, peeled and segmented
- ½ cup strawberries, hulled
- ¼ cup raspberry sherbet
- 1 cup ice cubes
- ¼ cup whey protein powder

Place all ingredients in a blender. Blend on high speed until smooth, about one minute. Adjust the consistency by adding more sherbet if it's too thin, or more cranberry juice if it's too thick. Pour into two glasses and use a straw!

Peanut Boost

- 1 scoop vanilla protein powder
- 6 ounces unsweetened almond milk (or milk of choice)
- 3 to 4 ice cubes
- 1 tablespoon natural, chunky peanut butter
- 1 tablespoon sugar-free instant butterscotch pudding mix

Put all of the ingredients into a blender, and blend until smooth.

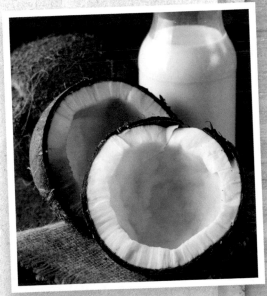

Coconuts and coconut milk (above); Coco-Mango Cooldown (opposite)

Power Protein Super Smoothie

- 2 cups mixed berries, fresh or frozen
- 1 cup silken tofu
- ¼ cup pomegranate juice
- 2 to 3 tablespoons honey
- 2 tablespoons ground flaxseed
- 1 teaspoon ginger, finely grated and peeled

In a blender, combine berries, tofu, pomegranate juice, 2 tablespoons honey, flaxseed, and ginger. Blend until smooth, 15 to 20 seconds.

Cranberry Protein Smoothie

- 1¼ cups unsweetened cranberry juice
- 2 scoops protein powder
- 5 ice cubes

Put all of the ingredients into a blender, and blend until smooth.

Fruit & Yogurt Smoothie

- 1½ cups plain nonfat yogurt
- ½ medium pear, chopped and peeled
- 1 small banana, sliced
- 2 tablespoons protein powder
- ¾ cup crushed ice

Wash all the produce, then put all of the ingredients into a blender, and blend until smooth.

Stay-Youthful Smoothie

- ½ cup frozen organic blueberries
- ½ cup frozen organic strawberries
- ½ cup chilled green tea
- ¾ cup plain low-fat yogurt
- 2 tablespoons ground flaxseed
- turbinado sugar or other natural sweetener, to taste

Wash all the produce, then put all of the ingredients into a blender, and blend until smooth. Garnish with fresh berries and serve.

Strawberry-Banana Tofu Shake

- 1 package (10 ounces) frozen, unsweetened strawberries, thawed
- 1 cup plain soy milk
- 1 small, ripe banana peeled and sliced
- ¼ cup honey
- 1 package (12 ounces) silken or soft tofu, drained
- 2 tablespoons fresh lemon juice
- a pinch of salt

In a blender, puree berries until smooth. Remove, and rinse blender. Combine the remaining ingredients, pureeing until smooth and thoroughly mixed, scraping down sides with rubber spatula as necessary. Divide among glasses and spoon strawberry puree on one side of each glass.

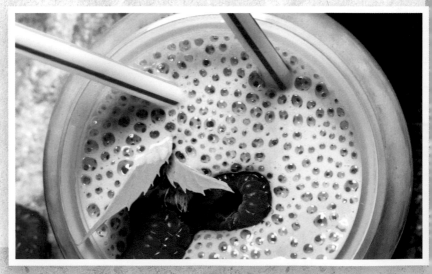

Strawberry-Banana Tofu Shake (above); Cherry-Tea Smoothie (opposite)

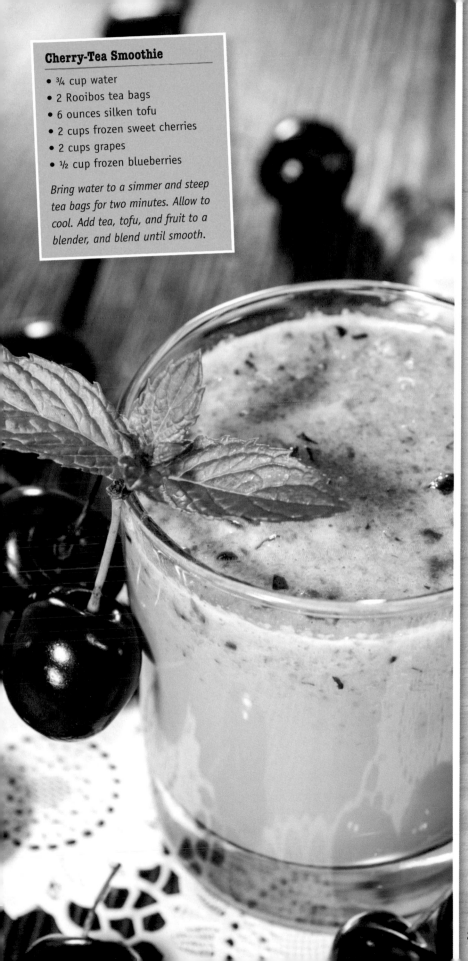

Cherry-Tea Smoothie

- ¾ cup water
- 2 Rooibos tea bags
- 6 ounces silken tofu
- 2 cups frozen sweet cherries
- 2 cups grapes
- ½ cup frozen blueberries

Bring water to a simmer and steep tea bags for two minutes. Allow to cool. Add tea, tofu, and fruit to a blender, and blend until smooth.

JUST FOR KIDS

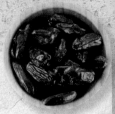

Dates

Growing kids need lots of nourishment and sustained energy throughout the day. Get them the nutrition they need with healthy smoothies.

CHILDREN'S UNIQUE NEEDS

Like adults, children need a balanced diet with plenty of fresh fruit and vegetables (two servings of fruit and at least five servings of nonstarchy vegetables per day); moderate amounts of protein, grains, and starchy carbohydrates; and small amounts of "good" fats, such as omega-3 fats. Depending on their age, gender, size, and level of activity, their energy needs will vary but will tend to be quite high.

Children need fiber, but not quite as much as adults. Too much can result in filling his or her small stomach quickly, resulting in a lack of other essential nutrients. In a balanced diet, which should also include plenty of water, most children will get sufficient fiber through fruits, vegetables, and whole grains without the need for fiber supplements.

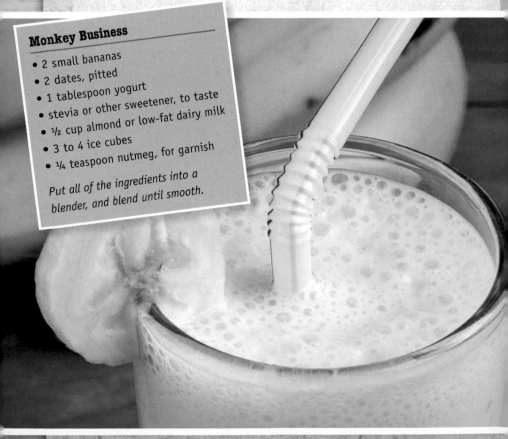

Monkey Business

- 2 small bananas
- 2 dates, pitted
- 1 tablespoon yogurt
- stevia or other sweetener, to taste
- ½ cup almond or low-fat dairy milk
- 3 to 4 ice cubes
- ¼ teaspoon nutmeg, for garnish

Put all of the ingredients into a blender, and blend until smooth.

Monkey Business

HEALTHY SNACKING

Kids are more likely than adults to need snacks between meals, or to require six smaller meals over the course of a day rather than three. This is partly because their small stomachs may not be able to take in sufficient nutrients to sustain them between meals. Children, especially energetic and fast-growing ones, may also need to eat between meals to maintain their blood sugar levels so that a drop does not make them tired and irritable. Some kids might simply feel hungry between meals and need a nutritious snack. A delicious and healthy smoothie is ideal for this purpose.

Children need all the vitamins and minerals that adults do, but have particularly high needs for calcium (for bones and teeth), vitamin D (which works with calcium to build strong bones), B-group vitamins (for metabolism, release of energy, and a healthy heart and nervous system). They also need vitamin E (to support the immune system and to keep blood vessels healthy), iron (to help red blood cells carry oxygen around the body), and zinc (for immunity).

HIDE THE VEGGIES

Many children don't like the taste of vegetables. Blending a few into a fruit-based smoothie is one way to introduce more of them into a child's diet, and if careful choices are made, the change in taste will be imperceptible. Spinach, for example, is wonderfully nutritious but seems to be one of the most hated vegetables among children, second only to brussels sprouts. A few baby leaves of spinach will blend into a child's smoothie unnoticed, immediately upping its nutritional value.

Smoothies are a fun way to help keep a child's diet nutritious—and they should look fun too. Few children are likely to be willing to consume a dark-green concoction that looks suspiciously like . . . liquefied spinach. A little bit of sweetener goes a long way, but use it only if necessary to introduce new flavors, and try to wean children off it as they become more accustomed to natural flavors. Give the drinks silly names, if that helps. Here are a few to get you started.

THINK ABOUT IT!

Many of these recipes call for milk, and in each case, either almond milk or low-fat dairy can be used. Low-fat dairy milk is an excellent choice because it is much higher in calcium than almond milk and also a good source of vitamin B12, which is so important for children. On the other hand, almond milk is generally lower in calories and is a good substitute for children who may not be able to tolerate dairy milk. Most commercial brands of almond milk are fortified with nutrients; look for ones that contain vitamins B12, A, and E, as well as calcium and other nutrients.

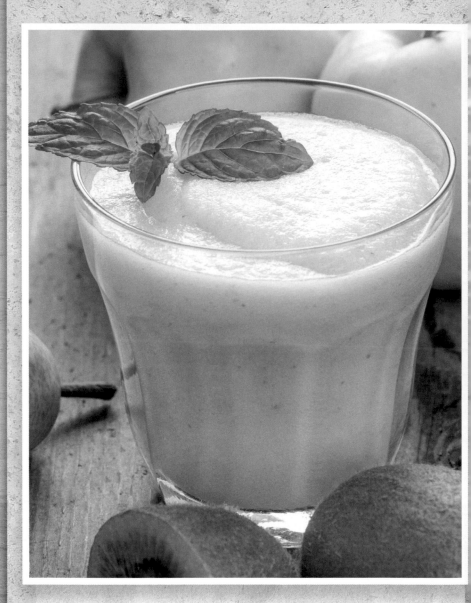

Tutti Frutti

- ¼ cup pineapple, peeled and cored
- 1 orange, peeled and deseeded
- 1 lemon, peeled and deseeded
- 1 apple, deseeded
- 1 kiwifruit, peeled
- ½ ruby grapefruit, peeled and deseeded
- 1 small handful baby spinach leaves
- ¼ cup mineral water
- 3 to 4 ice cubes

Wash all the produce, then put all of the ingredients into a blender, and blend until smooth.

Slimy Green Granny

- 4 kiwifruits, peeled
- 1 Granny Smith apple, cored and sliced
- 1 handful small spinach leaves, or other leafy green veggie
- stevia or other sweetener, to taste
- ½ cup water
- ½ cup ice cubes
- mint leaves

Wash all the produce, then put all of the ingredients into a blender, and blend until smooth.

Slimy Green Granny (above); Appattack (opposite)

Chocaberry Blitz

- 2 tablespoons cacao
- 1 tablespoon cannellini beans
- ½ cup strawberries
- ½ cup raspberries
- stevia or other sweetener, to taste
- ½ cup almond milk
- 3 to 4 ice cubes

Wash all the produce, then put all of the ingredients into a blender, and blend until smooth.

Manana Bango

- 1 mango, peeled and pitted
- 1 banana, peeled
- 1 tablespoon oats
- 1 tablespoon yogurt
- ½ cup almond milk
- nutmeg and lemon slice, for garnish

Wash all the produce, then put all of the ingredients into a blender, and blend until smooth.

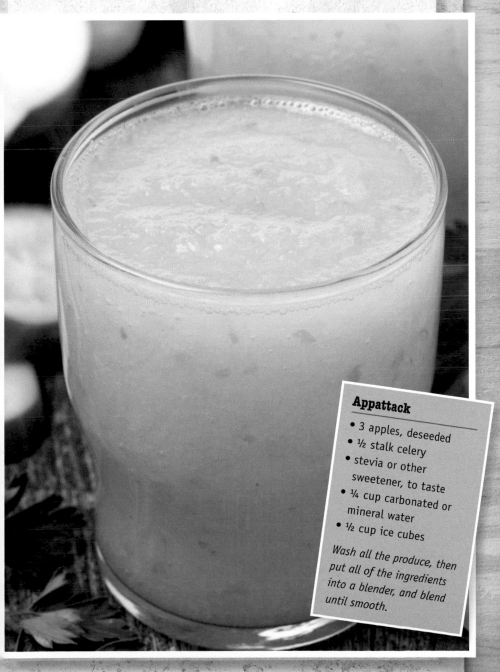

Appattack

- 3 apples, deseeded
- ½ stalk celery
- stevia or other sweetener, to taste
- ¼ cup carbonated or mineral water
- ½ cup ice cubes

Wash all the produce, then put all of the ingredients into a blender, and blend until smooth.

Bells of Saint Clemens

- 2 lemons, peeled and deseeded
- 2 oranges, peeled and deseeded
- ½ carrot
- 1 small handful cabbage leaves
- ½ cup mineral water
- 3 to 4 ice cubes

Wash all the produce, then put all of the ingredients into a blender, and blend until smooth.

Chocolate Milkshake

Chocolate Milkshake

- 2 tablespoons cacao
- 1 small handful baby spinach leaves
- 2 tablespoons yogurt
- stevia or other sweetener, to taste
- ½ cup almond milk
- 3 to 4 ice cubes
- berries, for garnish

Wash all the produce, then put all of the ingredients into a blender, and blend until smooth.

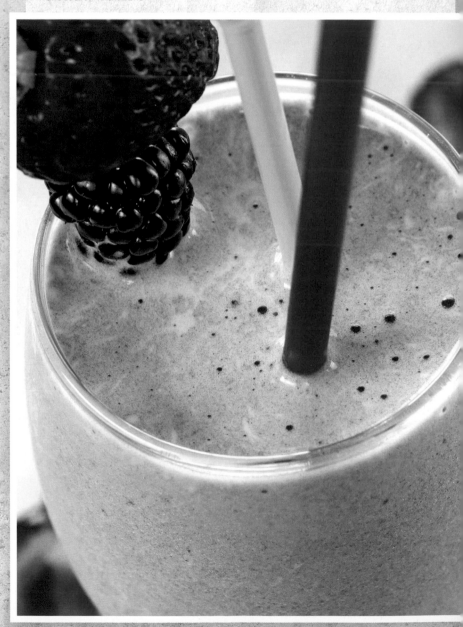

Orange Fizz

- 4 oranges, peeled and deseeded
- ½ small carrot
- ¼ cup carbonated or mineral water
- 3 to 4 ice cubes

Wash all the produce, then put all of the ingredients into a blender, and blend until smooth.

Raspberry Ripper

- 2 cups raspberries
- 1 small beet, peeled
- stevia or other sweetener, to taste
- ½ cup coconut water or water
- 3 to 4 ice cubes

Wash all the produce, then put all of the ingredients into a blender, and blend until smooth.

Pretty in Pink

- 1 cup strawberries
- 2 tablespoons yogurt
- ½ cup almond or low-fat dairy milk
- stevia or other sweetener, to taste
- 3 to 4 ice cubes

Wash all the produce, then put all of the ingredients into a blender, and blend until smooth.

Orange and Mango Spider

Ingredients for the syrup
- 1 tablespoon honey
- 1 orange, juice only
- ¼ cup water

Ingredients for the smoothie
- 1 mango, peeled and pitted
- 1 orange, peeled and deseeded
- ½ small carrot
- 2 tablespoons plain frozen yogurt
- 1 cup carbonated or mineral water

Wash all the produce, then put all of the ingredients into a blender, and blend until smooth.

TOP 10 SMOOTHIE TIPS

1. *Smoothie too thick?* If your smoothie is too thick, just add some extra water.
2. *Smoothie too thin?* Add some fibrous ingredients such as apple, banana, mango, avocado, or even oats, flaxseeds, or chia seeds.
3. *Get the most from your smoothie.* Ensure that the main ingredients are fresh fruits and/or vegetables.
4. *Try frozen fruit.* Mix in some frozen fruits and veggies instead of ice, or if certain fresh ingredients are not available—but always be sure the main ingredients are fresh fruit and vegetables.
5. *Wash the ingredients.* Always wash vegetables and fruit before using.
6. *If fiber is needed . . .* Seeds, such as chia and flaxseed, are great sources of dietary fiber.
7. *Make your own milk alternative.* You can make many of the nut milks on your own—homemade almond milk, for example, is both delicious and nutritious.
8. *Give a yogurt boost.* Yogurt added to smoothies can boost their nutritional value, improve digestion, and offer a huge range of benefits specific to yogurt.
9. *Add some grains and nuts.* Add grains to your smoothie—oats work particularly well, giving a smooth richness when blended with water. High-protein quinoa is also very nutritious.
10. *Tempt a fussy palate.* A healthier option than sugar is to sweeten smoothies naturally through the use of fruit. Some herbs, such as mint, can also have a sweetening effect without a significant calorie increase, as do small amounts of cinnamon and vanilla.

SMOOTHIE POPS

Get all the goodness of smoothies and juices in a frozen treat that kids (and adults) will love. You can hide the taste of healthy greens like spinach with sweet fruits, such as kiwi.

Strawberry

Strawberry & Blueberry Smoothie Pops

- 1 cup plain yogurt
- 1 medium banana
- ¾ cup strawberries, fresh or frozen
- ¼ cup blueberries, fresh or frozen
- ⅛ cup honey

Wash all the produce, then put all of the ingredients into a blender, and blend until smooth. Pour mixture into Popsicle molds, and freeze.

Very Berry Smoothie Pops

- ½ cup Greek yogurt
- ½ cup milk of your choice
- 1 cup mixed raspberries and blueberries, frozen

Put all of the ingredients into a blender, and blend until smooth. Pour mixture into Popsicle molds, and freeze.

Lemon-Lime Smoothie Pops

- ¼ cup lime juice
- zest of 1 lime
- ¼ cup lemon juice
- zest of 1 lemon
- 2 cups Greek yogurt
- ½ tablespoon vanilla extract
- 2 tablespoons honey

Put all of the ingredients into a blender, and blend until smooth. Pour mixture into Popsicle molds, and freeze.

Orange Juice Smoothie Pops

- 6½ ounces orange juice
- 2 teaspoons lemon juice
- 1 tablespoon honey
- ½ teaspoon vanilla essence

Put all of the ingredients into a blender, and blend until smooth. Pour mixture into Popsicle molds, and freeze.

Kiwichia Smoothie Pops

- 6 ounces vanilla yogurt
- 3 kiwis, peeled
- 1 banana, sliced
- 1 tablespoon chia seeds (optional)

Put all of the ingredients into a blender, and blend until smooth. Pour mixture into Popsicle molds, and freeze.

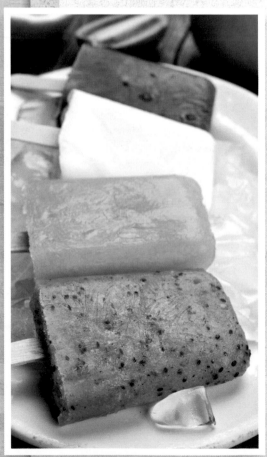

Assorted smoothie pops, from top to bottom: Very Berry, Lemon-Lime, Orange Juice, and Kiwichia

THINK ABOUT IT!

If you don't have Popsicle molds, it's easy to make your own. Just pour the smoothie mixture into paper cups, cupcake paper, plastic cups—just about any freezable container will do. Place in freezer. Once the mixture is partially frozen, insert sticks, and voila!

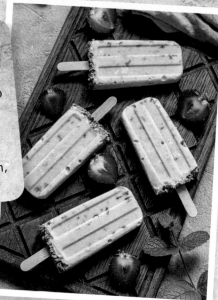

Striped Key Lime & Kiwi Smoothie Pops

Ingredients for the green layer

- 2 kiwis, peeled
- juice of 1 key lime
- ¼ cup spinach
- ½ avocado, stone removed
- ½ cup vanilla almond milk
- 1 teaspoon honey

Ingredients for the white layer

- ¼ cup key lime juice
- zest of 1 key lime
- 1½ cups Greek yogurt
- ½ tablespoon vanilla extract
- 1½ tablespoons honey

Wash all the produce, then put all of the ingredients into a blender, and blend until smooth. Pour mixture into Popsicle molds, and freeze.

Strawberries & Cream Graham Cracker Smoothie Pops

Strawberries & Cream Graham Cracker Smoothie Pops

- 2 cups frozen strawberries
- 1 container plain Greek yogurt
- 1 cup vanilla almond milk
- 1 tablespoon vanilla extract
- 1 tablespoon honey
- 1 cup graham crackers, crushed

Put all of the ingredients into a blender, and blend until smooth. Divide graham crackers evenly between Popsicle molds, then pour mixture over them, and freeze.

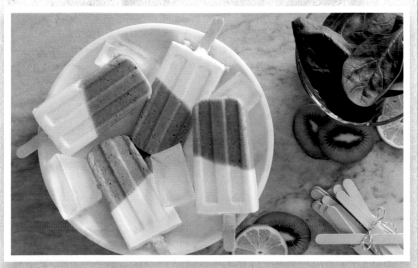

Striped Key Lime & Kiwi Smoothie Pops

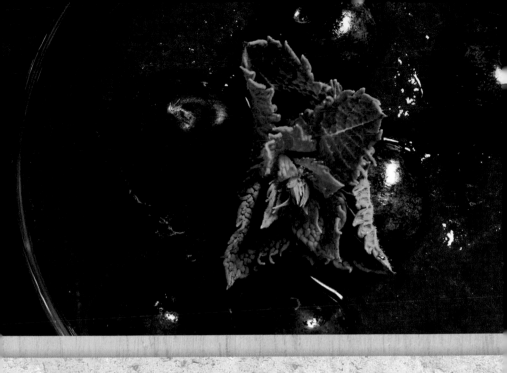

CHAPTER 7
TARGETED SMOOTHIES

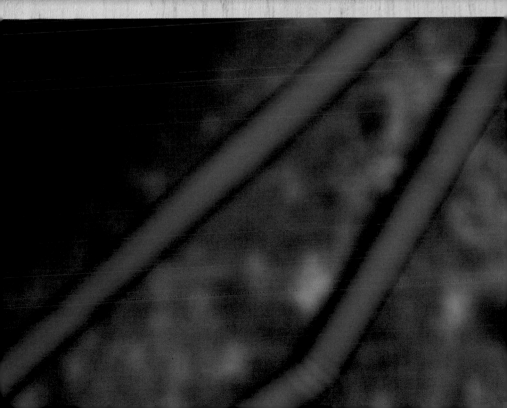

TARGETED
SMOOTHIES

Just like juices, smoothies can be created to target specific needs. The following pages give you smoothie recipes for eight categories. For example, the smoothies in the Beauty Box category might be of particular interest to those looking for ways to improve their skin. Red Hot Burners are for those trying to shed some pounds. But keep in mind that these drinks offer a range of benefits. So dip in, experiment, and have fun enjoying these smooth health boosters.

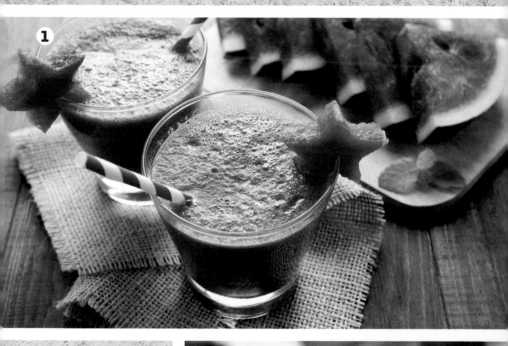

1 Watermelon Crush
2 Peaches 'n' Cream Smoothie
3 Over the Rainbow
4 Apple Pie Smoothie
5 Wicked Queen
6 Bright Eyes

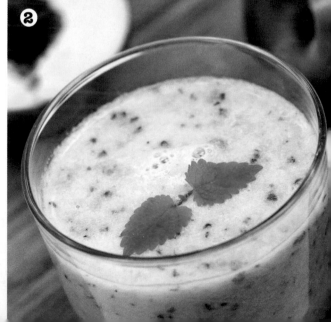

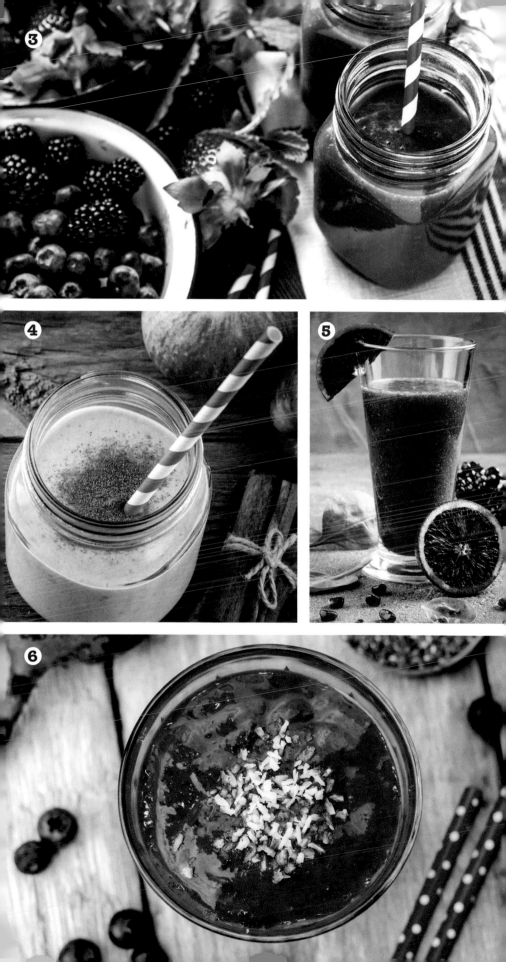

HAPPY DAYS

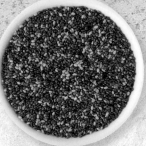

Chia seeds

Food has a major effect on how you think and on your mood. Certain vitamins, minerals, and phytochemicals can help keep you looking on the bright side.

FEEL-GOOD DIETS

There is a wealth of information about "feel-good" diets, some of it conflicting and some of it still in the early stages of research. Yet it does seem that smoothies containing nutrients like calcium, chromium, folate, iron, magnesium, omega-3 fats, vitamin B6, vitamin B12, vitamin D, zinc, and selenium will in some way improve your mood. A smoothie can also keep glucose levels stable so that you don't get those sugar highs and the subsequent crashes. This means lots of leafy greens, bananas, mangoes, berries, avocados, flaxseeds, and cinnamon. The following recipes can help you get started.

Mango Tango

- 1 large banana
- 1 mango, peeled, pitted, and diced
- 1 handful baby spinach leaves
- ½ cup water
- 2 tablespoons plain yogurt
- 3 to 4 ice cubes
- mint, for garnish

Wash all produce, then put all of the ingredients into a blender, and blend until smooth.

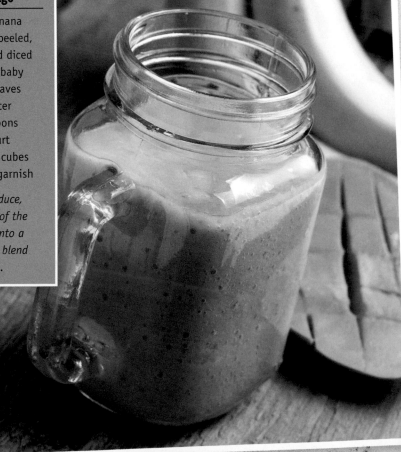

Easy as ABC

- ½ avocado, peeled and pitted
- 1 medium banana
- 2 tablespoons cacao
- ½ cup water
- 3 to 4 ice cubes
- stevia or other sweetener

Wash all produce, then put all of the ingredients into a blender, and blend until smooth.

3-B-Baby

- 1 cup blueberries
- 1 medium banana
- ½ cup broccoli
- ½ cup water
- 3 to 4 ice cubes
- stevia or other sweetener

Wash all produce, then put all of the ingredients into a blender, and blend until smooth.

Beet, Beet, Beetin' the Blues

- 1 beet, peeled
- ½ carrot
- 2 oranges, peeled and deseeded
- 1 to 2 thin slices ginger
- 1 tablespoon chia seeds
- ½ cup water
- 3 to 4 ice cubes

Wash all produce, then put all of the ingredients into a blender, and blend until smooth.

Kiwi-Kale-a-Cado

- 3 kiwifruits, peeled
- ½ avocado, peeled and pitted
- 1 handful baby kale leaves
- ½ cup water
- 3 to 4 ice cubes

Wash all produce, then put all of the ingredients into a blender, and blend until smooth.

Mango Tango (opposite)

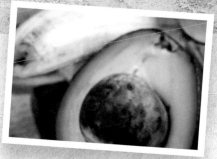

Avocado and banana

Flax Attack

- 1 handful baby spinach leaves
- 1 mango, peeled and pitted
- 1 medium banana
- 1 tablespoon flaxseeds
- ½ cup water
- 3 to 4 ice cubes
- stevia or other sweetener

Wash all produce, then put all of the ingredients into a blender, and blend until smooth.

Nutrition Bomb

- 1 orange, peeled and deseeded
- ½ medium banana
- 1 handful baby spinach leaves
- 1 mango, peeled and pitted
- 1 teaspoon sesame seeds
- 1 Brazil nut
- 1 tablespoon yogurt
- ½ cup water
- ½ cup ice cubes

Wash all produce, then put all of the ingredients into a blender, and blend until smooth.

Apple Pie Smoothie

- 1 cup water
- 1 large sweet apple
- 2 tablespoons chopped walnuts
- ½ teaspoon cinnamon
- ⅛ teaspoon nutmeg
- 1 date, ripe and soft
- 1 cup ice

Wash all produce, then put all of the ingredients into a blender, and blend until smooth.

FOUNTAIN OF YOUTH

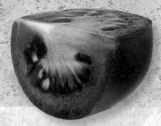

Tomato

Scientists can't yet promise eternal youth, but lots of nutrients found in food can enhance the quality of life. They have been proven to help keep us looking and feeling young, with a spring in our step. They can also keep your brain buzzing—or at least help you age well and get the most out of life through your senior years.

AGING WELL

While all nutrients help us age well, in one way or another, the big contributors are the antioxidants and omega-3 fats, particularly for their various associations with brain health, cardiovascular and heart health, anti-inflammatory properties, and perhaps cancer prevention. Other nutrients that also warrant a mention here are the B-group vitamins, necessary for a range of things that become of increasing concern as we age, including energy, healthy skin and eyes, and healthy brain function; calcium, for its ability to help prevent osteoporosis as we age; and magnesium and vitamin K, also needed for brain health, among other things. A diet full of essential nutrients is necessary throughout our lives—but we need even more of the "good stuff" as we age.

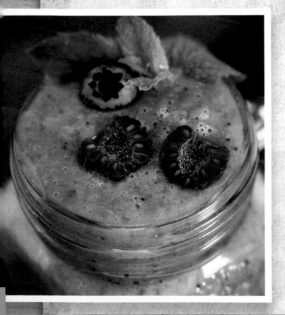

Brain Train

- ¼ cup blackberries
- ¼ cup strawberries
- ¼ cup raspberries
- ¼ cup blueberries
- 1 small handful baby spinach leaves
- ½ cup almond milk
- 3 to 4 ice cubes
- stevia or other sweetener
- mint for garnish

Wash all produce, then put all of the ingredients into a blender, and blend until smooth.

Brain Train

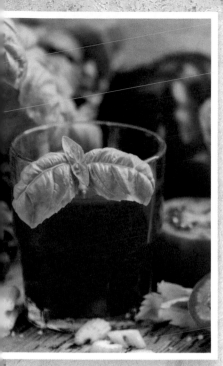

Hot Saucy Mama

Hot Saucy Mama

- 3 tomatoes
- ½ bell pepper
- ½ chili pepper, deseeded
- 1 cucumber, peeled
- ¼ onion, peeled
- 1 clove garlic
- 1 small handful parsley
- ¼ teaspoon turmeric, to taste
- a splash or two of water
- 3 to 4 ice cubes

Wash all produce, then put all of the ingredients into a blender, and blend until smooth.

123-OMG

- ½ honeydew melon, peeled and deseeded
- ½ papaya, peeled and deseeded
- ¼ cup water
- 1 tablespoon flaxseeds
- ½ teaspoon ground cloves
- 3 to 4 ice cubes

Wash all produce, then put all of the ingredients into a blender, and blend until smooth.

Forever Energetic

- 1 medium banana
- 1 mango, peeled and pitted
- ¼ cup strawberries
- 1 tablespoon oats
- 1 tablespoon yogurt
- ½ cup almond milk
- 1 tablespoon chia seeds

Wash all produce, then put all of the ingredients into a blender, and blend until smooth.

Over the Rainbow

- ¼ cup blueberries
- ¼ cup raspberries
- ¼ cup strawberries
- 1 orange, peeled and deseeded
- ½ mango, peeled and pitted
- ½ medium banana
- 1 apple, deseeded
- 1 kiwifruit, peeled
- ½ cup water
- 3 to 4 ice cubes

Wash all produce, then put all of the ingredients into a blender, and blend until smooth.

Bright Eyes

- 1 beet, peeled
- ¼ cup blueberries
- 1 orange, peeled and deseeded
- 1 small carrot
- 1 to 2 thin slices ginger
- 1 handful baby spinach leaves
- stevia or other sweetener
- ¼ cup water
- 3 to 4 ice cubes

Wash all produce, then put all of the ingredients into a blender, and blend until smooth.

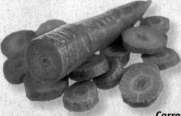

Carrots

NO MORE PRESSURE!

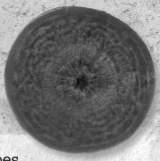

Carrot

Why all the pressure? Where does it come from? Why is it a problem? High blood pressure (hypertension) is often termed "the silent killer," because its symptoms are hardly, if at all, noticeable. At the same time, it predisposes us to stroke, heart attack, kidney damage, and other problems.

THE DASH DIET

This is a catchy name for what otherwise means "Dietary Approaches to Stop Hypertension," which has been proven to effectively reduce high blood pressure. It follows four main principles.

A healthy diet. This means eating a healthy diet that is rich in vegetables, fruit, low-fat dairy foods, nuts, and whole grains.

Monitor the fats. You should consume little or no saturated fats.

Include omega-3. Consume foods that are rich in omega-3 fats, including fish, flaxseeds, and chia seeds.

Junk the junk food. Eliminate empty calories from sugary foods and drinks, and delete junk food from your diet.

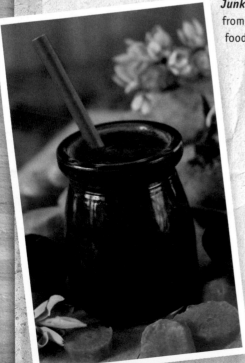

Royal Flush

- 1 beet, peeled
- ½ cucumber, peeled
- 1 stalk celery
- 2 oranges, peeled and deseeded
- ½ grated carrot
- 1 to 2 thin slices ginger
- 1 small handful parsley
- stevia or other sweetener
- ½ cup water

Wash all produce, then put all of the ingredients into a blender, and blend until smooth.

Royal Flush

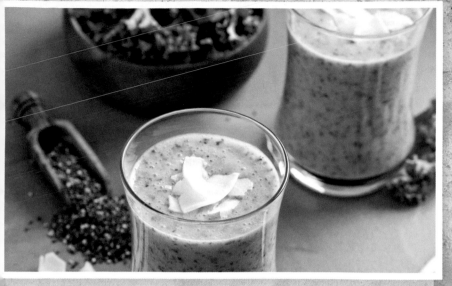

Fantastic Elastic

The Works

- 1 pomegranate, seeds and juice
- 1 apple, deseeded
- 2 oranges, peeled and deseeded
- ½ grapefruit, peeled and deseeded
- 1 tablespoon flaxseed
- stevia or other sweetener
- ¼ cup water
- 3 to 4 ice cubes
- lemon, for garnish (optional)

Wash all produce, then put all of the ingredients into a blender, and blend until smooth.

Fantastic Elastic

- 1 tablespoon flaxseeds
- 1 teaspoon chia seeds
- 1 medium banana
- ½ avocado, peeled and pitted
- a few small spinach leaves
- 1 Brazil nut
- ½ green apple
- ½ cup almond milk
- stevia or other sweetener
- 3 to 4 ice cubes
- coconut flakes, for garnish

Wash all produce, then put all of the ingredients into a blender, and blend until smooth.

Captain Avocado

- ½ avocado, peeled
- 1 stalk celery
- ½ cucumber, peeled
- ½ cup lime juice
- 3 fresh basil leaves
- 2 tablespoons yogurt
- stevia or other sweetener
- paprika, for garnish (optional)
- 2 teaspoons olive oil (optional)

Wash all produce, then put all of the ingredients into a blender, and blend until smooth.

Virgin Mary Smoothie

- 4 tomatoes
- 1 stalk celery
- ½ cucumber, peeled
- ½ lemon, peeled and deseeded
- ½ lime, peeled and deseeded
- a dash of low-sodium tabasco sauce
- a dash of low-sodium Worcestershire sauce
- a sprinkle of turmeric
- a sprinkle of cayenne pepper
- stevia or other sweetener
- leafy celery stalks, for garnish

Wash all produce, then put all of the ingredients into a blender, and blend until smooth.

BEAUTY BOX

Ginger

Not only do diets high in fresh fruit and vegetables provide numerous benefits to our overall health—they help us look good too.

LOOK GOOD AND FEEL GREAT

Nature offers a boundless array of nutrients to help us look and feel our best. Water, for instance, helps us look healthy. Well-hydrated skin looks plumper and fresher than less-hydrated skin. Vitamins, such as the antioxidants A, C, and E, are also important for supple skin and healthy hair, while B2 supports healthy skin and eyes. Don't forget about minerals, such as copper, silicon, calcium, and zinc, that also keep hair, skin, and nails in top shape. Finally, look for foods with omega-3 fats, such as those found in flaxseeds and walnuts, that help maintain the skin's natural oil barrier, keeping skin hydrated and maybe even giving it a healthy glow.

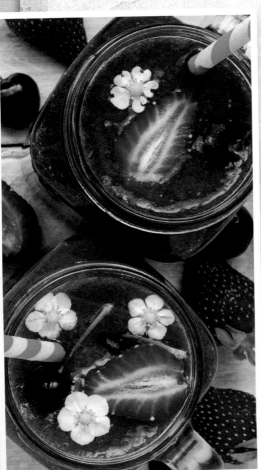

Peaches 'n' Cream Smoothie

- 3 peaches, peeled and pitted
- 2 tablespoons yogurt
- ½ cup almond milk
- stevia or other sweetener, to taste
- 3 to 4 ice cubes

Wash all produce, then put all of the ingredients into a blender, and blend until smooth.

Cherry Baby

- ½ cup cherries, pitted
- ½ cup strawberries
- 2 oranges, peeled and deseeded
- 1 small handful alfalfa sprouts
- ½ cup water
- 3 to 4 ice cubes

Wash all produce, then put all of the ingredients into a blender, and blend until smooth.

Cherry Baby

Forever Young

- 1 pomegranate, seeds and juice
- 1 teaspoon sesame seeds
- 1 lemon, peeled and deseeded
- ½ apple, peeled and deseeded
- 1 small handful cabbage
- ½ cup water
- 3 to 4 ice cubes

Wash all produce, then put all of the ingredients into a blender, and blend until smooth.

Skin Zinger

- ½ cup pineapple, peeled and cored
- ½ avocado, peeled and pitted
- 1 small handful alfalfa sprouts
- ½ cup coconut water
- 1 to 2 thin slices ginger
- 3 to 4 ice cubes

Wash all produce, then put all of the ingredients into a blender, and blend until smooth.

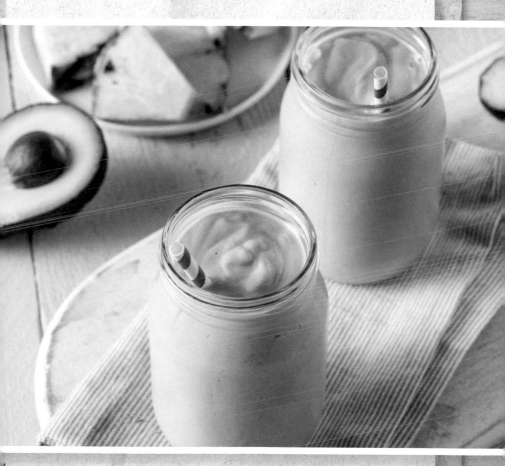

Hydrator

- 1 cup water
- 1 apple, peeled and deseeded
- ½ cup ice cubes
- mint, for garnish

Wash all produce, then put all of the ingredients into a blender, and blend until smooth.

Skin Zinger (above)

Wicked Queen

- 1 pomegranate, seeds and juice
- ½ cup cherries, pitted
- 1 blood orange, peeled and deseeded
- 1 small handful baby spinach
- 4 to 6 ice cubes

Wash all produce, then put all of the ingredients into a blender, and blend until smooth.

RED HOT BURNERS

Everyone wants a diet that not only gives them loads of energy, but also helps prevent weight gain and even encourages weight loss when needed.

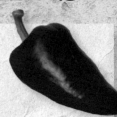

Chili pepper

THE 5:2 DIET

The 5:2 diet entails restricting calorie intake to 500 per day for women and 600 per day for men on two nonconsecutive days out of seven in the week, and then eating as one pleases on the remaining five days. Smoothies fit perfectly into a 5:2 diet plan, providing a quick, satisfying, and nutritious way to sustain the body on the two low-calorie days. The following sampling of smoothies is designed to complement a healthy weight-reduction diet and exercise plan. They are typically high in fiber, water, and nutrients, with a particular focus on nutrients the body needs for energy and satiety, such as low-GI carbohydrates, protein, and fiber. Most of them are a meal unto themselves. And, of course, all are quick, delicious, and fun.

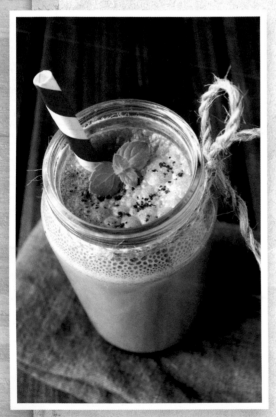

La Dolce Vita

La Dolce Vita

- ¼ cup cannellini beans
- 3 tablespoons cacao
- 1 medium banana
- ½ cup almond milk
- 1 tablespoon flaxseeds
- stevia or other sweetener
- 3 to 4 ice cubes

Wash all produce, then put all of the ingredients into a blender, and blend until smooth.

Lean & Peachy Keen

- 1 tablespoon oats
- 3 peaches, peeled and pitted
- 1 tablespoon flaxseeds
- 2 tablespoons yogurt
- ¼ cup almond milk
- stevia or other sweetener
- 3 to 4 ice cubes

Wash all produce, then put all of the ingredients into a blender, and blend until smooth.

Slim Jim

- 4 tomatoes
- 1 stalk celery
- ½ cup French beans
- ½ chili pepper, deseeded
- 1 tablespoon sesame seeds
- ½ clove garlic
- 6 basil leaves
- ¼ cup water

Wash all produce, then put all of the ingredients into a blender, and blend until smooth.

Call of the Wild

- 1 handful baby kale leaves
- 1 small handful baby spinach leaves
- ¼ cup peas, fresh
- 2 kiwifruits, peeled
- 2 oranges, peeled and deseeded
- ¼ cup fennel
- 1 tablespoon chia seeds
- ¼ cup water
- 3 to 4 ice cubes

Wash all produce, then put all of the ingredients into a blender, and blend until smooth.

Fiber Fantastic

- 1 tablespoon flaxseeds
- 1 tablespoon sunflower seeds
- 1 tablespoon chia seeds
- 1 mango, peeled and pitted
- 2 oranges, peeled and deseeded
- ½ small carrot
- 1 cup water
- 3 to 4 ice cubes

Wash all produce, then put all of the ingredients into a blender, and blend until smooth.

Smooth Moves

- ¼ cup cannellini beans
- 1 medium banana
- 2 kiwifruits, peeled
- 1 tablespoon flaxseeds
- 2 drops vanilla extract
- ½ cup almond milk
- 3 to 4 ice cubes
- mint, for garnish (optional)

Wash all produce, then put all of the ingredients into a blender, and blend until smooth.

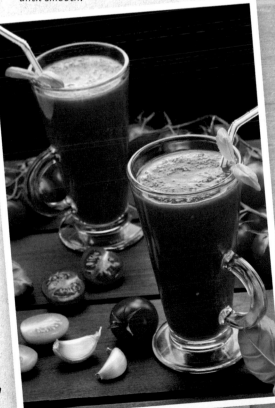

Slim Jim

COOL MOVES

The smoothies in this section are both refreshing and cooling. They might also feel in some way "cleansing," especially if integrated into a detox diet or liquid fast. The cleansing feeling itself is a powerful motivator that encourages healthy eating and positive feelings.

Pear

CLEAN EATING

There is uncertainty about the long-term benefits associated with intermittent fasting or very low-calorie diets, but from time to time they may have a place. If undertaken for only a short period and not too frequently, they can help give both the mind and body a rest from overnourishment, too often a problem in our society. Detox diets can also help people shift between overindulgence and "cleaner" eating, meaning a diet of fresh, unprocessed foods.

Watermelon Crush

- 3 cups watermelon, rind removed and deseeded
- 4 mint leaves
- ½ cup ice cubes
- ¼ cup water

Wash all produce, then put all of the ingredients into a blender, and blend until smooth.

Mint & Lime Crush

- 3 limes, peeled and deseeded
- 1 grapefruit, peeled and deseeded
- 1 handful baby spinach leaves
- stevia or other sweetener
- ½ cup mineral water
- 3 to 4 ice cubes

Wash all produce, then put all of the ingredients into a blender, and blend until smooth.

Peach 'n' Pear Fizz

- 2 pears, peeled and deseeded
- 2 peaches, peeled and deseeded
- 1 to 2 small slices ginger
- stevia or other sweetener
- ½ cup carbonated water
- 3 to 4 ice cubes

Wash all produce, then put all of the ingredients into a blender, and blend until smooth.

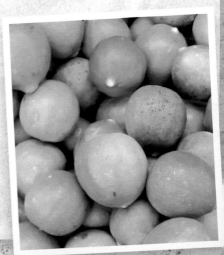

Limes

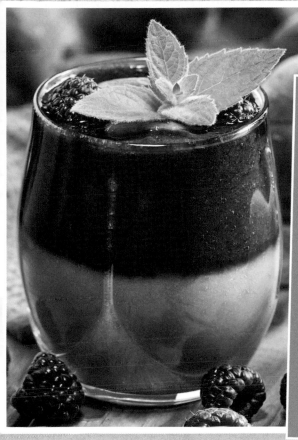

Peaches 'n' Berries Layered Smoothie

Peaches 'n' Berries Layered Smoothie

Ingredients for top layer
- ¼ cup raspberries
- 2 tablespoons yogurt
- stevia or other sweetener
- 2 ice cubes and splash of water

Ingredients for bottom layer
- 2 peaches, peeled and deseeded
- 1 to 2 small slices ginger
- 2 ice cubes and splash of water

For each batch, wash all produce, then put all of the ingredients into a blender, and blend until smooth. Layer each in a glass.

Peaches 'n' Berries Layered Smoothie

Green Tea Refresher

- 2 cups white grapes, frozen
- 1 cup green tea, strained and cooled
- stevia or other sweetener
- ½ cup ice cubes

Wash all produce, then put all of the ingredients into a blender, and blend until smooth.

Apple Teaser

- 3 green apples, cored and deseeded
- 1 stalk celery
- 2 small slices ginger
- ¼ cup water
- 3 to 4 ice cubes

Wash all produce, then put all of the ingredients into a blender, and blend until smooth.

Rainbow Melon Smoothie

Ingredients for first layer
- 2 cups honeydew, deseeded
- 2 ice cubes and splash of water

Ingredients for second layer
- 2 cups cantaloupe, deseeded
- 2 ice cubes and splash of water

Ingredients for third layer
- 2 cups watermelon, deseeded
- 2 ice cubes and splash of water

For each batch, wash all produce, then put all of the ingredients into a blender, and blend until smooth. Layer each in a glass.

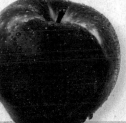

Honeycrisp apple (left) and Ambrosia (right)

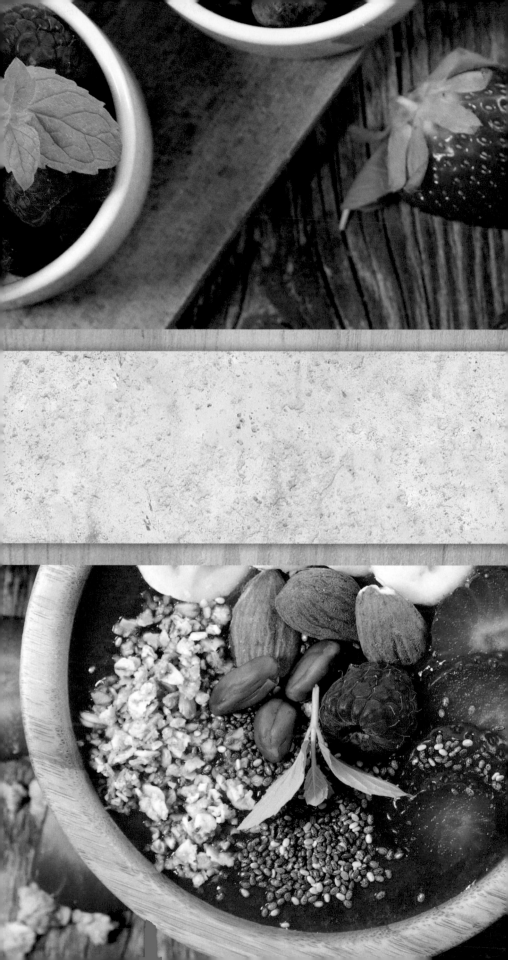

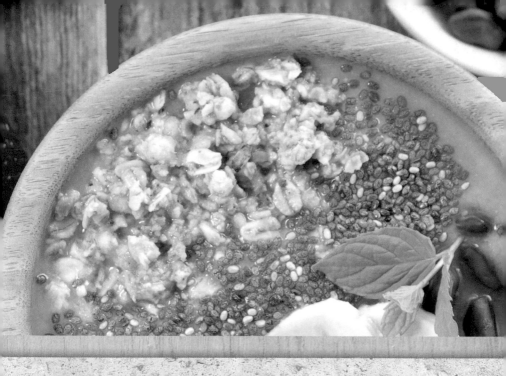

CHAPTER 8

SMOOTHIE BOWLS

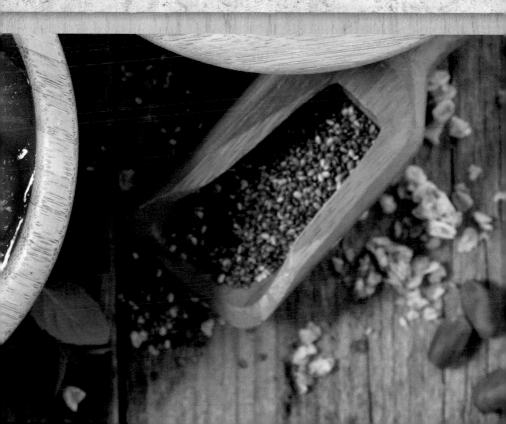

SMOOTHIE BOWLS

Bright, beautiful, and packed with the goodness of fresh fruits and veggies, smoothies bowls are a smart way to get essential vitamins, minerals, and other nutrients. The following pages offer a variety of recipes, but feel free to craft your own versions with your favorite ingredients and toppings.

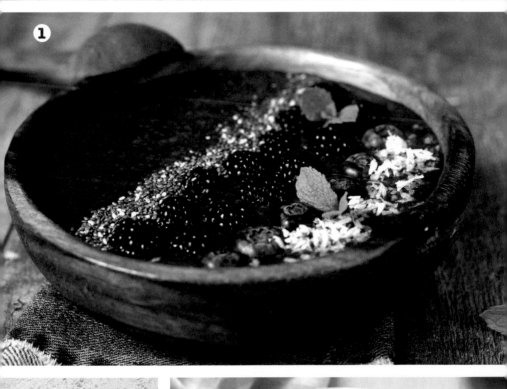

1 Royal Purple
  Breakfast Bowl
2 Autumn Pecan
  Smoothie Bowl
3 Goji Dragon
  Smoothie Bowl
4 Silken Chocolate
  Dessert Bowl
5 Blue Coconut
  Smoothie Bowl
6 Sweet Spinach
  Smoothie Bowl

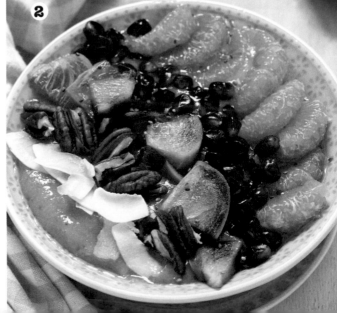

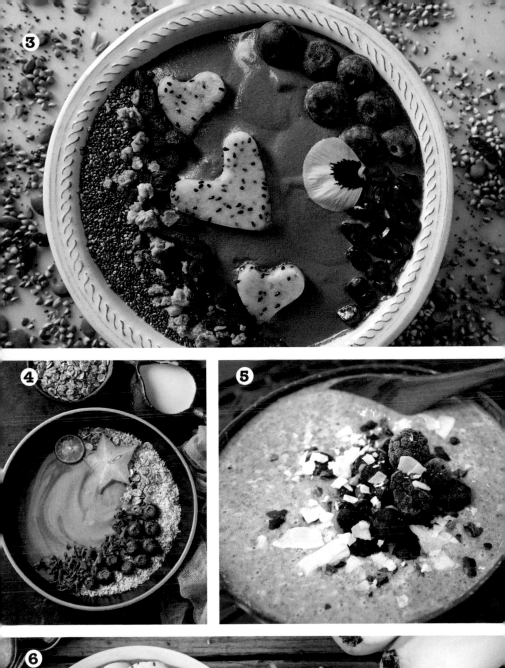
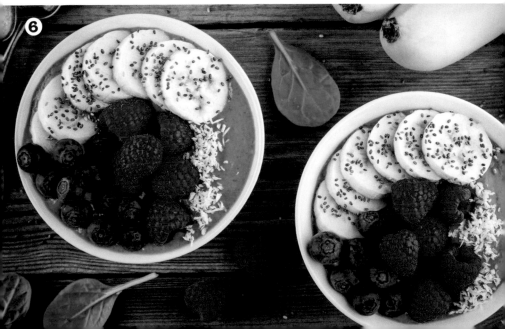

A MEAL IN A BOWL

Smoothie bowls have become a hot health trend. But being trendy doesn't mean they aren't good for you.

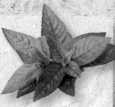

Mint leaves

DELICIOUS AND NUTRITIOUS

Just like classic smoothies, bowl versions are only limited by your imagination. Pack them with your favorite vitamin-rich veggies and fruits, and top them with extras that add value for a meal or snack any time of the day. With all their bright colors, smoothie bowls are not only full of nutrients, they are also beautiful to behold.

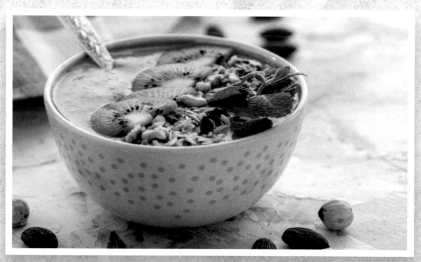

Kiwi-Mint Smoothie Bowl (above);
Cherry-Red Smoothie Bowl (opposite)

Kiwi-Mint Smoothie Bowl

- 2 ripe kiwis
- 1 large banana, frozen
- ½ cup coconut water
- 1 handful fresh mint leaves
- a squeeze of lime
- 1 small handful spinach

Suggested toppings
- sliced kiwis
- hazelnuts
- mint leaves

Put all of the ingredients into a blender, and blend until smooth. Pour into a bowl, and layer on toppings.

Cherry-Red Smoothie Bowl

- 1 cup cherries, pitted and frozen
- 1 cup red raspberries, frozen
- 1 medium banana, frozen
- ¾ cup coconut water

Suggested toppings
- cherries
- raspberries
- coconut flakes
- chia seeds
- sesame seeds
- pumpkin seeds

Put all of the ingredients into a blender, and blend until smooth. Pour into a bowl, and layer on toppings.

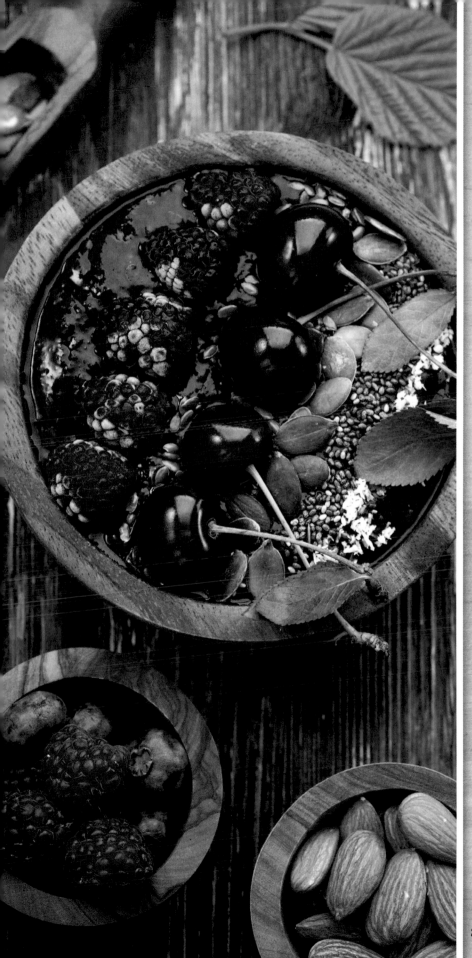

BREAKFAST BOWLS

Banana slices

Take a break from oatmeal and cereal, and fill your breakfast bowl with a healthy blend of fruits, veggies, nuts, and seeds.

START THE DAY RIGHT

The first meal of the day is arguably the most important one, stoking you with the nutrients you need to function at your best. Smoothie bowls are a delicious way to prepare for the day ahead.

Silky Yogurt Breakfast Bowl

- ½ avocado
- ½ medium banana, frozen
- ½ cup spinach
- 3 to 4 tablespoons almond milk yogurt
- ¼ cup coconut water
- ¼ cup ice
- ½ teaspoon maple syrup

Suggested toppings
- sliced strawberries
- sliced banana
- granola
- cinnamon

Put all of the ingredients into a blender, and blend until smooth. Pour into a bowl, and layer on toppings.

Silky Yogurt Breakfast Bowl

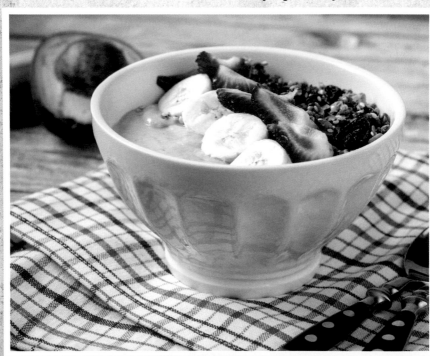

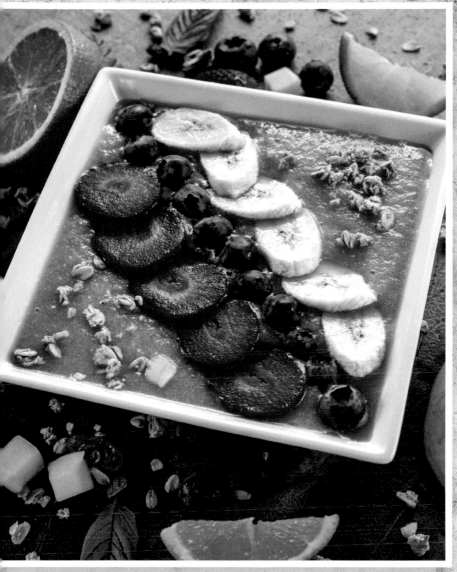

Morning Citrus Bowl

Oatmeal & Fruit Smoothie Bowl

- ¼ cup rolled oats
- 1 medium banana, frozen
- 1 cup raspberries
- ½ cup almond milk
- 1 tablespoon almond butter

Suggested toppings
- raspberries
- sliced banana

Microwave the oats with ¼ cup water for 1 minute, cool, then add to blender with the rest of the ingredients. Blend until smooth. Pour into a bowl, and layer on toppings.

Morning Citrus Bowl

- 1 medium banana, frozen
- 2 tablespoons lemon juice
- ¾ cup orange juice
- 1 to 2 teaspoons honey
- 1 to 2 ice cubes

Suggested toppings
- sliced strawberries
- sliced banana
- blueberries
- granola

Put all of the ingredients into a blender, and blend until smooth. Pour into a bowl, and layer on toppings.

Kiwi Dragon Breakfast Bowl

- 1½ cups pineapple juice
- 1 tablespoon honey
- 10 kiwis, peeled and diced
- 1 large dragon fruit, peeled and chopped
- 1 medium banana, frozen

Suggested toppings
- pineapple chunks
- dragon fruit balls
- coconut flakes
- pomegranate seeds
- chia seeds
- goji berries

Wash all produce, then put all of the ingredients into a blender, and blend until smooth. Pour into a bowl, and layer on toppings.

Goin' to Seed Breakfast Bowl

- 1½ cups frozen kiwi
- 1 medium banana, frozen
- 1 cups chopped spinach, frozen
- 1 cups almond milk
- 1 tablespoon almond butter
- 2 tablespoons acai powder
- 1 tablespoon ground flaxseed
- 2 tablespoons maple syrup
- a pinch of salt

Suggested toppings
- sliced strawberries
- pumpkin seeds
- chia seeds

Wash all produce, then put all of the ingredients into a blender, and blend until smooth. Pour into a bowl, and layer on toppings.

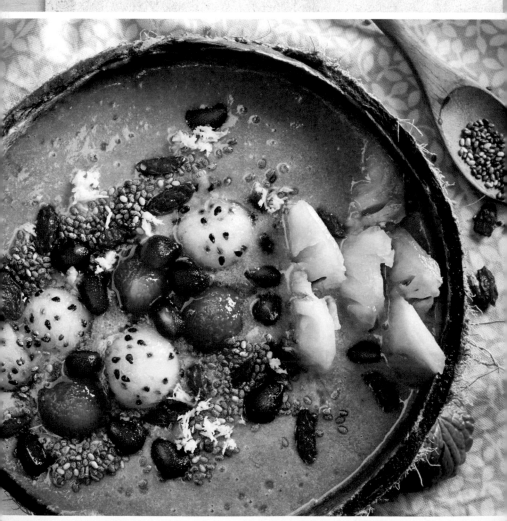

Kiwi Dragon Breakfast Bowl

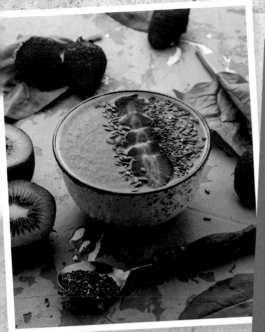

Goin' to Seed Breakfast Bowl

Nutty Banana Breakfast Bowl

- 1 medium banana, frozen
- 1 tablespoon almond butter
- 1 cup almond milk
- ⅓ cup rolled oats
- 1 tablespoon ground flaxseed
- 2 cups ice

Suggested toppings
- granola
- sliced almonds
- flaxseeds

Put all of the ingredients into a blender, and blend until smooth. Pour into a bowl, and layer on toppings.

Coconut Sesame Breakfast Bowl

- ½ cup coconut milk
- 2 tablespoons toasted black sesame seeds
- 1 large banana, frozen
- 1 cup ice

Suggested toppings
- toasted black sesame seeds
- toasted coconut flakes

Put all of the ingredients into a blender, and blend until smooth. Pour into a bowl, and layer on toppings.

SEEDY TOPPINGS

Seeds are very nutritious and packed full of the antioxidant vitamin E, fiber, healthy fats, B vitamins, and minerals. They also add a lot of flavor (especially if roasted).

- **Chia:** An ancient Aztec grain, chia rivals flaxseed as a plant source of omega-3s. Chia seeds are very high in soluble dietary fiber.

- **Flaxseed:** Also known as linseed, flaxseed is a good source of omega-3 fats.

- **Hemp seed:** This seed is another good source of omega-3 fats and fiber. Containing all essential amino acids, hemp seeds are a good-quality protein source for vegans.

- **Pumpkin seed:** Also called pepita, this seed is a good source of protein, fiber, and vitamin E. Rich in iron, zinc, magnesium, and copper, it is also high in essential fatty acids.

- **Sesame seed:** This tiny seed is an excellent plant source of protein and calcium. It has a mix of monounsaturated and polyunsaturated fats.

- **Sunflower seed:** This stripy seed is a rich source of omega-6 fats and a good source of vitamin E, as well as important minerals like magnesium, copper, and selenium.

Cherry Walnut Smoothie Bowl

- 2 cups cherries,
  pitted and frozen
- 1 medium banana, frozen
- ¾ cup coconut water

Suggested toppings
- cherries
- walnuts
- coconut flakes
- chia seeds
- pumpkin seeds

Put all of the ingredients into a blender, and blend until smooth. Pour into a bowl, and layer on toppings.

Cherry Walnut Smoothie Bowl (opposite); Coconut with Pomegranate Breakfast Bowl (below)

Coconut with Pomegranate Breakfast Bowl

- 1 cup plain Greek yogurt
- ¾ cup coconut milk
- 1 medium banana, frozen
- 1 teaspoon vanilla extract
- ¾ cup ice

Suggested toppings
- pomegranate seeds
- peach slices
- coconut flakes
- coconut chunks
- chia seeds
- mulberry
- carob powder

Put all of the ingredients into a blender, and blend until smooth. Pour into a bowl, and layer on toppings.

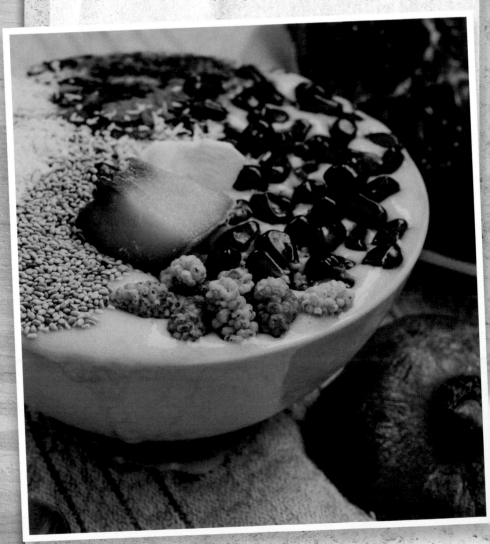

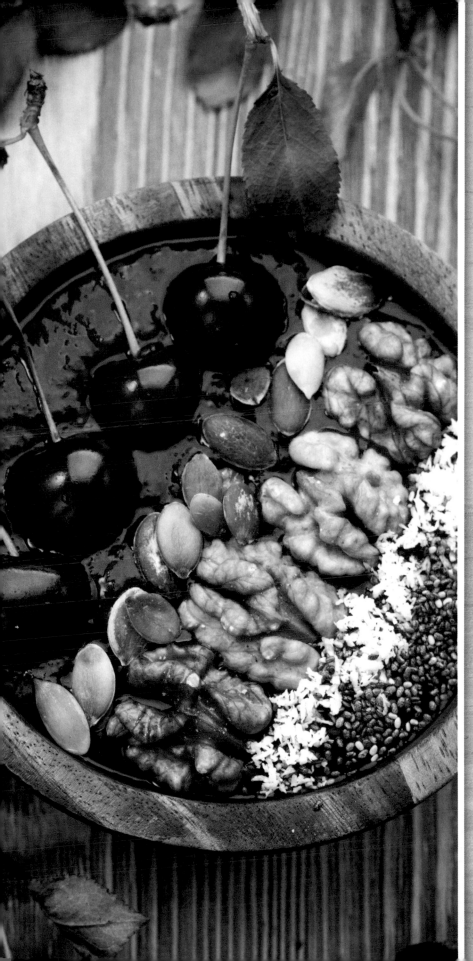

BENEFICIAL BERRIES

All kinds of berries—including raspberries, blueberries, strawberries, and blackberries—not only bring the taste of summer days to a breakfast bowl, they also bring high-quality nutrients. Less familiar berries, such as goji and acai, also pack a potent health punch. Acai, in particular, is a star in many bowl creations, lending a bright flavor, vibrant magenta color, and powerful antioxidant benefits.

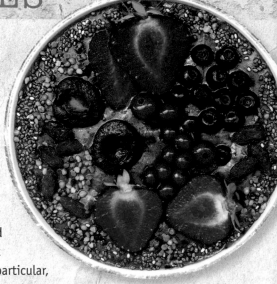

Peanut, Berry & Acai Smoothie Bowl

Peanut, Berry & Acai Smoothie Bowl

- 1½ cups mixed berries, frozen
- 1 medium banana, frozen
- 1 cup chopped spinach, frozen
- 1 cup almond milk
- 1 tablespoon peanut butter
- 2 tablespoons acai powder
- 1 tablespoon ground flaxseed
- 2 tablespoons maple syrup
- a pinch of salt

Suggested toppings
- strawberries
- goji berries
- blueberries
- redcurrants
- sliced plums
- chia seeds
- bee pollen

Wash all produce, then put all of the ingredients into a blender, and blend until smooth. Pour into a bowl, and layer on toppings.

Bee Berry Smoothie Bowl

- 2 cups blueberries
- 1 acai pack, frozen
- 1 medium banana, frozen
- ½ cup almond milk
- 1 teaspoon maple syrup
- 1 scoop whey protein
- ¼ teaspoon turmeric

Suggested toppings
- bee pollen
- chia seeds
- red pepper flakes

Put all of the ingredients into a blender, and blend until smooth. Pour into a bowl, and layer on toppings.

THINK ABOUT IT!
A dusting of bee pollen isn't just pretty. Bee pollen contains almost all of the nutrients required by the human body. It's rich in vitamins, minerals, proteins, and a host of other beneficial nutrients.

Hot Berry & Tofu Smoothie Bowl

- 1 pound fresh strawberries
- 2 cups blueberries
- 9 ounces tofu
- ½ teaspoon ground ginger
- 2 pinches of red pepper flakes
- ¼ teaspoon rum extract
- 1 tablespoon honey
- 1 teaspoon lemon juice
- ½ cup ice

Suggested toppings
- sliced strawberries
- blueberries
- red pepper flakes

Wash all produce, then put all of the ingredients into a blender, and blend until smooth. Pour into a bowl, and layer on toppings.

Vegan Berry Crunch Smoothie Bowl

- 1 cup chopped kale
  or baby spinach leaves
- 1 tablespoon chia seeds
- 1 cup unsweetened almond milk
- 1 cup mixed berries, frozen
- 1 medium banana, frozen
- 1 to 2 teaspoons light agave syrup

Suggested toppings
- sliced strawberries
- blueberries
- raspberries
- chia seeds
- sliced almonds

Wash all produce, then put all of the ingredients into a blender, and blend until smooth. Pour into a bowl, and layer on toppings.

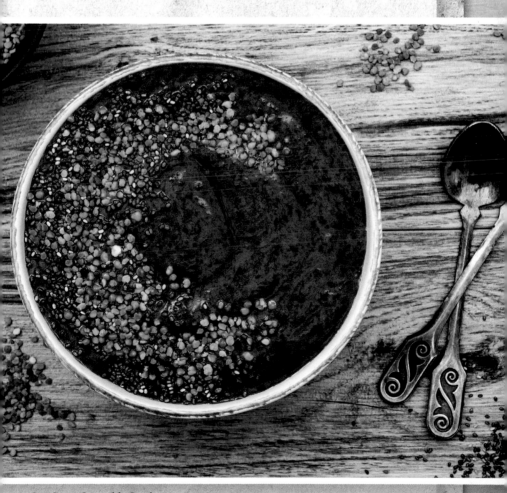

Bee Berry Smoothie Bowl

Coco-Nutty Strawberry-Raspberry Smoothie Bowl

- 1½ cups fresh strawberries
- 1 medium banana, frozen
- ¼ cup gluten-free rolled oats
- ½ cup almond milk
- ½ cup water
- 1 scoop protein powder
- ⅓ cup avocado
- 3 ice cubes
- ¼ cup unsweetened coconut
- 3 tablespoons raw pecans

Suggested toppings
- strawberries
- raspberries
- chia seeds
- sliced almonds
- pumpkin seeds

Wash all produce, then put all of the ingredients into a blender, and blend until smooth. Pour into a bowl, and layer on toppings.

Royal Purple Breakfast Bowl

- ½ banana, frozen
- ¾ cup fresh blueberries
- ½ cup fresh blackberries
- ¾ cup unsweetened almond milk
- 1 tablespoon chia seeds
- ¼ cup plain Greek yogurt
- ½ teaspoon raw honey

Suggested toppings
- blueberries
- blackberries
- chia seeds
- coconut flakes

Wash all produce, then put all of the ingredients into a blender, and blend until smooth. Pour into a bowl, and layer on toppings.

THINK ABOUT IT!
Plan ahead for a quick meal. Stock up on small freezer bags, and then fill them with berries. Or slice up bananas, and then freeze them in single servings. You'll always have a supply of healthy fruits to add flavor to your smoothie creations.

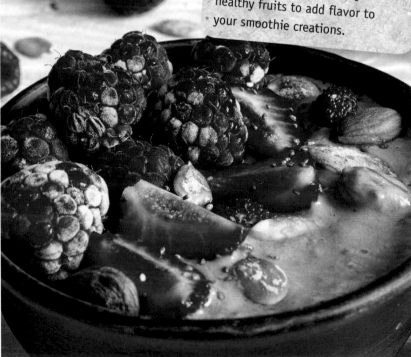

Coco-Nutty Strawberry-Raspberry Smoothie Bowl

Very Berry Smoothie Bowl

- 1 bag mixed berries, frozen
- 1 small ripe banana, frozen
- 2 to 3 tablespoons almond milk
- 1 scoop vanilla protein powder
- ½ teaspoon raw honey

Suggested toppings
- strawberries
- raspberries
- blueberries
- sliced almonds

Put all of the ingredients into a blender, and blend until smooth. Pour into a bowl, and layer on toppings.

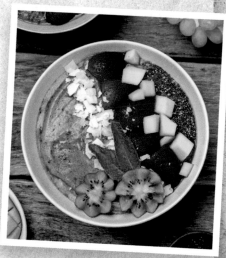

Strawberry Yogurt Breakfast Bowl

Strawberry Yogurt Breakfast Bowl

- 1 container low-fat strawberry yogurt
- ½ cup almond milk
- ¾ cup fresh strawberries
- ¾ cup crushed ice

Suggested toppings
- strawberries
- kiwis
- mango chunks
- chia seeds
- coconut flakes

Wash all produce, then put all of the ingredients into a blender, and blend until smooth. Pour into a bowl, and layer on toppings.

Blueberry Yogurt Breakfast Bowl

- 1 container low-fat blueberry yogurt
- ½ cup hazelnut milk
- ¾ cup fresh blueberries
- 1 teaspoon maple syrup
- ¾ cup crushed ice

Suggested toppings
- blueberries
- apple slices
- chia seeds
- hazelnuts

Wash all produce, then put all of the ingredients into a blender, and blend until smooth. Pour into a bowl, and layer on toppings.

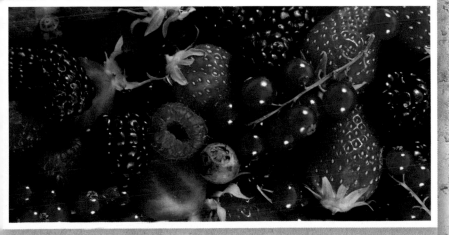

Mixed berries

SOMETHING FOR EVERYONE

Smoothie bowls are not just for breakfast. Enjoy them for lunch and dinner, as a midday snack, or a pre- or postworkout fortifier.

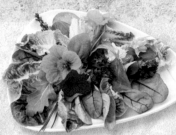

Edible flowers, including borage, pansies, lavender, and squash blossoms

SIZE MATTERS

Think about serving size when creating your bowl. You may want a heartier meal for breakfast than you will for dinner. Before a workout, go for a smaller bowl loaded with protein; after one, try potassium-rich ingredients like bananas to replenish lost nutrients.

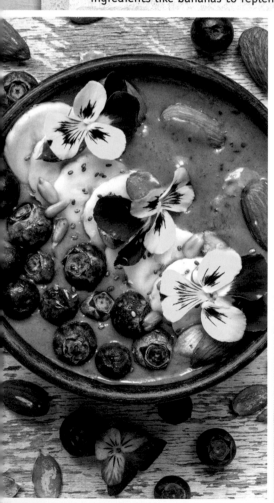

Berry & Banana Lunch Bowl

Berry & Banana Lunch Bowl

- 1 medium banana, frozen
- 1 cup blueberries, frozen
- ½ cup vanilla Greek yogurt
- ½ cup almond milk
- 1 tablespoon almond butter

Suggested toppings
- banana slices
- pansies
- blueberries
- pumpkin seeds
- sliced almonds

Put all of the ingredients into a blender, and blend until smooth. Pour into a bowl, and layer on toppings.

THINK ABOUT IT!

Smoothie bowls are meant to be visually tempting, so why not sprinkle on some edible flowers? Try pansies, violets, nasturtiums, chamomile, borage, calendulas, zucchini and squash blossoms, hibiscus, lavender, roses, sage flowers, or bee balm.

Super-Green Smoothie Bowl

- 1 medium banana, frozen
- 1½ cups chopped spinach, frozen
- 1 cup fresh pineapple cubes
- 1 cup coconut water
- 2 kiwis, peeled and sliced

Suggested toppings
- pansies
- spinach leaves
- blueberries
- pumpkin seeds
- sesame seeds

Put all of the ingredients into a blender, and blend until smooth. Pour into a bowl, and layer on toppings.

Super-Green Smoothie Bowl

Goji Dragon Smoothie Bowl

- 1 medium banana, frozen
- ¼ cup goji berries, dried
- ¼ cup blueberries, frozen
- ¼ cup strawberries, frozen
- ¼ cup almond milk
- ¼ cup pomegranate juice

Suggested toppings
- pansies
- goji berries
- blueberries
- granola
- dragon fruit
- pomegranate seeds
- chia seeds

Put all of the ingredients into a blender, and blend until smooth. Pour into a bowl, and layer on toppings.

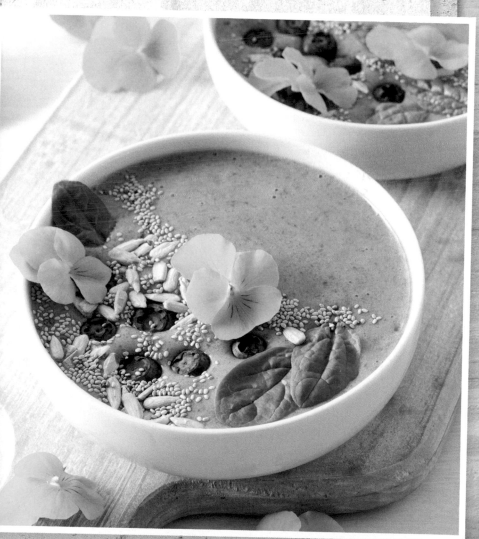

Pumpkin & Yogurt Smoothie Bowl

- ½ cup pumpkin puree
- 1 medium banana, frozen
- 1 cup vanilla Greek yogurt
- ½ teaspoon cinnamon
- ¼ teaspoon nutmeg
- ⅛ teaspoon allspice

Suggested toppings
- pecans
- goji berries
- blueberries
- pumpkin seeds
- chia seeds

Put all of the ingredients into a blender, and blend until smooth. Pour into a bowl, and layer on toppings.

Pumpkin & Yogurt Smoothie Bowl

Acorn Squash-Apple Smoothie

- 1 small acorn squash
- 1 large apple, peeled and cored
- 2 cups apple juice
- 1½ teaspoons fresh ginger, grated

Suggested toppings
- pineapple
- coconut
- mango
- chia seeds

Wash the squash, cut it in half, and scoop out the seeds. Place it, cut side down, in a dish with about ½ an inch of water. Microwave it for about 10 minutes. Scoop out the squash from the skin and add it into the blender with the other ingredients. Pour into a bowl, and layer on toppings.

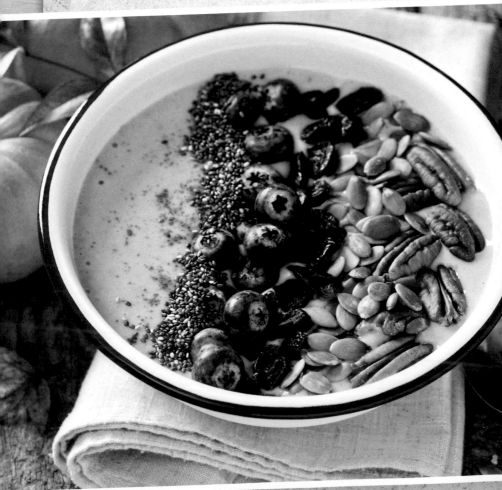

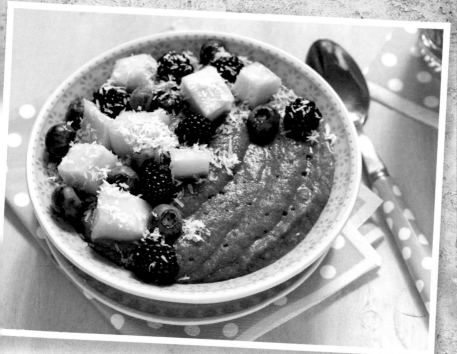

Fruity Broccoli Rabe Smoothie Bowl

Watermelon & Avocado Appetizer Smoothie Bowl

- 1 large ripe tomato
- ½ cup seedless watermelon, diced
- 1-inch-thick slice of day-old baguette, cut into pieces
- ½ cucumber, cut into chunks
- 2 tablespoons red onion, chopped
- 1 garlic clove
- ½ teaspoon kosher salt
- a dash of black pepper
- 1 ice cube
- 2 tablespoons extra virgin olive oil

Suggested toppings
- diced onion
- diced tomato
- diced cucumber
- watermelon slices

Put all of the ingredients, except olive oil, into a blender, and blend until smooth. Slowly drizzle in the olive oil. Pour into a bowl, and chill at least 30 minutes. Layer on toppings.

Fruity Broccoli Rabe Smoothie Bowl

- 2 cups broccoli rabe
- ½ medium banana, frozen
- 1 kiwi, peeled and diced
- 1 cup fresh pineapple cubes
- ½ teaspoon flaxseeds
- 1 cup coconut water
- 1 handful ice (optional)

Suggested toppings
- shredded coconut
- pineapple cubes
- blueberries
- raspberries

Put all of the ingredients into a blender, and blend until smooth. Pour into a bowl, and layer on toppings.

Chia seeds

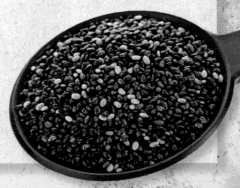

APPETIZING AVOCADO

Avocados are perfect for smoothie bowls. With a naturally creamy texture, they add body to a blend, along with a nutty flavor that works in both savory and sweet bowls.

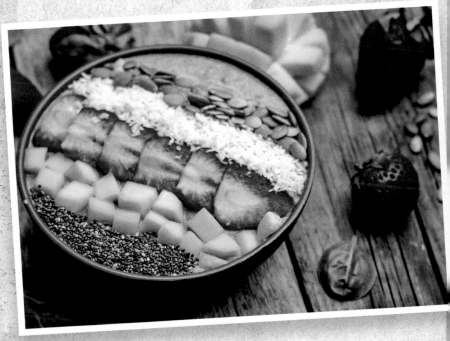

Fruity Avocado Smoothie Bowl (above); Nutty Avocado Smoothie Bowl (opposite)

Fruity Avocado Smoothie Bowl

- 2 cups spinach
- ½ cup unsweetened almond milk
- 1 tablespoon chia seeds
- 1 banana, frozen
- ½ avocado
- ice, as needed

Suggested toppings
- strawberries
- coconut
- mango
- pumpkin seeds
- chia seeds

Wash all produce, then put all of the ingredients into a blender, and blend until smooth. Pour into a bowl, and layer on toppings.

Tropical Avocado Smoothie Bowl

- 1 avocado
- 1 cup coconut milk
- 1 lime, peeled and deseeded
- 1 teaspoon spirulina powder
- 1 teaspoon agave syrup
- ice, as needed

Suggested toppings
- pineapple
- coconut
- mango
- chia seeds

Wash all produce, then put all of the ingredients into a blender, and blend until smooth. Pour into a bowl, and layer on toppings.

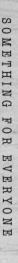

Nutty Avocado Smoothie Bowl

- ¼ ripe avocado
- 2 medium ripe bananas, sliced and frozen
- 2 large handfuls spinach
- 1 small handful kale
- 1½ to 2 cups almond milk
- 1 tablespoon flaxseed meal
- 2 tablespoons almond butter

Suggested toppings
- mango
- strawberry
- almonds
- pumpkin seeds

Wash all produce, then put all of the ingredients into a blender, and blend until smooth. Pour into a bowl, and layer on toppings.

PROTEIN BOOSTS

Smoothies, whether served in a glass or bowl, are a great way to boost your protein intake. Choose protein-rich ingredients like legumes, spinach, avocado, and broccoli, and top with high-protein nuts and seeds. You can also add a scoop of protein powder, and use tofu or soy as a base.

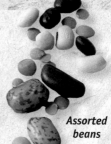

Assorted beans

Vegan Kiwi Protein Bowl

- ½ cup kiwi, frozen
- ½ cup mango, frozen
- 2 large handfuls baby spinach
- 1 medium banana, frozen
- 2 scoops soy protein powder
- ½ cup almond milk

Suggested toppings
- kiwi slices
- coconut flakes
- blueberries
- bee pollen

Wash all produce, then put all of the ingredients into a blender, and blend until smooth. Pour into a bowl, and layer on toppings.

Vegan Kiwi Protein Bowl

Sweet Spinach Smoothie Bowl

- 2 large handfuls baby spinach
- 1 medium banana, frozen
- ½ cup kiwi, frozen
- ½ cup pineapple, frozen
- 1 cup coconut milk
- 1 tablespoon almond butter
- 1 scoop protein powder

Suggested toppings
- banana slices
- coconut flakes
- blueberries
- raspberries
- chia seeds

Wash all produce, then put all of the ingredients into a blender, and blend until smooth. Pour into a bowl, and layer on toppings.

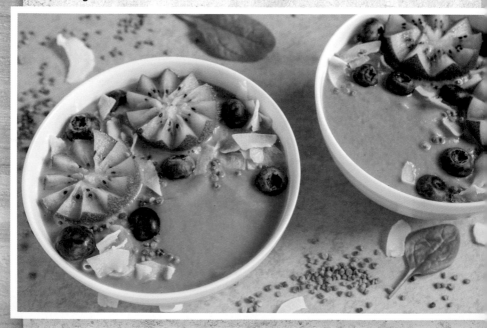

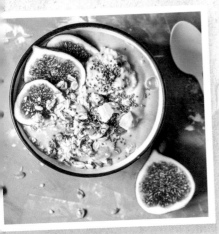

Figgy Nut Smoothie Bowl

Figgy Nut Smoothie Bowl

- 1 large banana, frozen
- 2 dried figs, chopped
- 2 tablespoons peanut butter
- ½ cup cashew milk
- 3 ice cubes
- ½ teaspoon agave syrup

Suggested toppings
- peanut butter
- fresh figs
- muesli
- chia seeds

Put all of the ingredients into a blender, and blend until smooth. Pour into a bowl, and layer on toppings.

Autumn Pecan Smoothie Bowl

- 1 cup pecan milk
- ½ cup raw pecan pieces
- ½ cup white beans
- ½ teaspoon vanilla
- 10 ice cubes
- 1 scoop vanilla protein powder

Suggested toppings
- clementine
- persimmon
- pomegranate
- pecans

Put all of the ingredients into a blender, and blend until smooth. Pour into a bowl, and layer on toppings.

GO NUTS

A sprinkling of nuts adds a bit of texture and a whole lot of flavor to a smoothie bowl. Each tree nut has its own unique nutrient makeup, but in general, they all include healthy fats, dietary fiber, arginine, plant sterols, and a range of vitamins and minerals known to be important for heart health.

- **Almond:** This tasty nut is one of the richest nut sources of vitamin E. Be sure to eat almonds with their brown skins, as the antioxidant properties are found in the skin.
- **Brazil nut:** This Amazon native is an excellent source of selenium, a vital mineral and antioxidant that may help prevent tissue damage.
- **Hazelnut:** This round nut is great source of dietary fiber, particularly the outer skin.
- **Macadamia:** Also called Hawaii nut, the macadamia is brimming with healthy monounsaturated fats and has been found to lower blood cholesterol.
- **Pistachio:** With a unique green color, the pistachio is rich in protein. About 60 pistachios make up an average nut serving.
- **Walnut:** A walnut is a rich source of alpha-linolenic acid (ALA). Research has shown that ALA from walnuts can reduce inflammation, like omega-3 fats from fish.

Hazelnuts, walnuts, and almonds

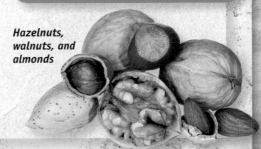

BLUE BOWLS

These beautiful bowls rely on spirulina for their color. And not only do they look good, the spirulina adds valuable protein and other nutrients.

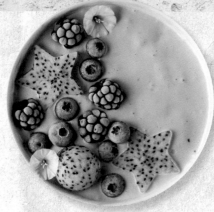

Blue Ocean Smoothie Bowl

Blue Coconut Smoothie Bowl

- 1 medium banana, frozen
- ½ small Fuji apple, cored and peeled
- ¼ cup unsweetened coconut
- 1 cup ice cubes
- ¼ cup coconut milk
- 1 teaspoon blue spirulina powder
- ¼ cup plain yogurt
- 1 splash almond milk

Suggested toppings
- raspberries
- cranberries
- blueberries
- coconut flakes
- cacao nibs

Put all of the ingredients into a blender, and blend until smooth. Pour into a bowl, and layer on toppings.

Blue Ocean Smoothie Bowl

- 1 large banana, frozen
- ⅓ cup blueberries, frozen
- ½ teaspoon blue spirulina powder
- 1 cup full-fat coconut milk

Suggested toppings
- dragon fruit
- blackberries
- blueberries
- nasturtiums

Put all of the ingredients into a blender, and blend until smooth. Pour into a bowl, and layer on toppings.

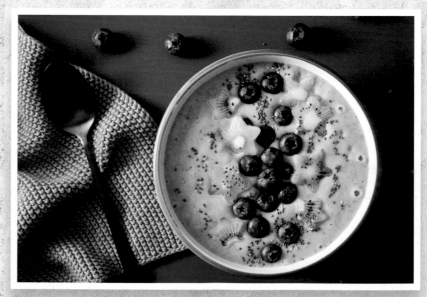

Blue-Green Smoothie Bowl

Blue-Green Smoothie Bowl

- 2 tablespoons blue spirulina powder
- 2 bananas, frozen
- 1 cup kiwi, frozen
- ¼ cup pineapple, frozen
- 1 cup almond milk

Suggested toppings
- kiwi slices
- blueberries
- chia seeds

Put all of the ingredients into a blender, and blend until smooth. Pour into a bowl, and layer on toppings.

Blue Banana Smoothie Bowl

- 2 bananas, frozen
- ½ kiwi
- 1 teaspoon blue spirulina powder
- ¼ cup almond milk

Suggested toppings
- banana slices
- coconut flakes
- kiwi slices
- pignolia nuts

Put all of the ingredients into a blender, and blend until smooth. Pour into a bowl, and layer on toppings.

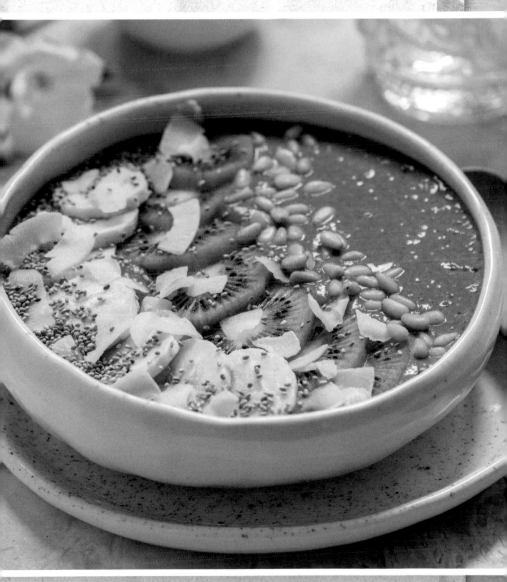

Blue Banana Smoothie Bowl

SWEET TREATS

Have a sweet tooth? Get the flavors you crave with healthier dessert options.

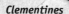
Clementines

A HEALTHIER OPTION

Smoothie bowls crafted from fruits and spices like vanilla, cacao, and cinnamon can soothe your cravings for something sweet. You can create bowls that taste as good as carrot cake or an oatmeal cookie, while still getting a healthy serving of fruits and vegetables.

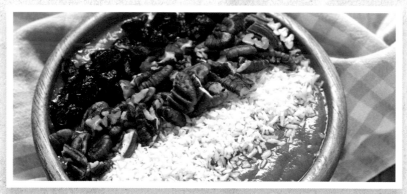
Carrot Cake Smoothie Bowl

Oatmeal Cookie Smoothie Bowl

- 1 medium banana, frozen
- 1 cup almond milk
- ½ cup rolled oats
- 1 tablespoon almond butter
- 1 to 2 tablespoons maple syrup
- ¼ teaspoon cinnamon
- 1 teaspoon vanilla extract
- a pinch of salt

Suggested toppings
- granola
- blueberries
- raisins
- cranberries
- coconut flakes
- sliced bananas
- toasted nuts

Put all of the ingredients into a blender, and blend until smooth. Pour into a bowl, and layer on toppings.

Carrot Cake Smoothie Bowl

- 2 cups carrots, chopped
- ½ cup pineapple chunks, frozen
- 1 medium banana, frozen
- 2 clementines, peeled
- ½ teaspoon vanilla extract
- ½ teaspoon cinnamon
- ¼ teaspoon ginger
- ¼ teaspoon nutmeg
- 2 tablespoons raw cashews
- 1 cup unsweetened coconut milk

Suggested toppings
- dried cranberries
- chopped pecans
- coconut flakes

Put all of the ingredients into a blender, and blend until smooth. Pour into a bowl and layer on toppings.

Coco-Hazel Dessert Bowl (opposite)

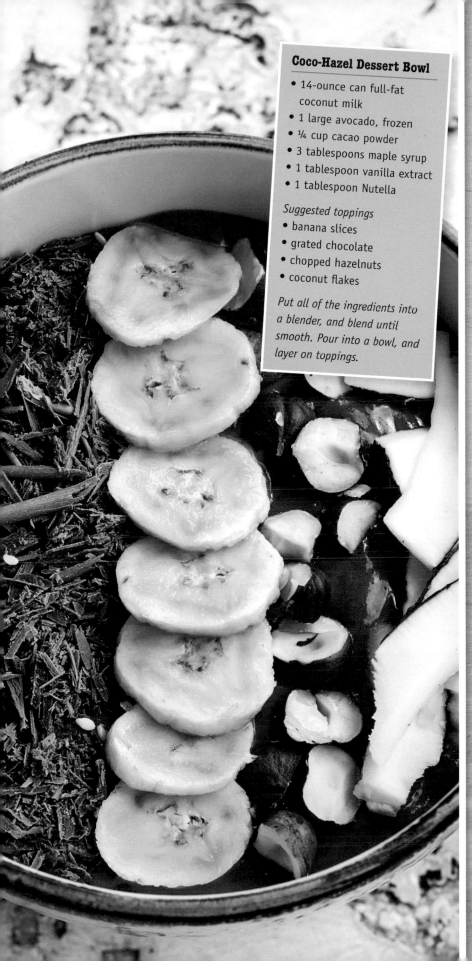

Coco-Hazel Dessert Bowl

- 14-ounce can full-fat coconut milk
- 1 large avocado, frozen
- ¼ cup cacao powder
- 3 tablespoons maple syrup
- 1 tablespoon vanilla extract
- 1 tablespoon Nutella

Suggested toppings
- banana slices
- grated chocolate
- chopped hazelnuts
- coconut flakes

Put all of the ingredients into a blender, and blend until smooth. Pour into a bowl, and layer on toppings.

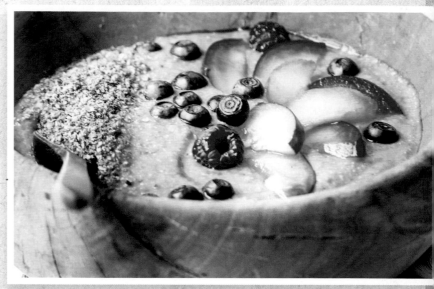

Plumini Smoothie Bowl (above); Summer Pink Smoothie Bowls (opposite)

Summer Pink Smoothie Bowl

- 6-ounce container low-fat yogurt (flavor of your choice)
- 1 cup raspberries, frozen
- 1 cup strawberries, frozen
- ½ cup pomegranate juice

*Suggested toppings
(choose your favorites)*
- strawberries
- raspberries
- blueberries
- sliced bananas
- sliced almonds
- mango chunks
- pomegranate seeds
- coconut
- lime
- star fruit
- dragon fruit

Put all of the ingredients into a blender, and blend until smooth. Pour into a bowl, and layer on toppings.

THINK ABOUT IT!
Prepare a family-sized batch of a smoothie, and then lay out a variety of toppings. Each family member can then customize their own bowl.

Silken Chocolate Dessert Bowl

- 1 cup vanilla low-fat Greek yogurt
- 1 medium banana, frozen
- 2 to 4 tablespoons almond milk
- 1 tablespoon cocoa powder
- 1 tablespoon maple syrup
- 4 to 6 ice cubes

Suggested toppings
- blueberries
- granola
- coconut
- lime
- star fruit

Put all of the ingredients into a blender, and blend until smooth. Pour into a bowl, and layer on toppings.

Plumini Smoothie Bowl

- 1 cup plums, frozen
- 1 cup peach yogurt
- 1 medium zucchini

Suggested toppings
- plum slices
- blueberries
- graham cracker crumbs

Put all of the ingredients into a blender, and blend until smooth. Pour into a bowl, and layer on toppings.

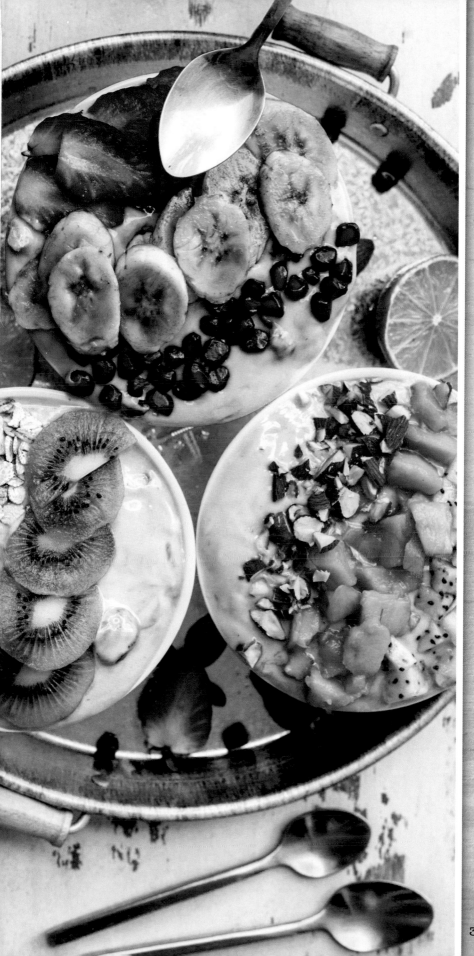

INDEX

PHOTO CREDITS

KEY

DT = Dreamstime.com   SS = Shutterstock.com

l = left   r = right   a = above   m = middle   b = below

Front cover: Leszek Czerwonka/SS; Yuliya Gontar/SS

Back cover: Artem Shadrin/SS; Peshkova/SS

Backgrounds: Paladin12/SS (paper); Brostock/SS; (wood); Peshkova/SS (granite); Daboost/SS (parchment); bsd/SS; Vector/SS; WonderfulPixel/SS (icons)

INTRODUCTION

2–3 Fortyforks/DT; 6 Boarding1now/DT; 7 Boarding1now/DT; 8 verca/SS; 9 Kondratova/DT; 10 Tannjuska/DT

CHAPTER 1

JUICE AND SMOOTHIE BASICS

12–13 113496721/DT; 14a 76917337/DT; 14b Olindana/DT; 15a Ittidech Pongpapas/DT; 15ml Tannjuska/DT; 15mr Piotr Adamowicz/DT; 15b Milovan Radmanovac/DT; 16 Anna1311/DT; 17 Alena Brozova/DT; 18b Marazem/DT; 18–19 Marko Valjak/DT; 19b Kondratova/DT; 20 Sataporn Jiwjalaen/DT; 21 Serhii Liakhevych/DT; 22a Georgii Dolgykh/DT; 22b Gordan Jankulov/DT; 23 Tanawat Bunyuen/DT; 25 Viktarm/DT; 26 Elena Veselova/DT; 27 Iuliia Nedrygailova/DT; 28 Sergii Koval/DT; 28al Angel Simon/SS; 29bl Matthew Barnes/DT; 29mr Itor/DT; 30a Sataporn Jiwjalaen/DT; 30–31 Viktor Bondariev/DT; 32a Bohuslav Jelen/DT; 32b Jörg Beuge/DT; 33a Tawan Jz//SS; 33b Jiri Hera/SS; 34a Voyagerix/DT; 34b bestv/SS; 35a Benoit Daoust/DT; 35b M. Unal Ozmen/SS; 36 Tatiana Mihaliova/SS; 37a nito/SS; 37b Antonio Delluzio/DT; 38l M. Unal Ozmen//SS; 38ar Radoslav Radev/DT; 38mr urbanbuzz/SS; 38br Shawn Hempel/SS; 39 djgis/SS

CHAPTER 2

INGREDIENTS A TO Z

40–42 Csaba Deli/DT; 42a Margouillat/DT; 42b Piliphoto/DT; 43a Peteer/DT; 43mr Istetiana/DT; 43ml omrodinka/DT; 43b Anastasiia Safronkina/DT; 44a Valentina Razumova/DT; 44b Oksanabratanova/DT; 45a Wieslaw Jarek/DT; 45b Gelia/DT; 46a Nevinates/DT; 46m Cynoclub/DT; 46b Nevinates/DT; 47 RGB Digital Ltd; 48a Tatiana Muslimova/DT; 48b Cherriesjd/DT; 49a Roman Samokhin/DT; 49b Yulia Mikhaylova/DT; 50a Valentyn75/DT; 50b Maxandrew/DT; 51 Batke82/DT; 52a Lepas/DT; 52b Liliya Kandrashevich/DT; 53 Denis Pogostin/SS; 54a Tatiana Muslimova/DT; 54–55 Alesyamakina/DT; 55 Vitalii Kit/DT; 56a Maskarad/DT; 56m Tomasz Resiak/DT; 56b Elena Schweitzer/DT; 57 Nataliya Arzamasova/DT; 58a Irochka/DT; 58b Africa Studio/SS; 59a Angel Luis Simon Martin/DT; 59b Sergio Delle Vedove/DT; 60a Nerss/DT; 60b Madeleinesteinbach/DT; 61a Michael Beckerman/DT; 61b Irinaorel/DT; 62a Katrinshine/DT; 62b RGB Digital Ltd; 63 Ramis Sabyrznov/DT; 64a Chuyu/DT; 64–65 Phasinphoto/DT; 66a Grublee/DT; 66b Tycoon751/DT; 67a Brooke Becker/DT; 67b Allnaturalbeth/DT; 68br Ivan Danik/DT; 68a, m, b Katerina Kovaleva/DT; 69 Anteromite/DT; 70a Melica/DT; 70b Africa Studio/SS; 71a Pongphan Ruengchai/DT; 71b Airubon/DT; 72a Hayati Kayhan/DT; 72–73 Foodpictures /SS; 73 Zerbor/DT; 74a Johnfoto/DT; 74bl CRuj/SS; 74m Evgeny Karandaev/SS; 75a Desislava Vasileva/DT; 75ml Max Lashcheuski/DT; 75bl schema/SS; 75mr schema/SS; 76a Valentina Razumova/DT; 76b Gabor Havasi/DT; 77m Yulia Davidovich/DT; 77a, m, b Yurakp /DT; 78a Inna Kyselova/DT; 78b RGB Digital Ltd; 79 Candus Camera/DT; 80a Phasinphoto/DT; 80–81 Jonathlee/DT; 81 Kaiskynet/DT; 82a Zigzagmtart/DT; 82b Ivansabo/DT; 83

Desislava Vasileva/DT; 84a Maya Kovacheva PhotographyDT; 84b Barbara Dudzinska/SS; 85 Artem Evdokimov/DT; 86a Kozzi2/DT; 86b Danelle Mccollum/DT; 87a Manon Ringuette/DT; 87b Konstantin KolosovDT; 88a Tatiana Muslimova/DT; 88b HandmadePictures/DT; 89a Digitalpress/DT; 89b Vladyslav Rasulov/DT; 90a Inna Kyselova/DT; 90b HandmadePictures/DT; 91a Ildipapp/DT; 91b Ildipapp/DT; 92a Atoss1/DT; 92b Nataliya Arzamasova/DT; 93 Luisa Leal Melo/DT; 94a Serhiy Shullye/DT; 94b Christian Jung/SS; 95 Anamomarques/DT; 96a artphotoclub/SS; 97m Katerina Kovaleva/DT; 97b HandmadePictures/DT; 98a Artem Samokhvalov/DT; 98b Photomailbox/DT; 99a Inna Kyselova/DT; 99b Piotr Wytrażek/DT; 100a Inna Kyselova/DT; 100–101 Samsandr/DT; 101m Kaiskynet/DT; 102a Luisa Leal Melo/DT; 102b Ildipapp/DT; 103 Piyachok Thawornmat/DT; 104a Yurakp/DT; 104b Story/DT; 105a Gita Kulinica/DT; 105b RGB Digital Ltd; 106 Elena Derevyagina/DT; 107 Ingridsi/DT; 108a Valentyn75/DT; 108b Al1962/DT; 109 Seth Anderson/DT; 110a Tbylka/DT; 110b Mariusz Blach/DT; 111ar Exopixel/DT; 111mr Lovelyday12/DT; 111al Anphotos/DT; 111ml Eric Krouse/DT; 111bl Kateryna Bibro/DT; 112a, m, b Max Lashcheuski/DT; 113 Odua/DT; 112–113 Woravit Vijitpanya/DT; 114a Shtraus Dmytro/DT; 114–115 Photomailbox/DT; 115 HandmadePictures/DT; 116a, n Anna Sedneva/DT; 116b Natika/DT; 117 Grafnata/DT; 117b Viter8/DT; 118a Melica/DT; 118b Eduardo Gonzalez Diaz/DT; 119 Photozirka/DT; 120a Binh Thanh Bui/SS; 120–121 Mohammed Anwarul Kabir Choudhury/DT; 121 HandmadePictures/DT; 122a Björn Wylezich/DT; 122b Zigzagmtart/DT; 123l Zigzagmtart/DT; 123ar Anphotos/DT; 123mr Elena Elisseeva/DT; 123br Elena Veselova/DT; 124a Anastasiia Skorobogatova/DT; 124b Photomailbox/DT; 125 Slavjonny/DT; 126a Melica/DT; 126m Anna Sedneva/DT; 126b Frui/DT; 127a Sergio33/SS; 127b Photomailbox/DT; 128a Anna1311/DT; 128b Oleg Golovnev/DT; 129a Subbotina/DT; 129b RGB Digital Ltd; 130a Le Thuy Do/DT; 130b Jochenschneider/DT; 131 Foodmicro/DT; 132a Enlightened Media/SS; 132b Marazem/DT; 133 Danil Chepko/DT; 134bl Chuyu/DT; 134br Shino Iwamura/DT; 134–135 Brent Hofacker/SS; 135 RGB Digital Ltd; 136a Max Lashcheuski/DT; 136b Inna Kyselova/DT; 136–137 Benoit Daoust/DT

CHAPTER 3
HIGH-ENERGY JUICES

138–139 Elena Veselova/DT; 140a chuckstock/SS; 140b Elena Schweitzer/DT; 141a lola1960/SS; 141ml anshu18/SS; 141mr Arkadiusz Fajer/DT; 141b maramicado/SS; 142a Boonchuay Iamsumang/DT; 142b vanillaechoes/SS; 143 Fotos43/DT; 144a Lev Kropotov/DT; 144b vanillaechoes/SS; 145a Melica/DT; 145b Msphotographic/DT; 146a Inna Yurkevych/DT; 146b Fotografaw/DT; 147 Lesya Dolyuk/SS; 148a sunsetman/SS; 148–149 Nicram Sabod/SS; 150a Inna Kyselova/DT; 150m Jean-louis Vosgien/DT; 151 thefoodphotographer/SS

CHAPTER 4
CLEANSING JUICES

152–153 Victorrustle/DT; 154a Inews77/DT; RGB Digital Ltd; 155a RGB Digital Ltd; 155ml RGB Digital Ltd; 155mr Dianearbis/DT; 155b Dianearbis/DT; 156 Alisali/DT; 157 RGB Digital Ltd; 158 RGB Digital Ltd; 159a Millafedotova/DT; /SS; 159b RGB Digital Ltd; 160 topseller/SS; 162–163 Joshua Resnick/DT; 161 RGB Digital Ltd; 163 RGB Digital Ltd; 164a Madlen/SS; 164b Millafedotova/DT; 165 RGB Digital Ltd; 166a Anastasiia Skorobogatova/DT; 166 Serhiy Shullye/DT; 167 RGB Digital Ltd; 168 Atoss1/DT; 168–169 RGB Digital Ltd; 170a Robyn Mackenzie/SS; 170b RGB Digital Ltd; 171 RGB Digital Ltd

CHAPTER 5
JUICE REMEDIES

172–173 Alina Yudina/DT; 174a Bat09mar/DT; 174b Odua/DT; 175al RGB Digital Ltd; 175ar Artanika/DT; 175mr Olga Lyubkin/SS; 175b Dimakp/DT; 176–177 Iquacu/DT; 178a Vitalii Kit/DT; 178b Valentyn Volkov/SS; 179 RGB Digital Ltd; 180 Alfio Scisetti/DT; 181 RGB Digital Ltd; 182 kviktor/SS; 183 Maxim Khytra/SS; 184a Max Lashcheuski/DT; 184b ER_09/SS; 185 vanillaechoes/SS; 186a Max Lashcheuski/DT; 186 Stryjek/DT; 187 elen_studio/SS; 188a Inna Kyselova/DT; 188b Maxim Khytra/SS; 189a Maskarad/DT; 189b Tycoon751/DT; 190a Boonchuay Iamsumang/DT; 190b Africa Studio/SS; 191 Maxim Khytra/SS; 192a Dumrongsak Songdej/DT; 192–183 Jarenwicklund/DT; 194 Oksana Ermak/DT; 195 RGB Digital Ltd; 196

Inna Kyselova/DT; 197 RGB Digital Ltd; 198a Atoss1/DT; 198b Pefkos/SS; 199 graphia/SS; 200a Grublee/DT; 200b RGB Digital Ltd; 201 RGB Digital Ltd; 202 Goldenleaf/DT; 202m Atoss1/DT; 203 RGB Digital Ltd; 204a Max Lashcheuski/DT; 204m Nataliia Melnychuk/SS; 205 RGB Digital Ltd; 206a Inna Kyselova/DT; 206m RGB Digital Ltd; 207a Anmbph/DT; 207 RGB Digital Ltd; 208a Inna Kyselova/DT; 208m Milovan Radmanovac/DT; 209 Subodh Sathe/DT

CHAPTER 6
SMOOTHIES FOR EVERYONE

210–211 Artem Shadrin/SS; 212a Czarnybez/DT; 212b Nitr/SS; 213a Ian Walker/DT; 213ml Igor Kovalchuk/SS; 213mr bitt24/SS; 213b Peteer/DT; 214a Sergey Kolesnikov/DT; 214bl Valentina Razumova/DT; 214br Vaclav Volrab/DT; 214–215 Alexandra Fedorova/DT; 215a Valentyn Volkov/SS; 215bl, br Sergey Kolesnikov/DT; 216a Hsagencia/DT; 216b Photomailbox/DT; 217 IrinaFedotova/SS; 218a Valentyn75/DT; 218b Ana Blazic Pavlovic/SS; 219 Mariana Romaniv/DT; 220a Jitkaunv/DT; 220b Jennifer Barrow/DT; 221a Goldenleaf/DT; 221b Elena Veselova/DT; 222a Melica/DT; 222m Sathit Plengchawee/DT; 223 Rawlik/DT; 224a Boarding1now3/DT; 224b Tasipas/DT; 225a Natika/DT; 225m Ian Andreiev/DT; 225b Sergii Korshun/SS; 226a Max Lashcheuski/DT; 226b Kondratova/DT; 227 Pigdevil Photo/SS; 228 Boyarkinamarina/DT; 229a Luisa Leal Melo/DT; 229b Fotoluminate/DT; 230a Luis Ramírez Kuthe/DT; 230b Iuliia Nedrygailova/DT; 231a Elena Derevyagina/DT; 231b TZIDO SUN/SS; 232a Anna Kucherova/SS; 232b 103622926/DT; 233 Kurylo54/DT; 234a Yurakp/DT; 234b Shebeko/SS; 235 stockcreations/SS; 236a Binh Thanh Bui/SS; 236b vanillaechoes/SS; 237a Anastasiia Skorobogatova/SS; 237b 240 HandmadePictures/SS; 241a Exopixel/DT; 241b vanillaechoes/SS; 242 DUSAN ZIDAR/SS; 2 244b sarsmis/SS; 245 jreika/SS; 246a Marek Uliasz/DT; 246b Farakos/DT; 247a Blackay/DT; 247b Picstudio/DT; 248a Anna Hoychuk /SS; 248b Layland Masuda/SS; 249 Africa Studio/SS; 250 Elena Schweitzer/DT; 251 Bhofack2/DT; 252 Nopphadon Jantranapaporn/SS; 253 Eugenia Lucasenco/SS; 254 Artem Shadrin/SS; 255 HandmadePictures/SS; 256a Georgii Dolgykh/DT; 256b Moken78/DT; 258 Zerbor/DT; 259

Yulia Davidovich/DT; 260 Lschirmbeck/DT; 262a Anastasiia Skorobogatova/DT; 262b Voltan1/DT; 263a Azurita/DT; 263b JeniFoto/SS

CHAPTER 7
TARGETED SMOOTHIES

264–265 Beataaldridge/DT; 266a Pravit Kimtong/DT; 266b Moniphoto/DT; 267a Marcin Jucha/DT; 267ml Kondratova/DT; 267mr Svitlana Tereshchenko/DT; 267b Nataliya Arzamasova/DT; 268a Reinis Bigacs/DT; 268b Natasha Mamysheva/DT; 269 Yulia Mikhaylova/DT; 270a Inna Kyselova/DT; 270b Maria Medvedeva/DT; 271a Viktoriia Panchenko/DT; 271b Shino Iwamura/DT; 272a Shino Iwamura/DT; 272b Oksana Chaun/DT; 273 Elena Veselova/DT; 274a Atoss1/DT; 274b Artem Evdokimov/DT; 275 Bhofack2/DT; 276a Tbylka/DT; 276b Oksanabratanova/DT; 277 Wideonet/DT; 278a Inna Kyselova/DT; 278b Azmanz/DT; 279a Nedim Bajramovic/DT; 279b Goldenleaf/DT

CHAPTER 8
SMOOTHIE BOWLS

280–281 Margouillat/DT; 282a Liliya Kandrashevich/DT; 282b Azurita/DT; 283a Lunamarina/DT;283ml NatashaBreen/DT; 283mr Karen Cucuzza/DT; 283b Kondratova/DT; 284a Alfio Scisetti/DT; 284b Marina Saprunova/DT; 285 Rozmarina/DT; 286a Artem Kutsenko/SS; 286b Yulia Mikhaylova/DT; 287 DronG/SS; 288 Alphonsine Sabine/SS; 289 Yulia Furman/SS; 290 Nina Firsova/DT; 291 Rozmarina/DT; 292 Svitlana Tereshchenko/DT; 293 Svitlana Tereshchenko/DT; 294 Artem Evdokimov/DT; 295a Nataliya Arzamasova/DT; 295b Margouillat/DT; 296a LiliGraphie/SS; 296b Artem Evdokimov/DT; 297 Duskbabe/DT; 298 Elena Veselova/DT; 299a Azurita/DT; 299b Madlen/SS; 300 Nataliya Arzamasova/DT; 301 Cristina Toth/DT; 302a Manon Ringuette/DT; 302b Azurita/DT; 303a Nina Firsova/DT; 303b Kguzel/DT; 304a Viennetta/DT; 304b Duskbabe/DT; 305 Azurita/DT; 306a Swapan Photography/SS; 306m Azurita/DT; 307 Svetlana Kolpakova/DT; 308 Anastasiia Vorontsova/DT; 309 Alena Ozerova/DT